Recent Results in Cancer Research 74

Fortschritte der Krebsforschung
Progrès dans les recherches sur le cancer

Cancer Chemo- and Immunopharmacology

1. Chemopharmacology

Edited by G. Mathé and F. M. Muggia

With 82 Figures and 150 Tables

Springer-Verlag
Berlin Heidelberg New York 1980

Professor Georges Mathé

Institut de Cancérologie et Immunogénétique, Hôpital
Paul-Brousse, 14–16 Avenue Paul-Vaillant-Couturier,
F-94800 Villejuif

Professor Franco M. Muggia

Institute of Environmental Medicine, New York University
Medical Center, Division of Oncology,
Department of Internal Medicine, 550 First Avenue,
USA – New York, NY 10016

Sponsored by the Swiss League against Cancer

ISBN-13: 978-3-642-81490-7 e-ISBN-13: 978-3-642-81488-4
DOI: 10.1007/ 978-3-642-81488-4

Library of Congress Cataloging in Publication Data. European Organization for Research on Treatment of Cancer. Cancer chemo- and immunopharmacology. (Recent results in cancer research; 74–75) "Communications presented at the 1979 EORTC annual plenary session on cancer chemo- and immunopharmacology." Bibliography: v. 1, p. Includes indexes. Contents: 1. Chemopharmacology. – 2. Relations and general problems. 1. Cancer – Chemotherapy – Congresses. 2. Antineoplastic agents – Testing – Congresses. 3. Cancer – Immunological aspects – Congresses. 4. Immunotherapy – Congresses. I. Mathé, Georges, 1922. – II. Muggia, Franco M. III. Title. IV. Series. [DNLM: 1. Neoplasms – Drug therapy – Congresses. 2. Immunotherapy – Congresses. 3. Antineoplastic agents – Congresses. W1 RE106P v. 74–75 / QZ267 E104c 1979] RC261.R35 vol. 74–75 [RC271.C5] 616.99'4s 80-18852 [616.99'4061]

Softcover reprint of the hardcover 1st edition 1980

Typesetting: Carl Ritter & Co., Wiesbaden

2125/3140–5 4 3 2 1 0

Preface

Local treatment cures about 30 to 40% of cancers, this proportion depending on the follow-up required to establish it. This means that 60 to 70% of the malignant neoplasias are disseminated either perceptibly (leukemias, visible metastases) or imperceptibly, forming a 'minimal imperceptible disease', which local treatment leaves, whether it consists of surgery, radiotherapy, or surgery plus radiotherapy.

When the neoplastic tissue is voluminous enough to be perceptible, cures can be obtained with chemotherapy or chemoimmunotherapy. When the neoplastic disease is imperceptible, made up of micrometastases, it apparently can be cured by systemic postsurgical chemotherapy, immunotherapy, or chemoimmunotherapy.

Hence there is the need for intensive development of these medical therapies which are applied by the medical oncologist and, at present, consist of chemotherapy, immunotherapy, or chemoimmunotherapy. These medical therapeutics can only grow with scientific development, the main weapon of which is experimental and clinical pharmacology.

These volumes report the communications presented at the 1979 EORTC Annual Plenary Session on Cancer Chemo- and Immunopharmacology.

Georges Mathé

Contents

List of Senior Authors

D. S. Alberts
Section Haematology and Oncology, University of Arizona, USA – Tucson, AR 85724

B. Ardalan
Biochemistry Section, Laboratory of Toxicology, Division Cancer Treatment, National Cancer Institute,
USA – Bethesda, MA 20205

M. Bayssas
ICIG, Hôpital Paul-Brousse, 14 avenue P.-V.-Couturier,
F-94800 Villejuif

M. Bobek
Department of Health, Roswell Park Memorial Institute, 666 Elm Street, USA – Buffalo, NY 14263

G. Bonadonna
Istituto Nazionale dei Tumori, Via G. Venezian 1,
I-20133 Milano

V. Bonfante
Istituto Nazionale dei Tumori, Via G. Venezian 1,
I-20133 Milano

N. Brock
Asta Werke AG, Postfach 140129, D-4800 Bielefeld

J. H. Burchenal
Sloan Kettering Institute, Cornell University Medical School, USA – New York, NY 10021

S. K. Carter
Northern California Cancer Program, 770 Welch Road,
Suite 190, USA – Palo Alto, CA 94304

H. Cortés-Funes
Cancer Chemotherapy Section, I. Octubre Hospital,
E-Madrid–26

D. Dantchev
ICIG, Hôpital Paul-Brousse, 14 avenue P.-V.-Couturier,
F-94800 Villejuif

R. Donehower
Division of Cancer Treatment, NCI, Bldg 10 Room 6N119,
USA – Bethesda, MD 20205

C. Erlichman
Clinical Pharmacology Branch, Division of Cancer Treatment,
National Cancer Institute, National Institute of Health,
USA – Bethesda, MD 20205

G. Fernbach
Department of Neoplastic Diseases, Mt. Sinai School of
Medicine, One Gustave L. Levy Place, USA – New York,
NY 10029

S. Garattini
Istituto Mario Negri, Via Eritrea 62, I-20157 Milano

F. A. Greco
Vanderbilt University, USA – Nashville, TN 37232

M. Hayat
ICIG, Hôpital Paul-Brousse, 14 avenue P.-V.-Couturier,
F-94800 Villejuif

D. L. Kisner
Clinical Investigation Branch, Division of Cancer Treatment,
NCI HIH, USA – Bethesda, MD 20205

P. Lelieveld
Radiobiological Institute TNO, 151 Lange Kleiweg,
NL-2280 HV Rijswijk

R. Maral
Centre Nicolas Grillet, 13 Quai Jules Guesde,
F-94400 Vitry/Seine

G. Mathé
ICIG, Hôpital Paul-Brousse, 14 avenue P.-V.-Couturier,
F-94800 Villejuif

F. M. Muggia
Institute of Environmental Medicine, New York University
Medical Center, Division of Oncology, Department
of Internal Medicine, 550 First Avenue,
USA – New York, NY 10016

N. I. Nissen
The Finsen Institute, 49 Strandboulevarden,
DK-2100 Copenhagen

S. Oka
Microbial Chemistry Branch Research Foundation, Institute
of Microbial Chemistry, 14–23 Kaminosaki, Tokyo, Japan

T. Oki
Central Research Laboratories, Sanraku-Ocean Co., Ltd.,
4-9-1-Johnan, Fujisawa, 251 Japan

C. Paoletti
Institut Gustave Roussy, 16 bis, avenue P.-V.-Couturier, F-94800 Villejuif

P. Ribaud
ICIG, Hôpital Paul-Brousse, 14 avenue P.-V.-Couturier, F-94800 Villejuif

M. Rozencweig
Institut Jules Bordet, 1 rue Héger Bordet, B-1000 Brussels

S. E. Salmon
Section of Hematology and Oncology, Department of Internal Medicine and the Cancer Center, University of Arizona College of Medicine, USA – Tucson, AZ 85724

J. L. Speyer
Clinical Pharmacology Branch, Division of Cancer Treatment, National Cancer Institute, National Institute of Health, USA – Bethesda, MD 20205

W. Wilmanns
Ludwig-Maximilians-Universität München, Klinikum Grosshadern, D-8000 München

J. Ziegler
Clinical Oncology, Evaluation Program, Division of Cancer Treatment, National Cancer Institute, USA – Bethesda, MD 20205

General Progress in Clinical Chemotherapy of Advanced Disease

F. M. Muggia, J. Henney, and V. DeVita, Jr.

Summary

Advanced cancer, because of its accompanying tumor burden, complex adverse host effects, and cellular heterogeneity, will prove much more difficult to control successfully than grave infectious diseases such as tuberculosis. This will likely be so, even when moderately successful chemotherapy is or will be available. Nevertheless, prospects for improving current results are present through application of chemotherapy alone or in combination with other modalities. Important developments include not only the availability of an increasing number of effective drugs, but also a better understanding of drug pharmacology, prediction of tumor cell cytotoxicity, locoregional drug delivery, exploitation of interactions with other forms of local therapy, and delineation of immunologic factors in tumor control. The single, most likely contribution to a curative approach to cancer, however, is likely to emerge from the application of aggressive systemic treatment in the circumstances of minimal residual disease. This topic is covered elsewhere.

Introduction

It has been accepted by even the most nihilistic physicians that drugs can cure certain forms of cancer. Awareness of this possibility began after the early observations utilizing nitrogen mustard, aminopterin, and methotrexate for the treatment of lymphomas, childhood leukemia, and choriocarcinoma, respectively. In the late 1950s, U.S. Congress appropriated sufficient funds for NCI to establish its drug development program. Such a radical concept, though readily adopted by legislators, has been slow in gaining acceptance, with disillusioned physicians sometimes being the worst enemies. Advanced cancer was and continues to be a most formidable opponent. The facts indicate that chemotherapy *can* lead to cures of patients with certain metastatic disease who had been destined to die. This knowledge should give us hope and encouragement. Furthermore, actual and conceptual advances in clinical chemotherapy give us confidence in a bright near future. We shall review these advances and briefly discuss how they lead to the combined modality approach, which is the topic of a subsequent chapter.

Anticancer Drug Development

The number of drugs introduced into clinical practice has proceeded at a steady pace (Table 1). These have usually had a period of testing within the NCI drug development

Table 1. Anticancer drugs which have received FDA approval for marketing in the United States

Alkylating agents – 6	*Synthetics – 6*
Nitrogen mustard (Mustargen)	Procarbazine (Matulane)
Thiotepa	Hydroxyurea (Hydrea)
Chlorambucil (Leukeran)	σ, ϱ'-DDD (Lysodren, mitotane)
Cyclophosphamide (Cytoxan)	DTIC (dacarbazine)
Pipobroman (Vercyte)	BCNU (carmustine, BiCNU)
Melphalan (L-PAM, Alkeran)	CCNU (lomustine, CeeNU)
Busulfan (Myleran)	
Uracil mustard	*Hormones and steroids – 14*
	Prednisolone
Antimetabolites – 6	Prednisone
Methotrexate	Diethylstilbestrol (DES)
Mercaptopurine (6-MP)	Tamoxifen (Nolvadex)
Thioguanine (6-TG)	Ethinylestradiol
Fluorouracil (5-FU)	Testosterone
Cytosar (ara-C)	Testolactone (Teslac)
FUDR	Fluoxymesterone (Halotestin)
	Dromostanolone
Plant alkaloids and antibiotics – 7	Methylprednisolone
Vinblastine (Velban)	Megestrol acetate (Megace)
Vincristine (Oncovin)	Methyltestosterone
Actinomycin D (Cosmegen)	Chlorotrianisene (Tace)
Mithramycin (Mithracin)	Triamcinolone
Doxorubicin (Adriamycin)	
Bleomycin (Blenoxane)	*Enzymes – 1*
Mitomycin (Mutamycin)	L-Asparaginase (Elspar)

program. In addition, investigational drugs have been introduced into clinical testing at a constant rate of about five to ten per year. These emanate from a flow of potential drugs through a "linear array," which represents a selective logical process with various decision points (referred to as "decision network") for ultimate advancement into clinical trial.

Since its inception in the 1950s, the drug development program has undergone several changes which represent important conceptual advances. Broadening the input of materials to be tested was a major concern. In 1975 the Division of Cancer Treatment (DCT) of the National Cancer Institute (NCI) set up an experimental screening program for the identification of new anticancer drugs. This program used panel matched pairs of spontaneous or transplanted syngeneic tumors and human tumor xenografts. In addition, efforts in identifying new natural products and in testing rationally selected compounds in the full panel were emphasized. Such changes will hopefully lead to identification of new structures with a different antitumor spectrum of activity [4].

Other important conceptual modifications are likely to have additional impact on drug development. The need to perform elaborate acute toxicologic studies has been an important rate-limiting factor in the development of drugs for clinical use. Such concern for elaborate routine large-animal toxicology studies to guarantee safety is misplaced in view of the high false-positive rates of such studies [11], coupled with the need for patients with advanced drug-resistant cancer to be exposed to totally new compounds. Moreover, phase I clinical studies may provide a more accurate source of information for defining specific toxicities that may require further evaluation either in animal models or man. This point is particularly relevant to the testing of analogues which are developed in order to overcome specific toxicities. It is becoming increasingly clear that modifications of currently active drugs are a fertile area of investigation, but one that must receive prompt and accurate clinical feedback [10]. Thus, a multidisciplinary approach for the development of analogues, couples with simplification of toxicologic studies, represents particularly crucial aspects in promulgating future advances in cancer chemotherapy at an accelerated rate. Nowhere is there a greater need for intimate communication between preclinical and clinical scientists than in the development of these second-generation anticancer drugs. Responsible and effective teams of investigators have the unique opportunity for advancing this aspect of chemotherapy.

Clinical Evaluation of Anticancer Drugs

From the preceding statements, it is apparent that an essential part of drug development is the clinical evaluation of anticancer drugs. For a number of years, various phases of investigation with anticancer drugs have been identified, designated by a nomenclature adapted from the Food and Drug Administration. Extensive organizational structures for conducting clinical trials with chemotherapeutic agents were developed under special grant programs of the NCI beginning in 1955. As requirements for the initial studies became better delineated and teams of investigators experienced in sophisticated clinical and pharmacologic observations were deemed essential, special contractual arrangements were developed with specific institutions via a competitive process [8]. Following determination of a maximal tolerable dose and delineation of toxicologic properties, drugs advance to efficacy trials with a built-in requirement for a minimum of clinical observations. This plan has served as a useful framework in which to ensure adequate evaluation of newly introduced drugs and a minimum of relevant clinical observations not subject to the whims or prejudice of investigators based on a brief clinical experience. Moreover, such a plan takes into account the complexity of human cancer, and the alterations in host and tumor biology that may take place by prior treatment and other relevant characteristics of afflicted patients. The plan of investigation that is followed consists of basically proceeding to phase II studies in patients with various carcinomas, leukemias, and lymphomas. A minimum number of studies is required to be performed in a clinical panel which includes diseases that are both common and readily evaluable for drug-related regression of tumor, or those uniquely responsive to a systemic approach. Moreover, by matching such evaluation to the preclinical screening panel, relevant correlates may be performed. Such correlates were the basis for the September 1978 meeting of our Division [8]. Acquiring an adequate clinical data base with each drug introduced by the linear array constitutes an important concept in the evolution of more efficient and sensitive screening systems. However, this plan of investigation needs to remain flexible, particularly when dealing with specific drugs such as analogues of well-established agents, or in order to follow leads developed

from biochemical and pharmacologic knowledge or from the initial clinical experience.
Subsequent steps of investigation do not lend themselves readily to such specific direction since much depends on the type of agent and on the initial observations. The NCI has relied on investigator-initiated research at grant-supported institutions where researchers possessing special expertise are free to develop their ideas in areas of their own choosing. More recently, under prompting by the FDA, the increasing interest of industry, and the pressures of maintaining drugs under investigation at an administratively manageable number, there has been an effort to channel suitable investigations toward the establishment of clinically useful indications that would lead to the marketing of the compound.

Impact of Chemotherapy

The initial dramatic susceptibility of certain rapidly fatal neoplastic diseases to chemotherapy introduced in 1948 provided considerable early hope followed by disappointment as drug-resistant relapses occurred. In the early 1950s, the initial experience with additional drugs provided evidence of refractoriness of most common cancers to chemotherapy. However, cure was achieved in choriocarcinoma and subsequently in Burkitt's lymphoma with use of single-agent chemotherapy. Dose combinations began to have an impact in advanced testicular carcinoma with approximately 10% long-term cures [7]. In addition, in malignancies of the hematopoietic system and in childhood neoplasms, substantial gains were being made beginning in the early 1960s. These achievements were translated into the development of effective combination chemotherapy programs which culminated in substantial survival benefit even in those patients who demonstrated far advanced metastatic disease at the time of diagnosis. It is important to recall that up to that time such diagnoses were synonymous with fatality! Five-year relative survival rates were demonstrated in a variety of diseases, and for the first time cure from cancer with chemotherapy became a reality.
A striking example, undisputably attributed to chemotherapy, is five-year survivals associated with leukemia in boys and girls less than 15 years old. Registry statistics reveal an increase from 0% in the 1950–1953 cohorts, to 5% and 4% in 1960–1963 cohorts, and finally to 23% and 33%, respectively, in the 1970–1973 cohorts. As a result of these improvements as well as those achieved through chemotherapy and combined modalities in other childhood solid tumors, such as rhabdomyosarcoma, Ewing's sarcoma, and Wilms' tumor, the mortality rate is declining sharply, beginning in 1970, for individuals less than 30 years old [4].
Cancer in adults less than 45 also indicates a decline in the mortality rate beginning in 1970, in spite of increasing or unchanged incidence. This can also be attributed in part to the impact of chemotherapy on the course of advanced testicular cancer and breast cancer. The results of combination chemotherapy of testicular cancer were presented in this conference last year. These studies constitute landmarks and indicate once again the magnitude of therapy progress that may be achieved by the introduction of new reproducibly effective drugs in circumstances where only moderate success had prevailed. These studies also reemphasize the importance of experienced investigators to follow up clinical observations.

There is every indication from the detailed analysis in one institute – that of Drs. Veronesi and Bonadonna – that the treatment of advanced breast cancer has been associated with substantially greater survival rates in this decade [1]. Treatment with combination chemotherapy is likely to be a factor responsible for declining mortality rate in breast cancer patients under age 45. It is possible that the impact of adjuvant chemotherapy is already perceptible; however, it is to be hoped that both adjuvant chemotherapy and refinements in hormonal treatment and defining the population of patients most likely to respond to a given therapy will have an additional beneficial effect on survival of the subsequent cohort.

Combined Modality Approaches

The concept that advanced cancer could be cured by drugs had a salutary effect on the general therapeutic approach to such patients. Eradication of visible cancer, even in its disseminated stages by surgery and/or radiation, was found to lead in certain well-defined instances to increased survival. The improvement in results often cannot be clearly attributed to any one therapeutic modality employed, and in some instances cannot be accepted uncritically as being due to the treatment itself, but on other factors such as patient selection. Nevertheless, solid scientific foundations exist for the strategy of diminishing tumor burden by surgery to enhance the ability of achieving cures with chemotherapy, where only "near cures" may be expected. Studies on the treatment of various stages of Wilms' tumor are a classic demonstration of such strategy [3]. In *osteosarcoma*, resection of pulmonary metastases has been associated with increasingly favorable survival [6]. The role of chemotherapy in these circumstances is actually in question. Similar trends have been observed in selected patients with a variety of other malignancies and pulmonary metastases. Aggressive local treatments coupled with systemic therapies have also been reported to be beneficial in advanced *breast cancer* [9] and in *malignant melanoma* (D. Morton, unpublished work). The simultaneous administration of radiation therapy to the primary site and combination chemotherapy has yielded favorable results in *small cell carcinoma* of the lung, although associated with considerable morbidity and mortality [2].

In other areas, exploitation of chemotherapy in advanced disease presentations is just beginning. In *ovarian cancer*, surgical resection of intraperitoneal metastases is associated with improvement in survival [5]. Resections followed by chemotherapy are being systematically studied. In *head and neck cancer*, *bladder cancer*, and *esophageal cancer*, the concept of chemotherapy complementing local therapies in regionally advanced tumors has finally been established. At present, however, one must still weigh the balance of achieving improvements by systemic treatment versus compromising our ability to deliver optimal local therapy. This must always be borne in mind when devising pertinent therapeutic experiments in conditions where local control is a crucial aspect of management.

Future Opportunities

It should be amply clear from the preceding that opportunities exist for improving the outlook of patients with advanced disease, even when the chemotherapy by itself has not shown curative potential. In common malignancies, such as squamous lung cancer and colon cancer, new agents must be sought which are more capable to selectively destroy these tumors than current drugs. However, one must not wait for the introduction of the "magic bullet" in order to test therapeutic concepts that may now be within reach. Clinical pharmacology has added a new dimension in the exploration of more effective measures with current anticancer drugs. Examples of such studies are listed in the summary and will be illustrated in many of the topics to be covered.

Dose rate is an important concept in improving the results from an effective cytotoxic regimen. Drug treatment may be administered via *peritoneal dialysis*: a greater than two increase in concentration relative to plasma levels has been achieved with 5-fluorouracil [13]. Similar studies are ongoing with adriamycin and may find applications in the treatment of predominantly intraabdominal malignancies. Pharmacologic monitoring not only provides a safety valve for monitoring these approaches, but also allows for the testing of cytotoxicity in model systems mimicking clinical circumstances. For example, clonogenic cell systems described by SALMON et al. can test the implications of dose rate in achieving cytotoxicity [12]. Such correlations, if substantiated, may also prove useful in intraarterial therapy. *Supportive measures* may have an important impact on our ability to effectively deliver chemotherapy. Nutritional support, although helpful in specific circumstances, needs to be systematically tested in circumstances where chemotherapeutic success is often achieved at a cost of some nutritional deprivation. *Blood component therapy* has become an essential support measure of any cancer treatment. Bolder experiments with autologous bone marrow reconstitution following profoundly myelotoxic regimens have been initiated in several institutions. Instances in which the additional dose response achievable will prove crucial needs to be identified. Finally, the proper clinical role of *immune reconstitution* continues to prove generally elusive, although specific studies reaffirm its importance.

Study of the interaction of drugs with other modalities is another important area of exploration. Hyperthermia, radiosensitization of tumor tissue, and radioprotection of normal tissue are just such examples. Opportunities for exploring these areas are currently available, in concert with experimental data.

References

1 Bonadonna G, Valagussa P, Rossi A, Zucali R, Tancini G, Bajetta E, Brambilla C, DeLena M, DiFronzo G, Banfi A, Rilke F, Veronesi U (1978) Are surgical adjuvant trials altering the course of breast cancer? Semin Oncol 5: 450

2 Brereton HD, Kent CH, Johnson RE (1979) Chemotherapy and radiation therapy for small cell carcinoma of the lung: A remedy for past therapeutic failure in lung cancer. In: Muggia FM, Rozencweig M (eds) Lung cancer: Progress in therapeutic research. Raven, New York, pp 575–586

3 D'Angio GJ, Evans AE, Breslow N, Beckwith B, Bishop H, Feigl P, Goodwin W, Leape LL, Sinks LF, Sutow W, Tefft M, Wolff J (1976) The treatment of Wilms' tumor: Results of the National Wilms' Tumor Study. Cancer 38: 633–645

4 DeVita VT, Oliverio VT, Muggia FM, Wiernik PW, Ziegler J, Goldin A, Rubin D, Henney J, Schepartz S (1979) The drug development and clinical trials programs of the Division of Cancer Treatment, National Cancer Institute. Cancer Clin Trials 2: 195–216

5 Griffiths CT, Parker CM, Fuller AF Jr (1979) Role of cytoreductive surgical treatment in management of advanced ovarian cancer. Cancer Treat Rep 63: 235–240
6 Muggia F, Catane R, Lee Y, Rozencweig M (1980) Factors responsible for therapeutic success in osteosarcoma: A critical analysis of adjuvant trial results. In: Salmon SE, Jones SE (eds) Adjuvant therapy of cancer, part II. North-Holland, New York, pp 383–390
7 Muggia FM, Jacobs EM (1979) Adjuvant chemotherapy of testicular carcinoma: The need for evaluation of curative strategies. In: Bonadonna G, Mathé G, Salmon SE (eds) Recent Results in Cancer Research, vol 68. Springer, Berlin Heidelberg New York
8 Muggia FM, Rozencweig M, Chiuten DF, Jensen-Akula MS, Charles LM, Kubota T, Bono VH Jr (1980) Phase II trials: Use of a clinical tumor panel and overview of current resources and studies. Cancer Treat Rep 64: 1–9
9 Nervi C, Arcangeli G, Concolino F, Cortese M (1980) Prolonged survival with postirradiation adjuvant chemotherapy in stage IV breast cancer. In: Salmon SE, Jones SE (eds) Adjuvant therapy of cancer, part II. North-Holland, New York, pp 311–317
10 Rozencweig M, DeSloover C, Von Hoff DD, Tagnon H, Muggia FM (1979) Introduction: Anthracycline derivatives in new drug development programs. Cancer Treat Rep 63: 807–809
11 Rozencweig M, Von Hoff DD, Staquet MJ, Guarino AG, Penta JS, Muggia FM (1979) Predictive value of animal toxicology with anticancer agents prior to early clinical trials. Clin Res 27: 391A
12 Salmon SE, Hamburger AW, Soehlen B, Durie BGM, Alberts DS, Moon TS (1978) Quantitation of differential sensitivity of human-tumor stem cells to anticancer drugs. N Engl J Med 298: 1321–1327
13 Speyer JL, Collins JM, Dedrick RL, Brennan MF, Londer H, DeVita VT Jr, Myers CE (1979) Phase I and pharmacological studies of intraperitoneal (I.P.) 5-fluorouracil (5-FU). Proc Am Assoc Cancer Res and Am Soc Clin Oncol 20: 352

Adjuvant Therapies of Postsurgical Minimal Residual Disease

G. Bonadonna, M. Gasparini, and A. Rossi

Summary

The review summarizes the most recent results obtained with present combined adjuvant strategy for the treatment of resectable cancer. Recent important randomized clinical trials, either unicentric or policentric, are discussed.
As fas as pediatric tumors are concerned post-surgical adjuvant chemotherapy was proved to play a useful role in prolonging the disease-free survival in Wilms tumor, rhabdomyosarcoma, Ewing sarcoma. Results obtained in the treatment of medulloblastoma and osteogenic sarcoma need further investigations.
In adult neoplasms the most important results with combined modality approach are presently being obtained in breast cancer and probably in melanoma. No consistent improvement by adjuvant chemotherapy has been observed in colorectal cancer.

Introduction

Combined-modality treatment is currently one of the most promising areas in cancer research and therapy, and relies heavily on sophisticated clinical trials involving all oncologic disciplines. As trials are increasing in number and scope, general reviews are useful to focus on the most promising and controversial results. The present review does not attempt to make an exhaustive analysis of all available publications on the subject of adjuvant therapy for resectable cancer. Ongoing trials are already innumerable, but too often the results are very preliminary and therefore difficult to compare with those of studies having longer follow-up. Thus, the data discussed in this review will be primarily those derived from recent studies that were randomized and had sufficient survival figures. Readers interested in further details are advised to consult our previous reviews [4, 43] as well as two recent books dealing specifically with the subject of adjuvant therapy [3, 34].

Pediatric Tumors

Adjuvant chemotherapy has been used extensively in the management of malignant disease in children and adolescents after surgical resection and/or radiotherapy for localized tumors. Its effectiveness in prolonging the relapse-free survival (RFS) has been demonstrated in numerous clinical trials, and its use has become routine in the management of most pediatric tumors. Clinical research in this field is undergoing important changes. Current clinical trials on treatment for localized and resectable tumors in children are being designed in order to establish the best chemotherapeutic regimen in terms of drug selection, optimal treatment duration, and minimal sequelae. Furthermore, cancer chemotherapy has become an important tool together with surgery and radiotherapy in the initial management of localized tumors (e.g., osteogenic sarcoma) with the goal of reducing morbidity from mutilating surgery. Some important prognostic factors are emerging that are being taken into account in the preparation of new clinical trials to answer specific questions. The most recent data of studies currently under evaluation about adjuvant treatment of childhood cancer will be summarized and the discussion will focus on questions that need an answer.

Wilms Tumor (Table 1)

In this tumor, combined surgery, radiotherapy, and chemotherapy have definitely improved the cure rate. Present directions involve controlled studies aimed at reevaluating the risk factors, the effectiveness of radiotherapy in different disease stages, the number of drugs to be administered, and the optimal duration of adjuvant therapy.

From the results of the three largest study groups on Wilms tumor, many important factors are emerging that could definitely influence the future treatment strategy [14, 38, 50]. First of all, the histologic features of primary tumor seem to be the most important factor influencing treatment results.

Regardless of stage and type of treatment, the sarcomatous and anaplastic patterns predict a poor prognosis. Children with favorable histology have better prognosis, and with current treatment programs about 90% of the patients with stages I and II are suviving disease-free at 2–3 years after nephrectomy. Other factors, such as age, tumor size, and presence of regional adenopathy, seem to play an important role in affecting treatment results [14, 38, 50]. All above-mentioned factors have to be considered in planning new trials in order to minimize treatment intensity in children with favorable prognostic factors.

Radiotherapy, in terms of dose and timing, needs to be reassessed. First of all, NWTSG-2 and SIOP-2 trials [14, 50] clearly seem to establish that postoperative radiotherapy is not necessary to improve the cure rate in stage I patients. There is also evidence that the incidence of local and distant relapse can be reduced when radiotherapy is started almost immediately after nephrectomy. As far as adjuvant chemotherapy is concerned, a short course, with vincristine (VCR) ± actinomycin D (Act-D), appears as effective as a long course, at least in patients with favorable histology. Adriamycin (ADM), which does not seem to improve the RFS in children with favorable histology, could be important in the treatment of high-risk patients. The NWTSG-3 was purposely designed to answer this question.

Rhabdomyosarcoma (Table 2)

The results of the Intergroup Rhabdomyosarcoma Study were recently updated in January 1979 during a meeting held in Orlando, Florida, and they confirmed what had been previously published [35, 36]. When radical resection of the primary tumor was

Table 1. Wilms tumor: recent results with systemic adjuvant treatment

Institution	Stage	No. of cases	Treatment regimen	% RFS ≥ 2 years	Remarks
NWTS-2 [14]	I	115	R < S+ACT–D, VCR × 6 months	98	Patients with favorable histology
			same × 15 months	98	
	II–III	196	R < S + RT + ACT–D, VCR	80	
			same + ADM	90	
SIOP-2 [50]	I	53	(RT) → S + ACT–D, VCR	93	No significant difference if chemotherapy is given for 6 or 15 months
	II	30	(RT) → S + RT + ACT–D, VCR	96	
	III	37	(RT) → S + RT + ACT–D, VCR	52	
MRC-2 [38]	I	61	S → RT + VCR < short course	91	
			long course	91	
	II–III	79	S RT + VCR < VCR, ACT–D	85–75	Differences not significant
			same + ADM		

R, random; S, surgery (nephrectomy); RT, radiotherapy

technically feasible (group-I disease), the 2-year RFS was more than 80% if adjuvant (VCR, Act-D, and cyclophosphamide (CTX) chemotherapy was administered. In this randomized study, the addition of postoperative chemotherapy failed to increase the percent of relapse-free survivors or the probability of local control, and the treatment was ineffective when the tumor was located in one of the extremities. In fact, six of seven children relapsed after amputation. In group-II disease (tumor resecton with microscopic residuals and/or extension into regional nodes or adjacent organs), 70% of the children were rendered disease-free for longer than 2 years by adjuvant

Table 2. Childhood rhabdomyosarcoma: Recent results of adjuvant chemotherapy in group I and II patients

Institution	Group	No. of cases	Treatment regimen	% RFS $\geqslant$ 2 years	Remarks
Intergroup	I	73	R < VAC + RT	86	RT seems unnecessary
			VAC	80	
	II	130	R < VA + RT	70	CTX does not improve results
			VAC + RT	70	
St. Jude Hospital	I	17	Various	71	Timing of ADM is probably important
	II	37	Various + RT	65	
Memorial Center	I–II	33	T_2 protocol ± RT	93	

U, UCR; A, ACT-D; C, CTX; R, random

radiotherapy and chemotherapy. Since no difference was observed between the two arms of the study protocol, it was concluded that a two-drug regimen (VCR and Act-D) was as effective as a three-drug regimen (the same plus CTX). The value of adjuvant chemotherapy was confirmed in Orlando by the experience also at St. Jude Children's Hospital in Memphis and at the Memorial Hospital in New York. In both centers, group-I patients were not administered postoperative irradiation. The therapeutic results summarized in Table 2 are of particular importance since very few patients show relapse beyond the second year.

The optimal dose of radiotherapy as well as the volume of tissue to be irradiated are not yet established. From the data of the Intergroup Rhabdomyosarcoma Study, there is evidence that a dose ranging from 3000 to 4000 rad may be sufficient to assure good local control. However, to reduce the incidence of long-term morbidity in the new study (to be activated), different doses and volumes of radiotherapy will be compared in group-II as well as in group-III (gross residual disease after resection) patients.

When evaluating the treatment results in children with localized rhabdomyosarcoma, many prognostic factors must be considered. The experience of the Intergroup showed clearly that the histologic subtype and the site of primary tumor are strongly related to prognosis. Alveolar subtype, primary tumor in the extremities, and parameningeal extension of head and neck rhabdomyosarcoma all involve a very poor prognosis. Therefore, all these situations require different, probably more intensive, treatment regimens.

Osteogenic Sarcoma (Table 3)

During the past 5 years, optimistic results have been reported in the treatment of this tumor [11, 28, 42, 47]. However, since the large majority of clinical trials were not randomized, considerations regarding some changes that may have occurred in the natural history of osteosarcoma, bias from patient selection, improved surgery, and short follow-up evaluation form the bases of current criticisms concerning present results. In fact, some or all above-mentioned factors may have favorably influenced the disease-free survival regardless of adjuvant chemotherapy. For this reason, some centers, such as the Mayo Clinic and the National Cancer Institute (NCI), are now conducting prospective randomized studies in which the results of amputation alone are compared with those of amputation followed by adjuvant chemotherapy (adriamycin plus high-dose methotrexate, or HDMTX). In fact, in these institutions, amputation followed by adriamycin, HDMTX, or both failed to achieve a 2-year RFS in more than 40% of the patients. Similar results were reported by the Milan Cancer Institute [19] after adriamycin, and by the EORTC group [29] after using two different forms of combination chemotherapy. Better results were reported by the Sidney Farber Cancer Center [28] and by the Memorial Hospital [42], where combined treatment is planned to avoid amputation in selected patients and to resect the tumor-bearing bone with prosthetic replacement. The good results obtained by the COMPADRI I regimen [47] were not confirmed by subsequent modification of the original combination (COMPADRI II, III, and IV). The CALGB is conducting a new randomized trial in which adjuvant adriamycin alone is compared with adriamycin plus HDMTX with late dose intensification. The updated results [12] show no difference between the two treatment regimens (approximately 50% 2-year actuarial RFS).

The importance of preoperative chemotherapy was stressed by Rosen et al. [42] at the Orlando meeting in January 1979. Patients whose tumor showed evidence of necrosis after preoperative chemotherapy had a very low incidence of distant relapse compared with patients whose tumor was not histologically affected by chemotherapy. Rosen et al. [42] suggested that this histologic assessment could represent a prognostic tool as well as a guide to drug selection for postoperative chemotherapy. Finally, the Karolinska study with interferon [46] administered as adjuvant after amputation suggests a possible role of immunotherapy in the management of osteosarcoma. These interesting results should be confirmed through an appropriate randomized trial.

Table 3. Osteogenic sarcoma: Current results with adjuvant treatment

Institution	No. of cases	Treatment regimen	RFS		Remarks
			%	Time (years)	
Sidney Farber [28]	12	A + VCR, HDMTX	41	4	
	22	A + VCR, HDMTX, ADM	59	2	
	37	S + VCR, HDMTX, ADM (with intensification)	73	0.5–1.5	RFS not influenced by type of S
Memorial Hospital	31	S + T_4 S + T_5	58	3	Poor results < 12 years of age
SWOG [47]	36	CONPADRI I	54	2	
CALGB [11]	46	A + ADM	55	4	RFS 27% in protocol violators
Milan [19]	13	A + ADM	31	3	ADM 75 mg/m² Q 4 weeks
Mayo Clinic	53	R ⟨ A A + RT (lungs) + ACT-D	35 35	4 4	
	?	R ⟨ A + transfer factor A + VCR, MTX, ADM	30 30	2 2	Skin test converters 58%
Karolinska [46]	24	A + interferon	64	2.5	
NCI	38	R ⟨ A + VCR, HDMTX A + VCR, HDMTX, BCG	40 40	2 2	RFS related to histologic grade

A, amputation; S, amputation or limb preservation; R, random

Ewing Sarcoma (Table 4)

During the past decade, the improvement of RFS and of local control has been well established. The most recent clinical trials report 40%–82% relapse-free survivors at 2–5 years. Some of the study groups updated their results at the meeting held in Orlando in January 1979. Among the important new findings, the Mayo Clinic and the Intergroup Ewing Sarcoma Study have reported a 12% local relapse after combined modality. Furthermore, when technically feasible, the addition of surgery favorably

Table 4. Ewing sarcoma: Current results with adjuvant treatment

Institution	No. of cases	Treatment regimen	% RFS 2 years	Remarks
Mayo Clinic	57	S + various drugs	65	
	205	RT + various drugs	40	12% Local recurrence
Intergroup	248	R ⟨ RT + VAC	35	12% Local recurrence; prognosis improved when S was utilized
		RT + VAC + lung RT	58	
		RT + VAC + ADM	74	
NCI [20]	79	RT + various drugs ± CNS prophyl.	45	No difference among various regimens
Memorial Hospital	20	RT + T_2	75	
	28	$T_6 \rightarrow RT \rightarrow T_2$	82	
Milan	30	RT + ADM + CTX + VCR	55	
EORTC/GTO [33]	12	RT + ADM + VCR + CTX + procarbazine	56	

S, surgical resection of primary tumor

affected the prognosis. As far as drug selection is concerned, the regimen of the Intergroup using a four-drug regimen (VCR, Act-D, CTX, ADM) yielded the best results, especially when intervals between cycles were shortened. Even more favorable results were recently published by LE MEVEL et al. [32] of the EORTC/GTO group. The treatment regimen included vincristine and cyclophosphamide during the radiation program while adriamycin and dactinomycin were added to the combination thereafter for a total of nine cycles. So far, no relapses have been observed, but the maximum reported follow-up was 24 months and the number of study patients was too small (11 cases) to draw meaningful conclusions. As far as adjuvant radiotherapy is concerned, in the Intergroup study, prophylactic lung irradiation failed to improve the RFS over adjuvant chemotherapy alone when given through a four-drug regimen. However, lung irradiation decreased the incidence of lung metastases and lengthened the time of their onset.

It should now be definitely recognized that treatment results are strongly influenced by the site of primary tumor. Primary involvement of distal bones is usually associated with longer free intervals compared with pelvic involvement, which almost invariably involves a very poor prognosis (20% disease-free survivors despite adequate combined regimens). The importance of the various prognostic factors [surgery, primary site, male sex, lactate dehydrogenase (LDH) level] was recently confirmed by the NCI group through a reevaluation of the studies by POMEROY and JOHNSON [20]. Each study was not homogeneous as far as prognostic factors were concerned. However, when the patient groups were balanced according to the various prognostic markers, no difference in the RFS was observed, regardless of whether single- or multiple-drug regimens were utilized as adjuvant to irradiation.

All above-mentioned findings must be considered in designing future trials. Pelvic primaries, unresectable tumors, male patients, and high values of LDH all represent unfavorable markers. Therefore, patients who belong to these categories are candidates for a more aggressive type of treatment. On the contrary, lesions in distal bones, partially or totally resectable, could be irradiated with lower doses and/or smaller fields. The importance of the initial successful treatment in Ewing sarcoma is also stressed by the knowledge of an almost invariably fatal outcome of relapsing patients. In fact, salvage treatment with some chance of success, such as in Wilms tumor and in osteogenic sarcoma, has proved so far to be ineffective in Ewing sarcoma.

Medulloblastoma (Table 5)

The two largest cooperative study groups on medulloblastoma planned a randomized trial with the objective to establish the actual role of adjuvant chemotherapy in the prolongation of the disease-free status after maximal surgical resection and neural axis radiotherapy [2, 9]. As yet, there is no significant evidence that adjuvant systemic chemotherapy has improved the therapeutic results over those obtained by surgery and radiotherapy. It is too early to draw significant conclusions, however, because the length of follow-up is still limited, i.e., less than 2 years. In fact, considering the natural history of medulloblastoma, relapses can occur also at many years after primary therapy.

At the Istituto Nazionale Tumori of Milan, 77% of 27 patients treated with surgery, radiotherapy, systemic chemotherapy, and intrathecal methotrexate are free of disease after a 4-year follow-up. Overall survival is 90%. In this group of patients, long-term sequelae were not observed, although a longer follow-up is required to critically ascertain this point.

Adult Tumors

Contrary to what has been observed for childhood neoplasias, systemic adjuvant therapy is not part of the routine management of resectable tumors in adults. At present, innumerable studies ongoing in major institutions of the world are attempting to establish the actual value of current drugs in subsets at high risk of early recurrence despite optimal local-regional modality. Most studies were started during the past 3 years, and therefore for many tumors available results are too premature [3, 4, 34, 43].

Breast Cancer (Tables 6 and 7)

In breast cancer with positive axillary lymph nodes, the new generation of clinical trials has produced a number of positive results. Adjuvant systemic therapy has been repeatedly shown significantly to prolong the RFS and, at least in two studies [5, 10, 44], also the overall survival. While the initial favorable results should be confirmed in a long-term analysis before combined-modality treatment with adjuvant chemotherapy can be considered as having absolute clinical value, newer studies are trying to answer some of the questions that emerged from the first report on CTX + MTX + 5-fluorouracil (FU) (CMF) and phenylalanine mustard (PAM) trials.

Table 5. Medulloblastoma: Recent results with systemic adjuvant treatment after surgery and craniospinal irradiation

Institution	No. of cases	Treatment regimen	RFS %	RFS Time (years)	Remarks
CCSG [9]	83	R < S + RT	59	2	Differences not significant
		R < S + RT + VCR, PRD, CCNU	64	2	
SIOP brain tumor trial [2]		S R < RT	67	2	Differences not significant
		S R < RT + VCR, CCNU	79	2	
Milan	27	S + RT + VCR, CCNU, MTX (IT)	77	4	No leukoencephalopathy

S, maximal surgical resection; IT, intrathecal; RRD, prednisone

Table 6. Recent results in operable breast cancer given adjuvant chemotherapy

Author or group	No. of cases	Disease extent	Drug therapy after RM	Follow-up (years)	Essential findings
Milan [5, 44]	386	T_{1-3A}, N +	CTR[a] vs 12 CMF	4	Increased RFS (pre + post) and survival
[48]	325 (pre)	T_{1-3A}, N +	12 vs 6 CMF	3	No difference related to duration of treatment
NSABP [18]	348	Stage II	CTR[a] vs PAM	4	Increased RFS pre 1–3 nodes over CTR
	672	Stage II	PAM vs PAM + FU	2	Increased RFS over HCTR[b]
COG [16]	254	N +	PAM vs CMF-V	4	Increased RFS in CMF-V especially in ≥ 50 years

[a] CRT, concomitant control group
[b] HCTR, historical control group

The first question deals with the therapeutic effect of single-agent versus combination chemotherapy. All published reports [3, 4, 34, 43] on this subject confirmed that polydrug therapy was superior to single-agent therapy in also an adjuvant situation. The second question deals with the role of postoperative radiotherapy in conjunction with adjuvant chemotherapy. Although the question has not yet been clearly answered, available results do not indicate that adjuvant radiotherapy plus adjuvant chemotherapy improved the RFS over adjuvant chemotherapy alone [3, 4, 34, 43]. In one study [10] for which the 8-year survival is available, the RFS was decreased when

Table 7. Recent results in operable breast cancer given adjuvant chemotherapy ± radiotherapy

Author or group	No. of cases	Disease extent	Drug therapy after RM	Follow-up	Essential findings
Cooper et al. [10]	100	N + $\geqslant$ 4	CMFVP ± RT	8 years	Increased RFS in nonirradiated patients
SWOG [21]	334	Stage II	CMFVP[a] ± RT vs PAM ± RT	26 months	CMFVP superior; high % of local recurrence
CALGB [49]	449	N +	CMFVP + RT vs CMF ± RT vs CMF + MER ± RT	3 years	No benefit from MER treatment
Mayo Clinic [1]	166	Stage II	PAM vs CFP vs CFP + RT	> 2 years	CFP ± RT superior to PAM in premenopause
Univ. Arizona [52]	98	Stage II	AC ± RT	4 years	No difference between pre and post; no negative effect of RT
M.D. Anderson [8]	222	Stage II–III	FAC + BCG + RT	3 years	Increased RFS and total survival (pre and post) over HCTR[b]

[a] Continuous administration
[b] HCTR historical control group
CMFVP: CMF, VCR, PRD; CFP: CTX, FU, PRD; AC: ADM, CTX; FAC: FU, ADM, CTX

radiation was combined with chemotherapy, probably because of immune suppression produced by radiotherapy. At any rate, the local control produced by combination chemotherapy such as CMF seems to be competitive with that usually achieved by postoperative radiotherapy [6].

An important aspect is the possible role of chemical castration as a factor contributing to the successful results reported in premenopausal compared with postmenopausal women [6]. Recent analysis of the RFS in women with and without CMF-induced amenorrhea [5] and with positive or negative estrogen receptors [7] have concluded that, although in a consistent fraction of women ovarian failure occurs as result of chemotherapy, the therapeutic benefit of CMF is not due to chemical castration. The comparative 4-year results indicated that adjuvant CMF chemotherapy was superior to adjuvant castration [6] and that this treatment was also effective in postmenopausal women when >75% of the optimal dose was administered [44]. Furthermore, practically none of the studies using polydrug regimens are showing a therapeutic difference between pre- and postmenopausal patients. Other relevant questions concern the optimal duration of drug therapy, the role of some drugs (e.g., ADM and corticosteroids), and the usefulness of adjuvant endocrine therapy and of immunotherapy when combined with chemotherapy. The optimal duration of therapy has not been established, but a general impression is that the prolongation of treatment beyond the first year is probably not necessary if drug therapy is sufficiently aggressive.

It is noteworthy that recent findings [48] have shown that RFS and total survival were comparable at 3 years after 12 or 6 cycles of CMF in premenopausal women. Adriamycin should be used cautiously in an adjuvant situation because of the potential risk of cardiomyopathy. At present, regimens containing adriamycin [34] do not appear to be clearly superior to those that do not use this drug. Several investigators are testing the value of adjuvant chemotherapy combined with endocrine therapy (especially tamoxifen) in postmenopausal women with positive estrogen receptors. No results are as yet available. On the contrary, initial evidence is that adjuvant chemoimmunotherapy, at least with BCG and MER [3, 34], is not improving the results over adjuvant chemotherapy alone. Further studies will probably be required before the relative merits of immunotherapy can be definitely assessed.

Malignant Melanoma (Table 8)

Current results on adjuvant treatment for malignant melanoma remain controversial [3, 34]. There is no convincing evidence that immunotherapy either alone or combined with chemotherapy has increased the RFS over surgery alone. The data of the randomized trials performed by CUNNINGHAM et al. [13] and by the WHO group (unpublished data) do not support the beneficial effects of BCG reported in nonrandomized trials. On the contrary, there is preliminary evidence of improved RFS at 2–3 years after adjuvant chemotherapy. Positive results were obtained either with dacarbazine (DTIC), such as in the large series by WHO, or with a complex polydrug therapy, as carried out in two different studies by the French group [27].

Gastrointestinal Cancer (Table 9)

In colorectal cancer, there seems to be minimal benefit from adjuvant FU [3, 4, 34, 43], but available results fail to show that this drug has made a consistent impact in the adjuvant situation. More recent studies utilizing nitrosourea derivatives such as methyl-CCNU, and immunotherapy with BCG or MER, confirmed that, at present, the available drugs cannot be used successfully in the treatment of colorectal cancer. The detailed analysis by DAVIS and KISNER [15] confirms this statement. An avenue worth considering is hepatic infusion plus systemic chemotherapy for patients at high risk.

Table 8. Current adjuvant results in malignant melanoma

Author or group	No. of cases	Disease extent	Drug therapy	Median Follow-up	Essential findings
COG [26]	165[a]	Stage I, II, III	DTIC for 1 year	30 months	Decreased RFS after DTIC
Kaufman et al. [31]	75	Clark III, IV, V	DTIC vs BCG vs DTIC + BCG for 2 years	18 months	Best results after DTIC + BCG
Jacquillat et al. [27]	117[a]	Clark III, IV, V	VLB + thiotepa + MTX + streptonigrin + PCZ ± IA DTIC for 1.5 years	4 years	Increased RFS over CTR especially in men; no benefit from IA DTIC
WHO	603[a]	N + and Clark III, IV, V	DTIC vs BCG vs DTIC + BCG for 2 years	25 months	Improved RFS after DTIC = BCG

[a] Including a randomized control group
IA: intraarterial; PCZ, procarbazine

No recent studies have been published concerning adjuvant treatment of gastric carcinoma. Most ongoing studies are using FAM (FU, ADM, and mitomycin) chemotherapy, which has been confirmed to be effective in 45%–50% of the patients with advanced disease.

Malignant Gliomas (Table 10)

Since neurosurgery followed by high-dose radiotherapy invariably fails to eradicate malignant brain gliomas, these tumors appear to be excellent candidates for adjuvant

Table 9. Current adjuvant results in colorectal cancer

Research group	No. of cases	Dukes class	Drug therapy	Follow-up	Essential findings
Grossi et al. [23]	500[a]	A–B–C	FU IL[b] + IV for 2 days	5 years	Trend in favor of Dukes' B and C
Higgins et al. [24]	338[a] 518[a]	A–B–C C	FU single course FU for 18 months	5 years 5 years	Improved survival (10%) No benefit over CTR
Grage et al. [22]	211[a]	B–C	FU for 1 year	Median 28 months	Improved RFS after FU in rectal cancer (C)
Lokich [33]	394[a]	B_2–C	MER-BCG vs FU + MeCCNU ± MER-BCG for 18 months	Median 13 months	No difference among treatments
Panettiere and Heilbrun [39]	295	B_2–C	FU + MeCCNU ± BCG for 12 months	Median 19 months	No benefit over CTR
McPherson et al. [37]	100[a]	B_2–C	BCG ± FU + MeCCNU for 1.5 years	Maximum 35 months	No benefit over CTR

[a] Including a randomized control group (CTR)
[b] IL: intraluminal

chemotherapy of the residual disease. Unfortunately, currently effective drugs, including nitrosourea compounds (BCNU, CCNU, MeCCNU), showed a low-grade activity on malignant gliomas. Therefore, the positive results so far published have not improved the cure rate of glioblastoma multiforme [3, 4, 25, 43]. Tumor grade (III or IV) and extent of surgical resection still remain important prognostic factors and should be used more systematically as stratification parameters in prospective studies.

Table 10. Recent results of adjuvant therapy in totally resected malignant gliomas

Author or group	No. of patients	Postoperative therapy[a]	Essential findings
SOLERO et al. [45]	102	RT + BCNU or CCNU	Improved survival after RT + CCNU
WALKER and STRIKE [51]	326	Radiotherapy + BCNU + MP ± PCZ ; additional corticosteroid	No difference in survival in the four treatment groups
EORTC [25]	81 93	RT ± CCNU RT ± VM 26 + CCNU	CCNU did not affect RFS; no improvement of early RFS after VM 26 + CCNU
PAOLETTI et al. [40]	168	RT + BCNU RT + CCNU	No difference in survival between the two groups

[a] MP, methylprednisolone

Table 11. Tumors in which adjuvant studies are ongoing, but results are not yet clearly evaluable

Site of disease	Stage	Current situation
Testicle	N+	Early vs late chemotherapy
Ovary	I–II	Single vs multiple-drug therapy
Endometrium	G 1–2–3	Value of medroxyprogesterone to be confirmed
Bladder	T_{1-3} N +	T_1: Local thiotepa, adriamycin N+: Value of chemotherapy is to be established
Head and neck	T_{2-3}	Value of preoperative chemotherapy
Lung	N–, N+	Value of chemotherapy remains to be clearly established
Stomach	N+	
Cervix	N+	
Soft tissue (adults)	Early	

Miscellaneous Tumors (Table 11)

In many tumors, combined treatment modality was started only a few years ago. Thus, present results are scanty and the value of chemotherapy remains to be established through appropriate trials. In other tumors (e.g., lung and gastric carcinomas), adjuvant chemotherapy was tried many years ago but, with very few exceptions [3, 4, 34, 43], the drug treatment applied has failed to improve significantly the RFS in the surgical adjuvant setting.

Testicular germ cell tumors are now curable, even in advanced stages [30]. Combination chemotherapy drug regimens, such as that with cisplatinum, vinblastine (VLB), and bleomycin [17], have made a major impact on survival of patients with testicular germ cell tumors, because these regimens can induce a high percentage of durable complete remissions, particularly in the absence of minimal advanced disease. The role of combined-modality therapy (chemotherapy and reductive surgery) needs to be further defined. In particular, prospective randomized studies should compare the value of adjuvant chemotherapy versus delayed chemotherapy, i.e., the same systemic treatment applied at the time of first relapse after radical surgery alone. In advanced (stages III and IV) ovarian cancer, Young et al. [53] have shown that combination chemotherapy with Hexa-CAF (hexamethylmelamine, CTX, MTX, and FU) is superior to PAM. Ongoing studies were designed with the intent to demonstrate that, also in the adjuvant situation, a polydrug regimen can yield better results than single-drug therapy. Compared with the situation in children, information on the usefulness of multimodal therapy for adult soft-tissue sarcomas is still limited [3, 4, 34, 43]. The NCI study conducted by Rosenberg et al. [43] has shown that both RFS and total survival were significantly improved by adjuvant combination chemotherapy over historical controls. A more properly designed prospective study was recently activated by the EORTC Soft-Tissue Sarcoma Group [41] where, after limb-sparing surgery, no further therapy is compared with combination chemotherapy containing CTX, VCR, ADM, and DTIC.

Conclusion

Present results indicate that adjuvant chemotherapy can be accepted as having absolute clinical value in only a few neoplastic diseases, particularly in pediatric tumors. However, it is logical to expect that, within the next decade, the results of well-designed studies will show a broader clinical application of multimodality therapy. In the meantime, some critical points must be kept in mind. As correctly stated by S. K. Carter (unpublished work), more detailed and sophisticated staging techniques have moved some patients, previously classified as having limited disease, into the extensive staging category. Therefore, these shifts have tended artificially to improve median survival for limited and for extensive disease when compared with earlier data, regardless of treatment. This has significant complications also for the use of historical controls [43]. Furthermore, many adjuvant trials use disease-free survival as a major end point for benefit analysis. There are, however, many clinical situations in which disease-free survival might not correlate with increased total survival. These clinical situations include the following: (a) where curative salvage therapy exists after first relapse (e.g., Hodgkin's disease and testicular cancer), (b) where prolonged survival can be achieved after first relapse (e.g., breast cancer and ovarian cancer), and (c) where adjuvant therapy would cause late complications such as chronic organ toxicity and the development of second tumors. Since many patients given adjuvant therapy are potentially cured by their primary surgery and/or radiation, the problem of late complications must be factored into the overall analysis of adjuvant trials.

References

1 Ahmann DL, Payne WS, Scanlon PW, O'Fallon JR, Bisel HF, Hahn RG, Edmonson JH, Ingle JN, Frytak S, O'Connell MJ, Rubin J (1978) Repeated adjuvant chemotherapy with phenylalanine mustard or 5-fluorouracil, cyclophosphamide, and prednisone with or without radiation, after mastectomy for breast cancer. Lancet 1: 893–896

2 Bloom HJG (1978) SIOP brain tumor trial. Proc Xth Meet Int Soc Pediatr Oncol, Bruxelles, pp 20–23
3 Bonadonna G, Mathé G, Salmon SE (eds) (1979) Recent results in cancer research. Adjuvant therapies and markers of post-surgical minimal residual disease, vol 68. Springer, Berlin Heidelberg New York
4 Bonadonna G, Tancini G, Rossi A, Gasparini M (1978) Chemotherapy in the prevention of the recurrence of resectable cancer. Ann Rev Med 29: 149–175
5 Bonadonna G, Valagussa P, Rossi A, Tancini G, Bajetta E, Marchini S, Veronesi U (1980) CMF adjuvant chemotherapy in operable breast cancer. In: Salmon SE, Jones SE (eds) Adjuvant therapy of cancer II. Grune and Stratton, New York, pp 227–235
6 Bonadonna G, Valagussa P, Rossi A, Zucali R, Tancini G, Bajetta E, Brambilla C, De Lena M, Di Fronzo G, Banfi A, Rilke F, Veronesi U (1978) Are surgical adjuvant trials altering the course of breast cancer? Semin Oncol 5: 450–464
7 Bonadonna G, Valagussa P, Tancini G, Di Fronzo G (1980) Estrogen receptor status and response to chemotherapy in early and advanced breast cancer. Cancer Chemother Pharmacol 4: 37–41
8 Buzdar AV, Blumenschein GR, Gutterman JU, Hortobagyi GN, Campos LT, Tashima CK, Smith TL, Hersh EM, Gehan EA (1980) Adjuvant therapy with 5-fluorouracil, adriamycin, cyclophosphamide and BCG (FAC-BCG) for stage II and III breast cancer. Prolongation of disease-free interval and survival. In: Salmon SE, Jones SE (eds) Adjuvant therapy of cancer II. Grune and Stratton, New York, pp 277–284
9 Children's Cancer Study Group: Evans AE, Jenkin RD, Ertel I, Wilson C (1979) Adjuvant chemotherapy for medulloblastoma, interim report from CCG 942. Proc Am Assoc Clin Oncol 20: 425
10 Cooper RG, Holland JF, Glidewell O (1979) Adjuvant chemotherapy of breast cancer. Cancer 44: 793–800
11 Cortes EP, Holland JF, Glidewell O (1978) Amputation and adriamycin in primary osteosarcoma: A 5 years report. Cancer Treat Rep 62: 271–278
12 Cortes EP, Necheles TF, Holland JF, Glidewell O (1979) Adriamycin (ADM) alone versus ADM and high dose methotrexate citrovorum factor rescue (HDMTX-CF) as adjuvant to operable primary osteosarcoma (OS): A randomized study by cancer and leukemia group B (CALGB). Proc Am Assoc Clin Oncol 20: 412
13 Cunningham TJ, Schoenfeld D, Nathason L, Wolter J, Patterson W, Cohen M, Kuperminc M, Carbone PP (1980) A controlled ECOG study of adjuvant therapy in patients with stage I and II malignant melanoma. In: Salmon SE, Jones SE (eds) Adjuvant therapy of cancer II. Grune and Stratton, New York, pp 507–517
14 D'Angio GJ, Beckwith JB, Breslow N, Sinks L, Sutow W, Wolff J (1979) Results of the second National Wilms' tumor study (NWTS-2). Proc Am Assoc Clin Oncol 20: 309
15 Davis HL, Kisner DL (1978) Analysis of adjuvant therapy of large bowel cancer. Cancer Clin Trials 1: 273–287
16 Davis HL, Metter GE, Ramirez G, Grage TB, Cornel G, Fletcher W, Moss S, Multhauf P (1979) An adjuvant trial of 1-phenylalanine mustard versus cyclophosphamide, methotrexate, 5-fluorouracil, and vincristine (CMF-V) following mastectomy for operable breast cancer. Proc Am Soc Clin Oncol 20: 358
17 Einhorn LH, Donohue JP (1977) Cis-diammine-dichloroplatinum, vincristine and bleomycin combination chemotherapy in disseminated testicular cancer. Ann Intern Med 87: 293–298
18 Fisher B (1980) Breast cancer: Studies of the National Surgical Adjuvant Primary Breast Cancer Project (NSABP). In: Salmon SE, Jones SE (eds) Adjuvant therapy of cancer II. Grune and Stratton, New York, pp 215–226
19 Fossati-Bellani F, Gasparini M, Bonadonna G (1979) Adriamycin in the adjuvant treatment of operable osteosarcoma. Recent Results Cancer Res 68: 25–27
20 Glaubiger D, Makuch R, Schwarz J, Levine AS (1979) Influence of prognostic factors on treatment results in Ewing's sarcoma. Proc Am Assoc Clin Oncol 20: 373

21 Glucksberg H, Rivkin S, Rasmussen S (1980) Adjuvant chemotherapy in stage II breast cancer. In: Salmon SE, Jones SE (eds) Adjuvant therapy of cancer II. Grune and Stratton, New York, pp 261–268
22 Grage T, Hill Y, Cornell G, Frelick R, Moss S (1980) Adjuvant chemotherapy in large bowel cancer. In: Salmon SE, Jones SE (eds) Adjuvant therapy of cancer II. Grune and Stratton, New York, pp 587–594
23 Grossi CE, Wolff WI, Nealon TF Jr, Pasternack B, Ginzburg L, Rousselot LM (1977) Intraluminal fluorouracil chemotherapy adjuvant to surgical procedures for resectable carcinoma of the colon and rectum. Surg Gynecol Obstet 145: 549–554
24 Higgins GA, Lee LE, Dwight RW, Keehn RJ (1978) The case for adjuvant 5-fluorouracil in colorectal cancer. Cancer Clin Trials 1: 35–41
25 Hildebrand J (1979) Adjuvant chemotherapy in malignant brain gliomas. Recent Results Cancer Res 68: 408–411
26 Hill GJ, Moss S, Fletcher W, Golomb F, Grage T (1978) DTIC melanoma adjuvant study: Final report. Proc Am Soc Clin Oncol 19: 309
27 Jacquillat C, Banzet J, Civatte J, Puissant P, Cottenot F, Israel L, Belarch S, Chastang C, Maral J (1979) Adjuvant chemotherapy or chemoimmunotherapy in the management of primary malignant melanoma of level III, IV, or V. Recent Results Cancer Res 68: 346–358
28 Jaffe N, Frei E III, Watts H, Traggis D (1978) High dose methotrexate in osteogenic sarcoma: A 5-years experience. Cancer Treat Rep 62: 259–264
29 Jasmin C (1979) Randomized trial of adjuvant chemotherapy in osteogenic osteosarcoma. EORTC Osteosarcoma Working Party Group. Recent Results Cancer Res 68: 28–32
30 Katz ME, Grosbach AB, Wein A, Glick JH (1978) Testicular germ cell tumors. Diagnosis, management, and the potential for cure. Cancer Clin Trials 1: 247–271
31 Kaufman SD, Cosimi AB, Wood WC, Carey RW (1979) Adjuvant therapy in malignant melanoma. A trial of immunotherapy, chemotherapy and combined treatment. Recent Results Cancer Res 68: 380–386
32 Le Mevel BP, Hoerni B, Durant D, Kenesi C, Salle M, Trifaud A, Liegey-Bagari D, Bainvel JV, Rogez JM, Fumoleau P, Mazabraud A, Dumont J, Tomend B, Brossel E, Garetta M, Guerrin D, Jasmin C, Sancho-Garnier H, Gimenez M (1979) EORTC/GTO adjuvant chemotherapy program for primary Ewing's sarcoma: Results at 5 years. Recent Results Cancer Res 68: 52–59
33 Lokich J (1978) Adjuvant therapy for surgically curable colon cancer. A controlled study of chemo- and immunotherapy. Proc Am Soc Clin Oncol 20: 423
34 Salmon SE, Jones SE (eds) (1980) Adjuvant therapy of cancer II. Grune and Stratton, New York, pp 1–663
35 Maurer HM (1978) Intergroup Rhabdomyosarcoma Study (IRS): Current status. Proc Xth Meet Int Soc Pediatr Oncol, Bruxelles, p 23
36 Maurer HM, Moon T, Donaldson M, Fernandez C, Gehan EA, Hammond D, Hays DM, Lawrence W Jr, Newton W, Ragab A, Raney B, Soule EH, Sutow WW, Tefft M (1977) The Intergroup Rhabdomyosarcoma Study. A preliminary report. Cancer 40: 2015–2025
37 McPherson TA, Young D, Lim C, Dewar G, McMurray G, Bone G (1980) Adjuvant chemoimmuno- and immunotherapy in B_2 and C colorectal cancer. In: Salmon SE, Jones SE (eds) Adjuvant therapy of cancer II. Grune and Stratton, New York, pp 603–612
38 Morris-Jones PH (1978) M.R.C. Second Nephroblastoma Trial. Proc Xth Meet Int Soc Pediatr Oncol, Bruxelles, pp 7–9
39 Panettiere FJ, Heilbrun L (1980) Effectiveness of postoperative adjuvant therapy with methyl CCNU plus 5-FU with or without oral BCG in an attempt to prevent recurrence of Dukes B_2 or C colon cancer. Interim report of a continuing SWOG study. In: Salmon SE, Jones SE (eds) Adjuvant therapy cancer II. Grune and Stratton, New York, pp 595–602
40 Paoletti P, Butti G, Casotto A, Grunta F, Knerich R, Marini G, Mazza C, Robustelli della Cuna G, Schiffer D, Soffietti R (1979) Italian multicenter study on malignant brain tumor

therapy. Proceedings of the international symposium on multidisciplinary aspects of brain tumor therapy. Gardone Riviera, Italy, June 8–10, 1979, p 68
41 Pinedo HM, Vandrik CPJ, Bramwell VHC, Slooten EA van, Deakin DP, Unnik JAM van, Staquet M, Sylvester R, Bonadonna G (1979) Evaluation of adjuvant therapy in soft tissue sarcoma. A collaborative multidisciplinary approach. Eur J Cancer 15: 811–817
42 Rosen G, Murphy ML, Huvos AG, Gutierrez M, Marcove RC (1976) Chemotherapy, en bloc resection and prosthetic bone replacement in the treatment of osteogenic sarcoma. Cancer 37: 1–11
43 Rossi A, Bonadonna G (1979) Current impact of adjuvant chemotherapy in resectable cancer. Cancer Chemother Pharmacol 3: 7–16
44 Rossi A, Bonadonna G, Tancini G, Bajetta E, Marchini S, Valagussa P, Veronesi U (to be published) Trials of adjuvant chemotherapy in breast cancer. The experience of the Istituto Nazionale Tumori of Milan. Eur J Cancer
45 Solero CL, Monfardini S, Brambilla C, Vaghi A, Valagussa P, Morello G, Bonadonna G (1979) Controlled study with BCNU vs CCNU as adjuvant chemotherapy following surgery plus radiotherapy for glioblastoma multiforme. Cancer Clin Trials 2: 43–48
46 Strander H, Adamson U, Aparisi T, Broström A, Cantell K, Einhorn S, Hall K, Ingimarsson S, Nilsonne V, Söderberg G (1979) Adjuvant interferon treatment of human osteosarcoma. Recent Results Cancer Res 68: 40–44
47 Sutow WW, Gehan EA, Dyment PG, Vietti T, Miale T (1978) Multidrug adjuvant chemotherapy for osteosarcoma: Interim report of the Southwest Oncology Group Studies. Cancer Treat Rep 62: 265–269
48 Tancini G, Bajetta E, Marchini S, Valagussa P, Bonadonna G, Veronesi U (1979) Operable breast cancer with positive axillary nodes (N+): Results of 6 vs 12 cycles of adjuvant CMF in premenopausal women. Proc Am Assoc Cancer Res 20: 172
49 Tormey D, Falkson G, Weiss R, Perloff M, Glidewell O, Holland JF (1980) Postoperative chemotherapy with/without immunotherapy for mammary carcinoma. Salmon SE, Jones SE (eds) Adjuvant therapy of cancer II. Grune and Stratton, New York, pp 253–260
50 Voûte PA, Tournade MF, Lemerle J, Rey A, Perry HJM, Sekaly F (1978) Results of studies conducted by the International Society of Pediatric Oncology (SIOP) from 1971–1978 concerning Wilms' tumor. Proc Xth Meet Int Soc Pediatr Oncol, Bruxelles, pp 3–14
51 Walker MD, Strike TA (1979) An interim analysis of methylprednisolone, procarbazine, BCNU or BCNU plus methylprednisolone in the treatment of malignant glioma. Proc Am Assoc Cancer Res 20: 200
52 Wendt AG, Miller RC, Heusinkveld RS, Giordano GF, Jackson RA, Salmon SE, Jones SE (1980) Adjuvant treatment of breast cancer with adriamycin-cyclophosphamide ± radiotherapy. In: Salmon SE, Jones SE (eds) Adjuvant therapy of cancer II. Grune and Stratton, New York, pp 285–293
53 Young RC, Chabner BA, Hubbard SP, Fisher RI, Bender RA, Anderson T, Simon RM, Canellos GP, De Vita VT Jr (1978) Advanced ovarian adenocarcinoma. A prospective clinical trial of melphalan (L-PAM) versus combination chemotherapy. N Engl J Med 299: 1261–1266

Limits of Animal Models in Cancer Chemotherapy

S. Garattini

Summary

In animal models used in cancer chemotherapy, there is a low variability in terms of sensitivity of cancer cells in vitro, plasma levels of anticancer drugs, and interhost immune responses. In contrast, human tumors (e.g., ovarian carcinoma) show much greater variability. It is suggested that greater attention should be given to the study of the variables which distinguish the clinical setting from the animal models.

Extensive literature now exists detailing the animal models available for studies on cancer chemotherapy, and there is no need here to recall that these comprise a large spectrum of neoplasms of inbred or outbred animals, originating from most of the body organs and possessing different rates of growth and varying in their capacity to disseminate and give metastases and to elicit host responses. It is also well known that a sizable number of such tumors have been characterized in some depth as regards their sensitivity and resistance to the most commonly used antitumoral drugs. Even if there is still large ground and urgent need for the development of more sensitive and specific models, one may argue that there exists at the experimental level a number of models which reasonably mimic a relatively large number of clinical conditions.

Indeed it is undeniable that knowledge obtained in experimental models has been crucial in much of the progress made in clinical cancer treatment over the last 25 years. It has also been long recognized, however, that even with experimental models which are quite close to the human condition, there are results obtained in animals which are difficult or impossible to reproduce in the reality of the clinical situation.

In this report, some data obtained by this laboratory is presented which may have a bearing on this problem. Obviously there is no ambition to discuss here every possible reason for the difficulties in the transfer of data from experimental models to man, but rather it has been preferred to concentrate on three specific points.

Experimental tumors can be cultured in vitro and therefore it is relatively easy to establish the cytotoxic effects of antitumoral drugs on the same cells growing in vitro and in vivo. Table 1 summarizes data obtained using C3H mammary tumor cells in vitro [4]. A marked cytotoxic effect occurs after exposure to adriamycin at relatively low doses and the effect increases in relation to the length of the incubation period. The coefficient of variation is low, indicating that the cytotoxic effect of adriamycin is reproducible and that, within 0.3 and 1.3 μg/ml, this drug is active in 95% of the experiments when 24 h of incubation with the drug and 120 h of recovery are used. Similar data could easily be described for other experimental tumors as well as for other drugs, leading to a conclusion of relative uniformity of tumor cells in this respect

Table 1. ED_{50} (μg/ml and 95% confidence limits) of adriamycin on murine mammary carcinoma cells in vitro [4]

Time of treatment (h)	ED_{50} after the end of treatment (h)		
	0	24	120
1	> 100	88 (18–44)	3 (1–5)
8	24 (17–35)	7 (4 11)	3 (1–10)
16	21 (14–33	4 (3–5)	2 (1–4)
24	3 (2–5)	2 (1–4)	1 (0.3–1.3)

under the chosen experimental conditions. In contrast, Table 2 indicates that human tumor cells originated from the same organ (ovary) and, showing the same histologic features, exhibit a marked difference in sensitivity to several antitumoral drugs. For instance, considering the effect of adriamycin, it may be concluded that the only way to obtain a cytotoxic effect in most of the tumors would be to use a range of concentrations between 0.16 and 40 μg/ml. In addition, tumors of certain individuals are insensitive even to 40 μg/ml of adriamycin. One may therefore suggest that whereas experimental models show a relatively uniform sensitivity to adriamycin, human tumors (at least ovarian serous carcinomas) can be quite heterogeneous in their response to the same drug.

The active concentration of a drug in vitro is not a reliable parameter for deciding the degree of efficacy in vivo because it is necessary to know which concentrations of the drug can be reached in vivo without obtaining toxic effects on normal organs and functions of the host. Data on the levels of antitumoral drugs in blood and tissues after their administration in vivo offer another possibility of analysis of possible differences between experimental and clinical tumors. In C3H mice bearing mammary tumors, the administration of various doses of adriamycin results in dose-related peak levels of this drug in blood and tissues. The blood levels obtained are compatible with the concentrations necessary in vitro to exert a cytotoxic effect (Table 3). There is therefore a reasonable agreement between the concentrations of adriamycin effective in vitro and those present in blood at drug doses effective in reducing the growth of the same tumor in vivo. In contrast, studies in ovarian cancer patients indicate that the blood levels of adriamycin are highly variable, making it almost impossible to predict the blood levels of this drug in any given patient on the basis of the administered dose (Table 4). Indeed, peak values between 2.6 and 11.5 μg/ml can be obtained with doses ranging between 40 and 50 mg/m^2 IV. The range of levels obtained in these patients do not always cover the range of concentrations necessary to obtain an effect in vitro on the same tumors. It may be therefore concluded that whereas in experimental animals the drug is distributed, metabolized, and excreted in a relatively homogeneous manner in different hosts, in cancer patients there is a much larger variability.

Attention has been focused recently on the host immunologic reactivity as one of the factors possibly explaining the different outcome of therapeutic treatments. Table 5 shows that the cytotoxic effect of macrophages on experimental cancer cells is quite reproducible for a given tumor. For instance, macrophages isolated directly from the nonmetastasizing FS6 fibrosarcoma growing in isogenic C57Bl/6 mice are significantly cytotoxic in vitro for cancer cells. On the contrary, macrophages obtained from a subline (mFS6) of the same tumor which spontaneously metastasizes, rather than

Table 2. In vitro sensitivity of human ovarian carcinoma cells after 24 h incubation with adriamycin [3]

Patient	ED_{50} (μg/ml)
1	40
2	0.16
3	> 40
4	0.16
5	1
6	10
7	10
8	1

Table 3. Plasma level of adriamycin in mammary-carcinoma-bearing C3H mice [5]

Time after adriamycin	Adriamycin plasma levels (μg/ml ± SE) after	
	3.75 mg/kg IV	15 mg/kg IV
1 min	8.7 ± 0.6	22.3 ± 1.0
5 min	2.4 ± 0.2	7.4 ± 0.9
15 min	1.5 ± 0.2	2.6 ± 0.3
30 min	1.0 ± 0.1	1.8 ± 0.1
60 min	0.7 ± 0.3	1.2 ± 0.08
3 h	< 0.05	< 0.05
C_0[a] (μg/ml ± SE)	8.2 ± 0.4	35.8 ± 0.4
AUC[b] (μg/ml × min ± SE)	31 ± 3	237 ± 25

[a] Concentration at time zero
[b] Area under the curve

Table 4. Pharmacokinetic parameters of adriamycin in ovarian cancer patients [6]

No. of patients	Dose of adriamycin mg/m² IV	Plasma C_0[a] (μg/ml)	AUC[b] (μg/ml × min)
8	40[c]	6.32 ± 2.82 (2.6 – 11.0)	93 ± 25 (61 – 130)
8	50[c]	7.07 ± 2.67 (3.4 – 11.5)	127 ± 60 (75 – 269)
8	40[d]	3.77 ± 1.46 (1.6 – 4.8)	90 ± 39 (38 – 159)

[a] Concentration at time zero
[b] Area under the curve
[c] Monochemotherapy
[d] Polychemotherapy

Table 5. Effect on in vitro mFS6 tumor cell growth of tumor-associated macrophages isolated at different times after implantation of the FS6 and mFS6 sarcomas [1]

Tumor	Days after tumor transplantation	% Inhibition (−) or stimulation (+) of mFS6 tumor cell DNA synthesis
FS6	15	− 52 ± 2
	21	− 59 ± 2
	30	− 45 ± 1
mFS6	17	+ 85 ± 1
	24	+ 79 ± 4
	30	+ 83 ± 5

Table 6. Growth inhibitory (−) or stimulatory (+) activity of macrophages obtained from ovarian cancer patients on E cells in vitro [2]

Patient	Attacker-target cell ratio	% Inhibition (−) or stimulation of tumor cell DNA synthesis
1	7 : 1	− 63 ± 2
2	7 : 1	− 20 ± 3
3	35 : 1	− 39 ± 6
	7 : 1	− 28 ± 7
4	7 : 1	+135 ± 5
5	35 : 1	− 49 ± 3
	7 : 1	− 22 ± 3

reducing the growth of cancer cells in vitro, are capable of stimulating the growth of these cancer cells. It would seem that for a given tumor model and stage thereof, the behavior of macrophages is uniform. In contrast, ascitic macrophages obtained from ovarian cancer patients show much greater heterogeneity when assayed for their effects on the in vitro growth of cancer cells. In fact, macrophages from certain individuals will be nonspecifically cytotoxic for a given type of target cell (Table 6), whereas macrophages obtained from other ovarian cancer patients at the same stage of disease progression are capable of stimulating the in vitro growth of the same type of target cell.

Even on the basis of the limited examples reported above, one may be led to conclude that in cancer patients there is a considerable heterogeneity as far as sensitivity of cancer cells in vitro to chemotherapeutic agents, levels of the antitumoral agents in plasma, and effect of host responses as exemplified by macrophage-mediated cytotoxicity. Different combinations of these three heterogeneous parameters in given individuals might be responsible, at least in part, for the relatively large differences in the individual therapeutic response. It seems therefore important to emphasize this heterogeneity in cancer patients vis-à-vis the relative homogeneity of the models utilized in experimental cancer chemotherapy. Accordingly, it seems logical to recommend that more attention be given in future to recognize and analyze the components of this heterogeneity. This knowledge, besides hopefully allowing an optimization of existing therapy for individual patients, may in turn provide useful information to improve the use of experimental models even as far as permitting discovery of better therapeutic approaches.

References

1 Mantovani A (1978) Effects on "in vitro" tumor growth of murine macrophages isolated from sarcoma lines differing in immunogenicity and metastasizing capacity. Int J Cancer 22: 741–746

2 Mantovani A, Peri G, Polentarutti N, Bolis G, Mangioni C, Spreafico F (1979) Effects on "in vitro" tumor growth of macrophages isolated from human ascitic ovarian tumors. Int J Cancer 1980 23: 157–164

3 Morasca L, Balconi G, Erba E, D'Incalci M, Ottolenghi L, Salmona A, Garattini S (1980) Pharmacokinetic approach to "in vitro" testing of ovarian cancer cell sensitivity. Oncology 37: 169–173

4 Morasca L, Fogar-Ottaviano EG, Garattini S (1976) Time dependent cytotoxicity of adriamycin and daunomycin in primary cultures of normal and neoplastic mammary glands. Eur J Cancer 12: 107–111

5 Pacciarini MA, Barbieri B, Colombo T, Broggini M, Garattini S, Donelli MG (1978) Distribution and antitumor activity of adriamycin given by a high-dose and a repeated low-dose schedule to mice. Cancer Treat Rep 62: 791–800

6 Piazza E, Donelli MG, Broggini M, Sessa C, Natale N, Ottolenghi L, Marsoni S, Libretti A, Mangioni C, Morasca L (to be published) Early phase pharmacokinetics of adriamycin in plasma of cancer patients during single or multidrug therapy. Cancer Treat Rep

Clinical Chemotherapy: Its Correlation with Experimental Models

S. K. Carter

Summary

The inputs into clinical trials are many and the possibilities for study are nearly infinite. The only way rational choices and priorities can be established is through the use of experimental models. Clinicians and experimentalists must develop a continuous dialogue so as to mutually develop their questions of importance for study.

The clinician approaches the design of therapeutic trials with myriad possible choices. These choices are largely empiric, based on the clinician's rational analysis of past clinical experience and his feelings about what might have the best chance of success. He looks to the experimentalist for aid in making these choices and has at his disposal a vast amount of experimental data that have accumulated over many years of laboratory study. Unfortunately, in many cases the clinician and experimentalist work parallel to each other with only a few meager bridges of interaction that generally do not cross the clinical-experimental gap at the critical juncture. Figure 1 illustrates the potential inputs into an experimental or clinical trial and the potential parallel and/or interactive aspects of the two systems.

The potential clinical protocols that could be undertaken in oncology are nearly infinite. Currently there are more than 30 anticancer drugs with established activity against at least one type of human cancer [3]. In addition, more than 50 drugs are under active clinical investigation to establish their activity spectrum. For all of these drugs, there are variabilities of schedule, intensity, route, and duration. For example, a drug such as methotrexate can be given long term daily, daily × 5, weekly, twice weekly, or as a single dose every 2–3 weeks. Methotrexate can be given orally, intravenously, intramuscularly, and interathecally; by intravenous push or by infusion

Experimental data base	Clinical data base
Experimentalist's intuition	Clinican's intuition
Experimentalist's interest	Clinican's interest
Clinical data base	Experimental data base
Clinical need	
↓	↓
Experimental trial	Clinical trial

Fig. 1. Inputs to clinical and experimental trials

of varying durations; at the range of doses up to 15 g/m^2, and even higher combined with "rescue" with calcium Levcovorin (Leucovorin) which can be given on varying schedules either intravenously or orally. It is now established that cancer is not one but a multiplicity of diseases and that each disease must be tested individually for drug activity. Therefore it would be possible to design literally hundreds of protocols to test methotrexate completely with all the variables mentioned elucidated.

When drug combinations are contemplated, the complexity of possible protocol studies increases by log orders of magnitude. Starting from a minimal base of 30 actives the number of two-, three-, four-, and five-drug combinations that could be devised requires a computer to calculate. All of the single-drug variables still exist and to those are added the combination variables of sequence and ratio.

Increased complexity also arises when drugs are combined with other modalities. Two effects can occur when drugs are combined with irradiation. The drugs can be adjuvant to the irradiation killing tumor cells outside the range of the beam, or the drugs can either synergise or add to the irradiation cell kill. Radiation has variables of fractionation schedule, port size, equipment utilized, and intensity. These variables plus all the drug variables must interact with the additional variables of sequence and ratio of intensity. The same complexities exist with surgery and drugs and when cytotoxic drugs are combined with attempts at immune modulation.

With this complexity of clinical trial possibilities, how does the clinician choose what to do? Ideally the clinician would like to be rationally designing his studies based on questions that have been posed to and answered by experimental model systems. Unfortunately this is not the case for most clinical studies. One of the sadder realities of oncology today is that clinicians are undertaking studies beyond the scope of established model systems. While the experimentalists are utilizing model systems that test a single dose of X-ray with a single drug on a variety of sequences, the clinician is empirically putting together four-drug combinations with multiple-fraction X-ray. In many situations the experimentalist is not out in front of the clinical experiments helping to define some choices among the myriad of possibilities. The experimentalist and the clinician have been working in parallel to each other without true bridges of interactive communication.

Any clinical protocol has four major variables that have to be considered: the modalities chosen, the disease under study, the strategy under test, and the design utilized. A relatively simple example involves new drug evaluation. The modality is single-drug chemotherapy. The initial strategy is phase I evaluation. The design is an uncontrolled sequential testing of patients on escalating doses, and the disease is relatively unimportant except that it is advanced cancer refractory to all other standard treatment. When the strategy becomes phase II testing the disease becomes much more critical. Multiple phase II studies will be designed for individual tumor types. Where the phase II testing can be done, within the overall therapeutic flow of options, will differ between lung cancer and lymphomas. The most common design is an uncontrolled treatment of sequential patients, utilizing the historical data base in decision making as to whether phase III studies are indicated. Alternate prospectively randomized controlled phase II study designs also exist and have been utilized [2].

With phase III studies of new drugs the multitude of possibilities increases. Drugs found to be active in a phase II setting are often moved immediately into combination studies. These combination studies make single-drug efficacy vs single-drug toxicity difficult to successfully interpret. The designs become muddled because strategies begin to overlap. The strategy becomes dominated by how best to treat a given tumor, at a given clinical and pathologic stage, and this tends to overwhelm the strategy of new drug evaluation.

One example of overlapping strategies making interpretation difficult can be seen with the drug cis-platinum diammine dichloride (DDP), which has recently been commercially approved for sale in the United States with its indications being testicular cancer and ovarian cancer. Data indicate that the drug is also active against squamous cell head and neck cancer [5]. A variety of uncontrolled disease-oriented phase II studies have indicated that DDP can give an objective regression ratio in excess of 30% in advanced patients beyond the hope of cure with X-ray or surgery. This compares favorably with the historical data base of single-agent activity with methotrexate and bleomycin, which are the other two drugs felt to be active in this disease setting [1].

What is the phase III strategy for DDP in head and neck cancer? The ideal trial from a pure new drug testing strategy viewpoint would be the following:

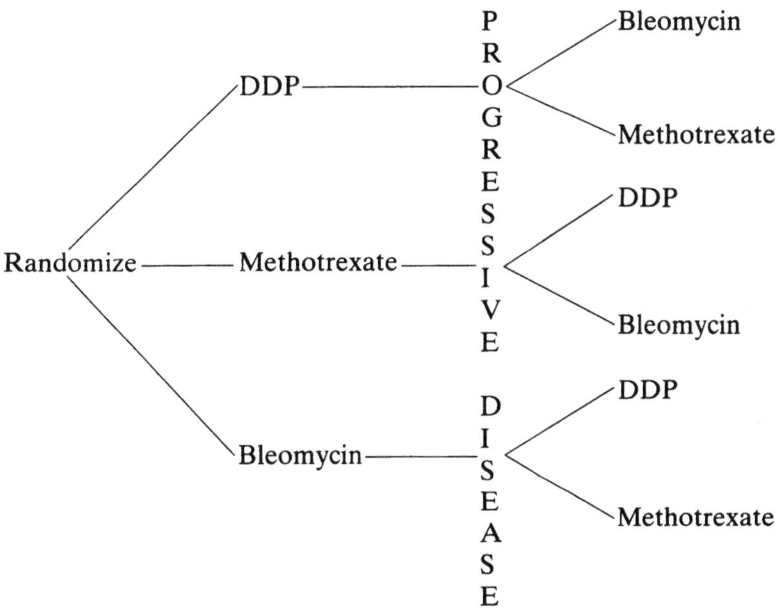

This trial, adequately executed with large numbers of patients, would fully elucidate the value of DDP in comparison with the other two actives, and would lead to a recommendation of whether DDP should be given as first-line single-agent therapy or as a second- or third-line drug.

The above trial conflicts, however, with an overall combined modality strategy for advanced-stage head and neck cancer. DDP has been combined with bleomycin, or with methotrexate, or with both drugs in what can only be described as phase II type trials. For example, studies at the Memorial Sloan-Kettering Cancer Center have indicated, in a phase II fashion, that the combination of DDP plus bleomycin may have a response rate of 70% [4]. This needs to be confirmed in phase III studies. One approach could be to treat larger numbers of patients with this regimen in an uncontrolled fashion. If the response rate stays in excess of 70%, relate it to the historical data base and decide the combination is superior. If the response rate should fall to 50%–60%, this would pose a problem since that would not be significantly higher than the 50% response rate that has been reported with methotrexate alone. An idealized, prospectively randomized, controlled trial would be as follows:

Randomize	DDP + bleomycin	PROGRESSIVE DISEASE	Methotrexate
	DDP		Methotrexate
	Bleomycin		Methotrexate
	Methotrexate		DDP + bleomycin

As yet, neither of these types of trials have been undertaken and the true role of DDP in head and neck cancer still remains to be elucidated. Despite this, a national study in the United States has been begun for operable stage III and IV head and neck cancer (Fig. 2). Now DDP alone and combined with bleomycin is part of a triple-modality protocol. The drug combination is given preoperatively and the single drug is given after postoperative irradiation in an adjuvant fashion. On what basis was this study designed? How were the modalities chosen and how were the schedules and sequences arrived at? The only honest answer that can be given is rational empiricism. No experimental models for head and neck cancer exist that allow for the complexities of two-drug combination chemotherapy, surgery, and multiple-fraction irradiation to be prospectively elucidated.

A major problem in correlating experimental data's predictiveness for clinical results is that only a tiny fraction of the studies done experimentally can be undertaken clinically. The capacity in clinical research is minute in relation to that in the experimental laboratory. This results in only the most positive experimental studies being attempted clinically. Thus some ability to develop the true- and false-positive predictive ability of experimental systems exists. There is no way to gauge prospectively the true- and false-negative rate. Since clinicians often work independently of experimentalists, retrospective correlation sometimes enables the true- and false-negative rate to be explored. It is worth pointing out that in general the clinician is out in front of the experimentalist. Almost all of the major combination chemotherapy regimens were developed empirically although the conceptual rationale for combining drugs was inherent in the experimentally developed cell-kill hypothesis. Despite this, combinations such as MOPP, vincristine-prednisone, Velban (vinblastine) + bleomycin + DDP, CMF(VP), and ara-C + daunomycin were not developed from experimental synergism studies.

What is needed is a consensus meeting of clinicians and experimentalists regarding which questions the clinician could use help with which would be feasible for the experimentalist to undertake to answer prospectively. A priority needs to be put on the existing experimental resources that are allocated to immediately clinically relevant questions as apart from exploratory basic research. For example, a vast number of combination chemotherapy studies are being performed in murine

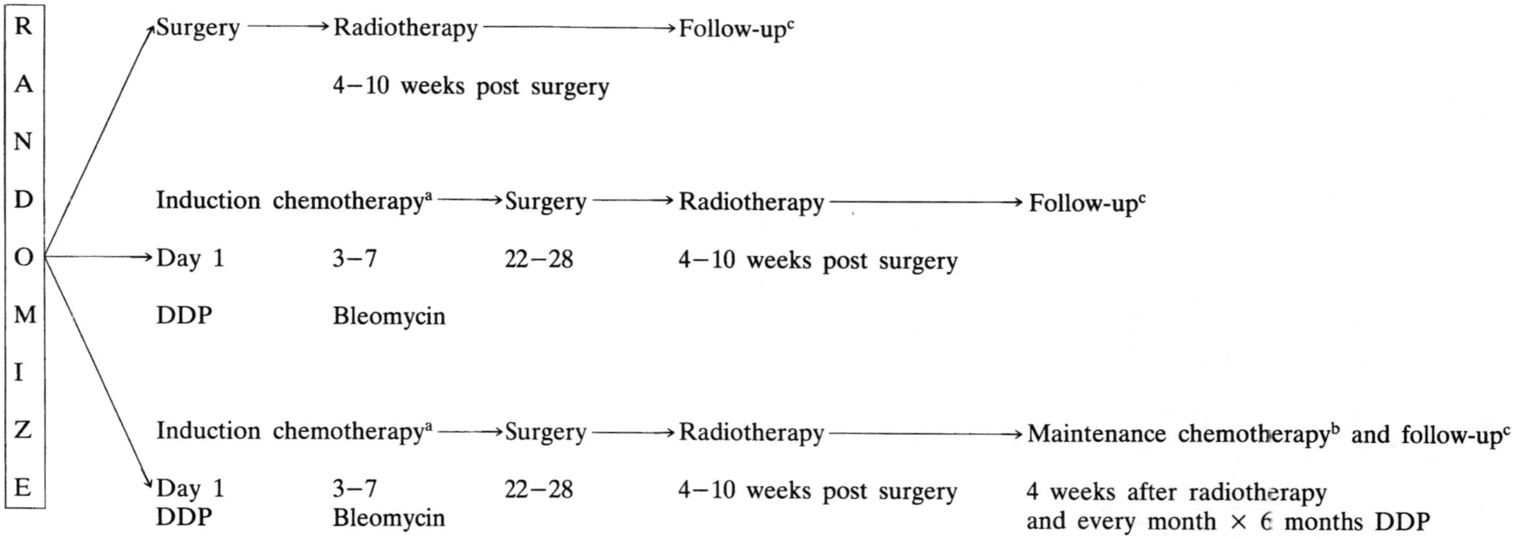

[a] Induction chemotherapy: DDP, 100 mg/m^2 IV push day 1
Bleomycin, 15 mg/m^2 IV push, then 15 mg/m^2/day × 5 continuous infusion, days 3–7
[b] Maintenance chemotherapy: DDP, 80 mg/m^2 continuous infusion for 24-h period
[c] Follow-up: Monthly for first year; every 2 months for second year; every 3 months for third year

Fig. 2

transplantable systems. What is the strategy of the testing being done? A variety of approaches are possible: (a) Screening could be done so that every possible two- and three-drug combination derived from the existing clinical drugs would be studied on a few schedules, ratios, and sequences. The idea would be to find unusually synergistic combinations that could be further studied. (b) A modification of this approach would be to choose an important reference drug, e.g., DDP, and run it in combination with all other drugs to find unusual synergism. (c) Pick a few critical combinations, e.g., DDP + adriamycin ± Cytoxan (cyclophosphamide), vinblastine + bleomycin ± DDP, or VP-16 + adriamycin, and study them in great detail. Explore the full range of possibilities for ratio, sequence, and schedule with the aim of elucidating some optimal way of putting these drugs together. The only way a rational choice can be made among these various approaches is to have the clinicians and the experimental biologists meet to explore each other's needs and resources.

References

1 Carter SK (1977) Chemotherapy of head and neck cancer. Semin Oncol 4: 413–424
2 Carter SK (1977) Clinical trials in cancer chemotherapy. Cancer 40: 544–557
3 Carter SK, Bakowski M, Hellmann K (1977) Chemotherapy of cancer. John Wiley & Sons, New York
4 Randolph UL, Vallejo A, Spiro R, Shan J., Strong, EW, Huvos AG, Wittes, GE (1978) Combination therapy of advanced head and neck cancer. Cancer 41: 460–467
5 Wittes RE, Cvitkovic E, Shah J, Gerold FP, Strong EW (1977) Cis-dichlorodiammine dichloride in the treatment of epidermoid carcinoma of the head and neck. Cancer Treat Rep 61: 359–366

Metabolic Conversion of Methotrexate in Man

R. C. Donehower

Summary

Metabolism of methotrexate (MTX) to closely related analogues has been increasingly recognized in recent years. 7-Hydroxymethotrexate, 2,4-diamino-N^{10}-methylpteroic acid, and methotrexate poly-γ-glutamates have been established as products of metabolic conversion in man. The significance of the formation of these metabolites has not been firmly established. Certain of these compounds may play a role in the development of the renal failure syndrome associated with high-dose infusions, contribute to the chronic toxicity of MTX administration, and cross-react to a significant degree in radioimmunoassay methods for measurement of MTX concentrations.

Introduction

Aspects of the biochemical and clinical pharmacology of methotrexate (MTX) have been fruitful areas of investigation for many years. Progress has been made along many diverse avenues of investigation enabling clinical chemotherapy to be based on clearly defined pharmacokinetics, mechanism of action, determinants of cytotoxicity, and possible mechanisms of resistance. Perhaps the most notable current result is the clinical use of infusions of high-dose MTX which require Leucovorin (calcium folinate) or other exogenous "rescue" to prevent serious toxicity. Although the clinical indications and usefulness of high-dose MTX regimens remain to be fully established, their use has led to increased recognition and understanding of important aspects of MTX pharmacology. One such aspect is the metabolic conversion of methotrexate to related analogues in patients receiving high-dose infusions. This report will review information on the metabolic products of MTX which have been identified, and consider the implications these metabolites may have for the toxicity and therapeutic efficacy of high-dose MTX regimens.

Discussion

Although small quantities of a metabolic product had been found in the urine of patients who had received conventional doses of MTX (30 mg/m^2) [4], significant metabolism of MTX was first reported by Jacobs and co-workers, who identified 7-hydroxymethotrexate (7-hydroxyMTX) in the urine of patients receiving high-dose infusions (> 50 mg/kg) [7]. These authors demonstrated that 7-hydroxyMTX made up 7%–33% of MTX-derived material excreted in the time interval between 18 and 24 h after the start of the infusion. The presence of 7-hydroxyMTX has subsequently been confirmed and characterized further by other workers [9, 14, 15]. WATSON et al. identified 7-hydroxyMTX concentrations by high-pressure liquid chromatography (HPLC) that exceed those of MTX in plasma samples drawn 24 h after high-dose drug administration [15]. WANG and co-workers have demonstrated that the peak plasma levels of 7-hydroxyMTX in children occur within 3 h after completion of a 6-h MTX infusion (50–250 mg/kg) [14]. In five patients receiving 200 mg/kg of MTX, peak plasma levels of 7-hydroxyMTX reached were 180 ± 90 μ*M* as compared with 410 ± 220 μ*M* for MTX. At 12 and 24 h after the start of the infusions, levels of this metabolite exceeded those of MTX. A biphasic disappearance was observed for 7-hydroxyMTX with apparent half-lives of 4.5 h and 28 h. But perhaps most surprising are the studies by LANKELMA et al., who have shown significant plasma levels of 7-hydroxyMTX as compared with those of MTX during infusions at several dosage levels (25 mg/24 h, 378 mg/24 h, and 950 mg/6 h) [9]. These data suggest that 7-hydroxyMTX is formed in measurable quantities at sustained plasma levels of MTX as low as 0.1 μ*M*. Additionally, these authors demonstrated that conversion of MTX to 7-hydroxyMTX appeared to increase in a given patient after the initial infusion, suggesting the enzyme responsible for this conversion was inducible. Although the oxidation of MTX to 7-hydroxyMTX by hepatic aldehyde oxidase has been shown to occur readily in other species [8], it has been difficult to demonstrate this reaction with homogenates of human liver. Despite this difficulty, an aldehyde oxidase is still felt to be the enzyme responsible for this oxidation in man.

The clinical significance of this metabolite is uncertain. Despite the magnitude of the metabolism of parent drug to 7-hydroxyMTX that has been observed in recent studies [9, 14], it seems unlikely that the therapeutic potential of high-dose regimens will be compromised on the basis of this conversion to a less effective inhibitor of dihydrofolate reductase. However, studies of the effect of 7-hydroxyMTX on determinants of MTX cytotoxicity, such as membrane transport, have not been done and may be warranted. More importantly, the presence of this metabolite in high concentrations may play a role in the development of renal failure on the basis of precipitation of MTX-derived material in the renal tubules, as the aqueous solubility of 7-hydroxyMTX is three- to fivefold less than that of MTX (Table 1) [7].

A second metabolite of MTX has recently been identified on the basis of significant cross-reactivity in the radioimmunoassay, one of the commonly used methods for clinical monitoring of MTX levels [3]; 80% of plasma samples drawn from patients 48 or 72 h after the start of a 6-h drug infusion and assayed for MTX concentrations gave

Table 1. Aqueous solubility of MTX and metabolites

Compound	mg/ml		
	pH 5.0	pH 6.0	pH 7.0
MTX	0.39	1.55	9.04
7-hydroxy MTX	0.13	0.37	1.55
DAMPA	0.05	0.10	0.85

results by radioimmunoassay which were greater than twofold those measured by a competitive dihydrofolate reductase binding assay [11]. This finding suggested the presence of one or more compounds in plasma following high-dose infusions of MTX which were detected with greater sensitivity by MTX radioimmunoassay. One such component was identified in both urine and plasma; the ultraviolet absorbance spectrum and chromatographic characteristics of this compound identified it as 2,4-diamino-N^{10}-methylpteroic acid (DAMPA). Although this compound is present as a contaminant in the commercial preparation which these patients received [2], cumulative urinary excretion of this compound determined by HPLC exceeded the amount which would have been expected on that basis alone [3]. This metabolite had previously been identified in the urine and intestinal contents of mice receiving MTX [13], and its presence in man was not surprising. In man, it is believed that this metabolite is formed in the intestine during enterohepatic circulation of the drug, since no mammalian carboxypeptidase capable of the cleavage of glutamate from the MTX molecule has been identified. A bacterial carboxypeptidase with a high affinity for MTX has been well characterized [10].

Since the cross-reactivity of DAMPA in the available radioimmunoassay techniques has been found to be variable [3], it is important that clinicians be aware of the specificity of assays being used in their institutions. Like 7-hydroxyMTX, DAMPA has more limited aqueous solubility than MTX, as shown in Table 1. The limited solubility of this compound again raises the possibility that renal precipitation might occur under selected circumstances. This must be considered as a potential complication in regimens employing intravenous infusions of purified carboxypeptidase G_1 as a means of rescue in high-dose MTX therapy [1], in which MTX is cleaved enzymatically to glutamine and the less soluble metabolite.

MTX may also be converted to polyglutamate forms. Significant quantities of MTX poly-γ-glutamyl derivatives have been found in human liver [6], and there is accumulating evidence that other tissues, including perhaps tumor cells, may form polyglutamates [12]. Jacobs et al. have demonstrated that, unlike the other metabolites identified, MTX (+ G_1) is an equally potent inhibitor of dihydrofolate reductase activity and of cell replication [5]. A role of MTX polyglutamates in chronic forms of MTX toxicity such as hepatotoxicity has been proposed but remains largely speculative at this time. MTX polyglutamates may remain in liver months after drug administration. Whether their presence results in continued inhibition of dihydrofolate reductase and produces the hepatic lesion has not been established. MTX (+ G_1) has recently also been identified in the plasma of children following high-dose MTX infusions [14], probably a result of efflux of small quantities from cells in which it was formed. The peak levels attained and time course of the presence of polyglutamates in plasma have not been further examined.

Conclusion

The formation of methotrexate metabolites in man is summarized in Fig. 1. Although the formation of these metabolic products does not appear to be unique to high-dose MTX regimens, the recognition of their presence has largely been a result of the use of these dosage schedules. The importance of MTX metabolites in the clinical care of patients receiving high-dose infusion remains to be fully established. Although there is no clinical or laboratory evidence to suggest that formation of these metabolites has

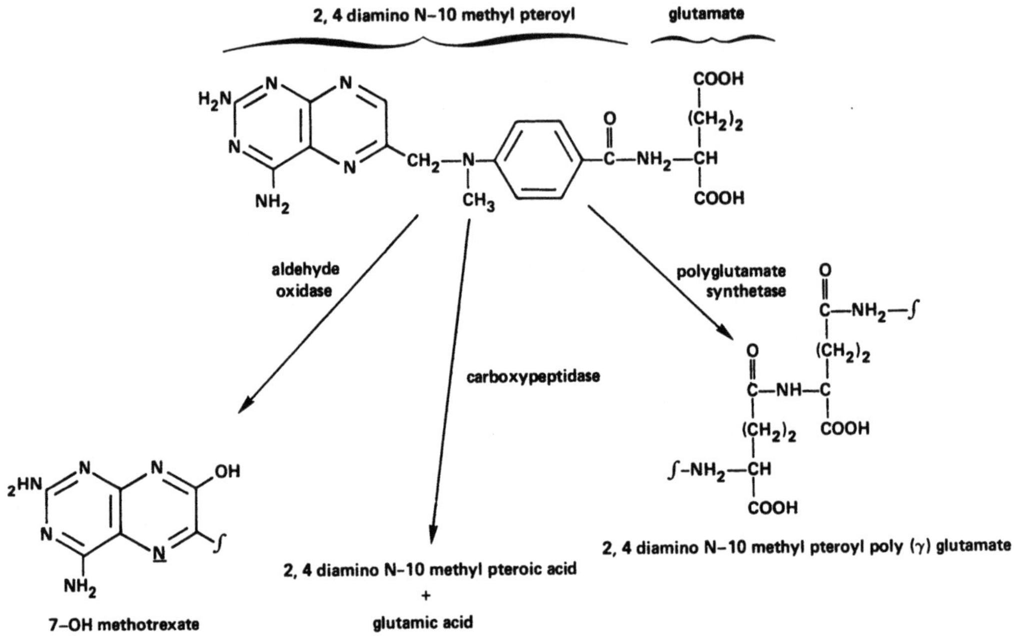

Fig. 1. Methotrexate metabolites in man. Methotrexate has been shown to be converted in vivo to 7-hydroxymethotrexate, 2,4-diamino-N^{10}-methylpteroic acid, and polyglutamate derivatives

any effect on the chemotherapeutic results with MTX, this has not been adequately studied. A role in the acute and chronic toxicities of MTX therapy is more likely on the basis of the limited solubility of 7-hydroxyMTX and DAMPA, and the long-term presence of polyglutamate in liver and other tissues.

Further studies on the clinical and biochemical pharmacology of these compounds will be necessary before definitive conclusions can be reached as to their importance in clinical chemotherapy.

References

1 Abelson HT, Ensminger W, Rosowsky A, Uren J (1978) Comparative effects of citrovorum factor and carboxypeptidase G_1 on cerebrospinal fluid methotrexate pharmacokinetics. Cancer Treat Rep 62: 1549–1552
2 Chatterji DC, Frazier AG, Gallelli JF (1978) Identification and quantitation of impurities in methotrexate. J Pharm Sci 67: 622–624
3 Donehower RC, Hande KR, Drake JC, Chabner BA (1979) Presence of 2,4-diamino-N^{10}-methylpteroic acid after high-dose methotrexate. Clin Pharmacol Ther 26: 63–72
4 Huffman DH, Wan SH, Azarnoff DL, Hoogstraten B (1973) Pharmacokinetics of methotrexate. Clin Pharmacol Ther 14: 572–579
5 Jacobs SA, Adamson RH, Chabner BA, Derr CJ, Johns DG (1975) Stoichiometric inhibition of mammalian dihydrofolate reductase by the γ-glutamyl metabolite of methotrexate, 4-amino-4-deoxy-N^{10}-methylpteroyl glutamyl-γ-glutamate. Biochem Biophys Res Commun 63: 692–698

6 Jacobs SA, Derr CJ, Johns DG (1972) Accumulation of methotrexate diglutamate in human liver during methotrexate therapy. Biochem Pharmacol 26: 2310–2313
7 Jacobs SA, Stoller RG, Chabner BA, Johns DG (1976) 7-Hydroxymethotrexate as a urinary metabolite in human subjects and rhesus monkeys receiving high-dose methotrexate. J Clin Invest 57: 534–538
8 Johns DG, Valerino DM (1971) Metabolism of folate antagonists. Ann NY Acad Sci 186: 378–386
9 Lankelma J, Van der Kleijn E, Termond EFS (1978) Assay of methotrexate and 7-hydroxymethotrexate by high-pressure liquid chromatography and its application to clinical pharmacokinetics. In: Pinedo HM (ed) Clinical pharmacology of anti-neoplastic drugs. Elsevier/North-Holland, New York, pp 13–28
10 McCullough JL, Chabner BA, Bertino JR (1971) Purification and properties of carboxypeptidase G_1. J Biol Chem 246: 7207–7213
11 Myers CE, Lippman ME, Eliot HM, Chabner BA (1975) Competitive protein binding assay for methotrexate. Proc Natl Acad Sci USA 72: 3683–3686
12 Rosenblatt DS, Whitehead VM, Dupont MM, Vuchich M-J, Vera N (1978) Synthesis of methotrexate polyglutamates in cultured human cells. Mol Pharmacol 14: 210–214
13 Valerino DM, Johns DG, Zaharko DS, Oliverio VT (1972) Studies of the metabolism of methotrexate by intestinal flora I. Biochem Pharmacol 21: 821–831
14 Wang YM, Howell SK, Smith RG, Hosoya R, Benvenuto JA (1979) Effect of metabolism on pharmacokinetics and toxicity of high-dose methotrexate therapy in children. Proc Am Soc Clin Oncol 20: 334
15 Watson E, Cohen JL, Chan KK (1978) High-pressure liquid chromatographic determination of methotrexate and its major metabolite, 7-hydroxymethotrexate, in human plasma. Cancer Treat Rep 62: 381–389

Biochemical Control of High-Dose Methotrexate/Leucovorin Rescue Therapy

W. Wilmanns, H. Sauer, and A. Schalhorn[1]

Summary

High-dose methotrexate/Leucovorin rescue therapy is based on the assumption of differences in the transport system for folate compounds between normal and malignant proliferating cells. Thus, under normal conditions, methotrexate (MTX) and Leucovorin (citrovorum factor, CF) in low doses can enter the cells by an active transport system, whereas in some malignancies – such as osteosarcoma – these substances only penetrate through the cell membrane by passive diffusion if they are given in very high doses. Therefore, after high-dose MTX treatment, the cytotoxic effect of the folate antagonist is compensated for by rescue with Leucovorin in low doses only in the normal cell system. The consequence of this kind of treatment is a selective antitumor effect.

To avoid cytotoxic side effects, this therapeutic regimen must be monitored carefully. The decrease of the ratio of ^{3}H-deoxyuridine (dUR)/^{3}H-thymidine (dTR) incorporation into the DNA of the cells is a good biochemical parameter for estimating the MTX effect on rapidly proliferating cell systems. Using this indicator, it was shown that the usually administered dose of Leucovorin is not sufficient for an effective rescue of the bone marrow cells as long as the MTX serum concentration is equal or higher than $10^{-6}M$. If in critical cases the MTX elimination is retarded, a rescue can only be achieved by Leucovorin at doses tenfold higher than the actual amount of MTX in the whole body system. The Leucovorin rescue doses under such circumstances can be calculated according to the formula

$$\text{Leucovorin (mg)} = 10 \times \text{MTX (mg/l)} \times 0.76 \times \text{body weight (kg)}.$$

Introduction

High-dose methotrexate (HDMTX) therapy followed by Leucovorin (citrovorum factor, CF) rescue is based on the assumption that primary resistant tumors have an impaired active membrane transport system for folate compounds which is normally shared by methotrexate (MTX) (Fig. 1). At very high MTX serum concentrations, however, the drug can enter these cells by passive diffusion independent of the active

* This work was supported by the Deutsche Forschungsgemeinchaft. We thank Mrs. K. Heil, Mrs. R. Sarkar, Mrs. G. Stupp-Poutot, and Mrs. U. Wünsch for their skillful technical assistance

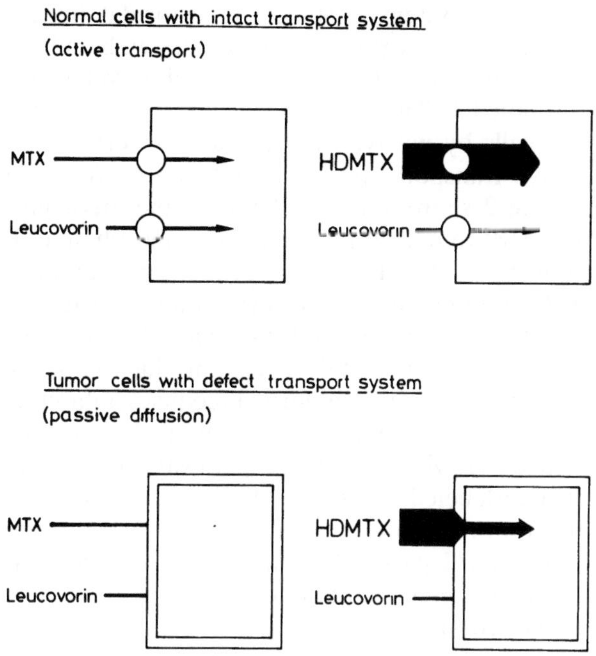

Fig. 1. Principle of high-dose methotrexate (HDMTX) therapy

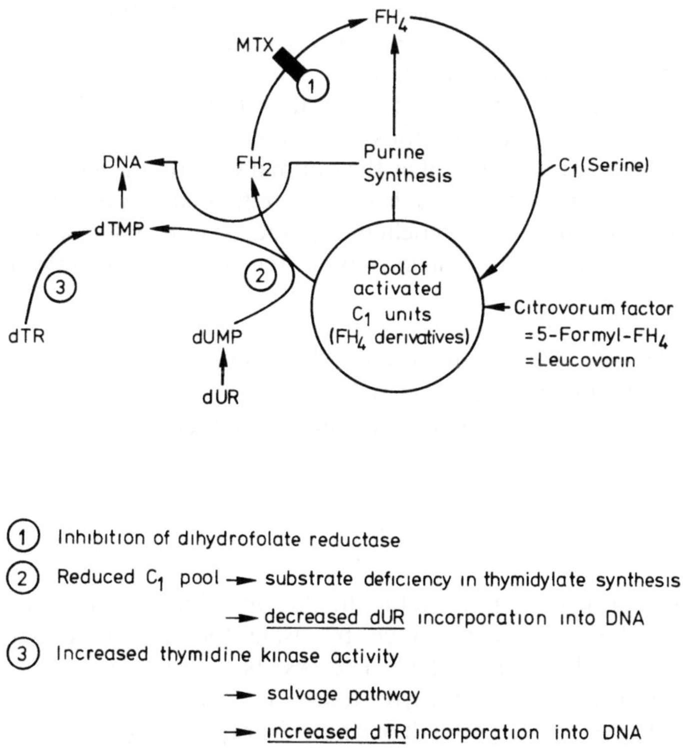

Fig. 2. Biochemical effects of methotrexate (MTX)

transport system, resulting in cytocidal intracellular MTX concentrations [2, 5]. Normal, rapidly proliferating tissues with an intact active transport system for folates can be protected from death caused by MTX by applying relatively small doses of the antidote CF. This is the so-called rescue effect of CF. Since essentially no CF can enter the cells by passive diffusion at low serum concentrations, tumor cells lacking the active transport system do not benefit from the rescue effect.

Figure 2 shows that MTX affects the methylation of deoxyuridine monophosphate (dUMP) to deoxythymidine monophosphate (dTMP) by inhibiting the dihydrofolate reductase. Therefore, if exogeneous tritium-labeled deoxyuridine (dUR) is offered to MTX-treated cells, its incorporation into the DNA is reduced. Thus, the effect of MTX can be monitored biochemically [10, 15].

As a consequence of decreased production of thymidine triphosphate (dTTP) via the de novo pathway, the normal feedback inhibition of the thymidine kinase reaction is released. Activation of the thymidine kinase results in increased production of dTMP and dTTP via the salvage pathway. This explains the increased incorporation of tritium-labeled dTR in MTX-treated cells. Thus, both the decrease of dUR incorporation and the increase of dTR incorporation into the DNA serve as biochemical parameters of the MTX effect [14].

Different rescue techniques for the correction of cytocidal MTX effects have been described [1]:

1) The intravenous (IV) continuous infusion of thymidine (8 g/qm) over a 3-day period.
2) The enzymatic degradation of MTX by carboxypeptidase G_1, a technique which still is experimental.
3) The administration of CF as the antidote for MTX.

This activated folate derivative enters directly the pool of activated one-carbon units (Fig. 2) [8]. Thus, dTMP synthesis and de novo purine synthesis can resume, although the dihydrofolate reductase is still inhibited by MTX. Biochemically, the rescue effect of CF is indicated by the normalization of the dUR/dTR ratio [10, 15].

However, some questions as to the length of the interval between MTX and CF administration, as well as the optimal CF dose necessary to protect the normal tissues from undesired MTX side effects, remained unanswered. To answer these questions, we have studied the biochemical aspects of the CF rescue in normal bone marrow cells in patients with osteosarcoma receiving an HDMTX/CF rescue therapy after operation.

Methods. The details of the dUR- and dTR-incorporation studies, the estimation of the thymidine kinase activities, and the determination of serum MTX levels by inhibition of purified dihydrofolate reductase are described elsewhere [9, 11].

Results

The principles of the metabolic changes which are characteristic for the effects of MTX and CF were determined by using the model system of a permanent growing lymphoblast culture LS_2. The results are shown in Fig. 3. In comparison with the control, 5-formyltetrahydrofolate (citrovorum factor) alone has no significant effect either on the cell growth or on the incorporation rates of ^{3}H-dTR and ^{3}H-dUR. Under

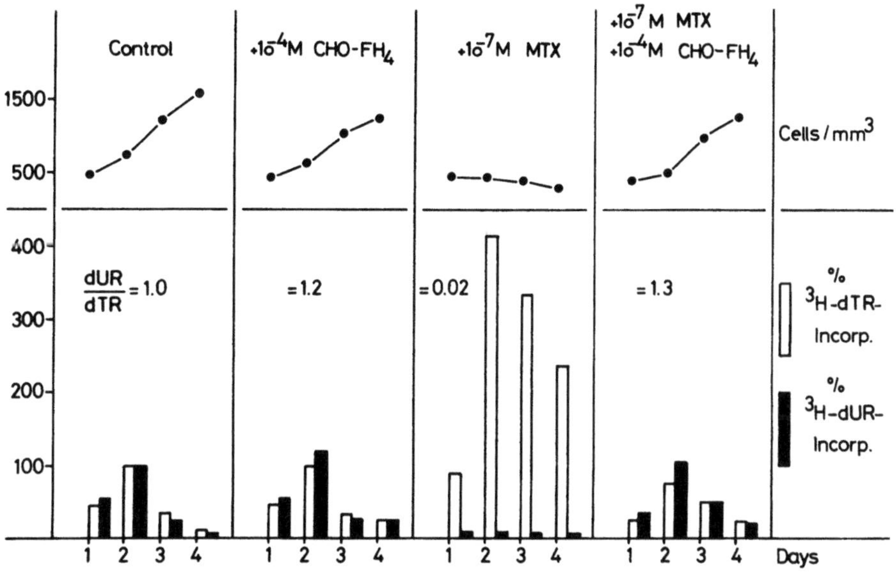

Fig. 3. DNA metabolism in cultured human lymphoblasts (LS_2). Effects of methotrexate (MTX) and citrovorum factor (Leucovorin = $CHO\text{-}FH_4$)

normal conditions, the incorporation rates of these two nucleosides are nearly equal. The normal range of the dUR/dTR ratio is 0.7–1.3. Under MTX – as expected from the biochemical mechanism – the dUR incorporation falls almost to zero, whereas the dTR incorporation increases considerably. As a sign of the MTX effect on DNA synthesis, the dUR/dTR ratio falls below 0.1. The DNA metabolism of the cells is so much disturbed that reproduction can no longer occur. The addition of CF normalizes the incorporation rates. The dUR/dTR ratio rises again to the normal value of 1.3. Cultures growth is then regular again.

Figure 4 shows that the incorporation rates of dUR and dTR can be normalized only if the CF concentration is at least tenfold higher than the MTX concentration. After incubation of the cells with 10^{-6} *M* MTX, the dUR/dTR ratio is corrected by addition of 10^{-5} *M* CF to the medium and normalized by 10^{-4} *M* CF. A MTX concentration of 10^{-7} *M* is ineffective under these conditions. At a very high concentration of 10^{-5} *M* MTX, there is no rescue effect with 10^{-4} *M* CF.

The same parameters as in the model culture were estimated in bone marrow cells of patients under MTX therapy. Figure 5 presents schematically the regimen of HDMTX/CF treatment. MTX is infused permanently over a 6-h period; 2 h later, a 15-mg dose of CF is given i.v. every 3 h (eight times) and then every 6 h (eight times). This treatment is repeated every 2 weeks. During the first three applications, the MTX dose is increased from 3 g/m^2 to 6 g/m^2 and to 7.5 g/m^2. Then it is held at the latter dose for the following courses.

Figure 6 shows the results of the dUR/dTR ratio and the corresponding MTX serum levels in a patient with metastatic osteosarcoma who received 3.8 and 14.0 g of MTX, respectively. Even 24 h after the end of the MTX infusion, the DNA metabolism in the bone marrow shows a clear MTX effect in both cases, although up to that time seven doses of CF (15 mg each) already have been injected. At this time, the values of the dUR/dTR ratios are considerably below normal, and the activity of thymidine kinase

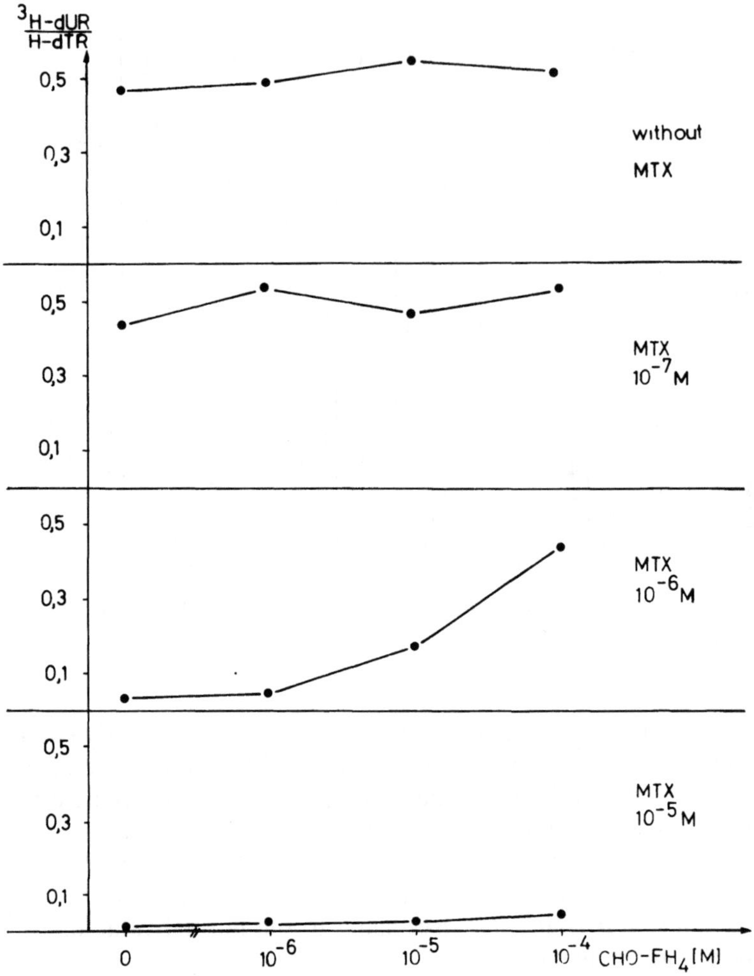

Fig. 4. Reversal of MTX effect by citrovorum factor (Leucovorin = CHO-FH$_4$) in LS$_2$ cultures

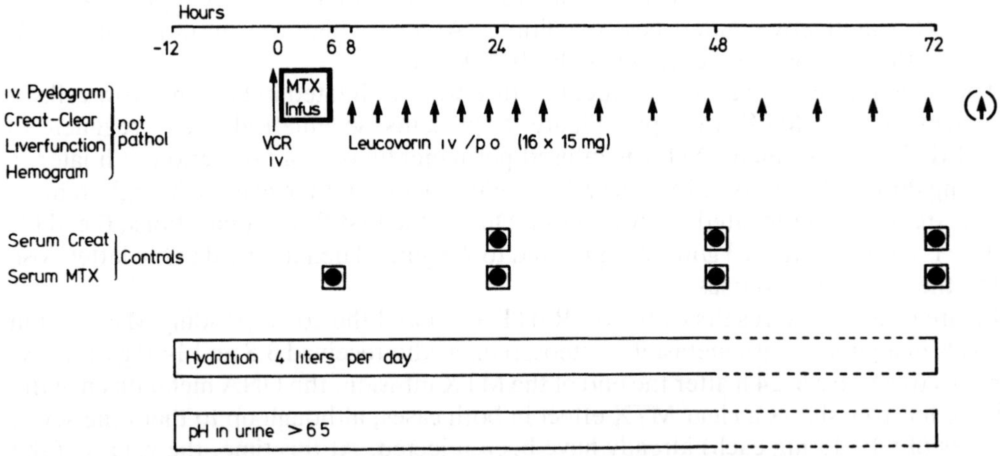

Fig. 5. High-dose methotrexate/citrovorum factor (HDMTX/CF) regimen

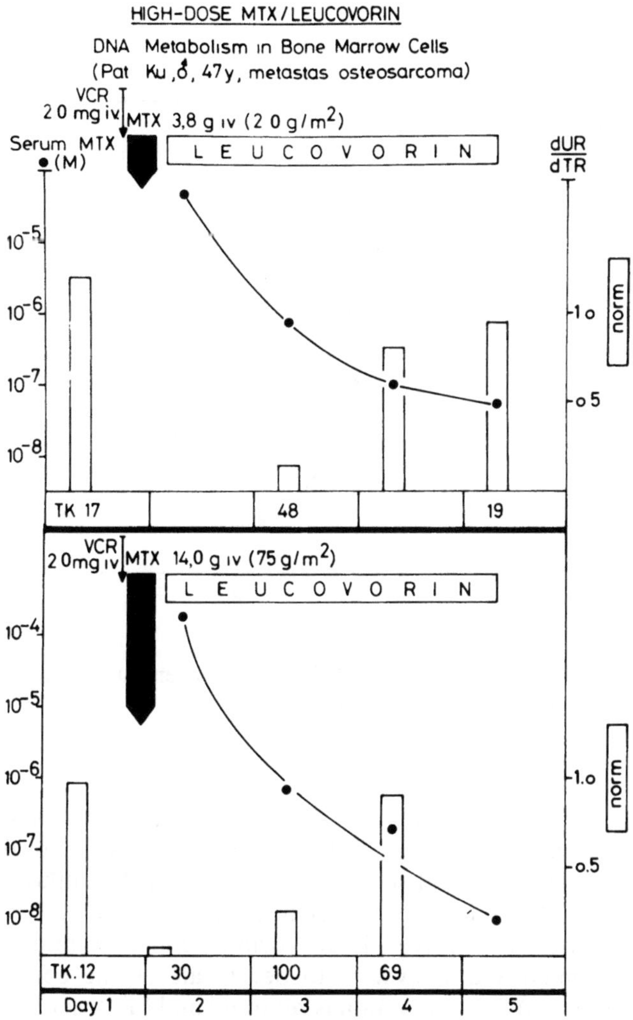

Fig. 6. MTX serum concentrations and DNA metabolism in bone marrow cells of a patient under HDMTX/CF therapy

(TK) responsible for the increased dTR incorporation is elevated significantly. Only after 48 h, when the MTX serum concentration decreased to 10^{-7} *M*, did the dUR/dTR ratios and DNA metabolism return to normal. Similar results were obtained in other patients treated according to the methods described.

Figure 7 summarizes the correlation between MTX serum levels and the normalization of DNS synthesis under Leucovorin rescue after HDMTX therapy in different patients. It is remarkable that conventional Leucovorin doses can correct DNA synthesis only at MTX serum levels below 10^{-6} to 10^{-7} *M*.

Discussion

The results show that the usually administered doses of about 100 mg CF/day are not sufficient as an effective rescue for protecting the bone marrow cells as long as the MTX serum concentration is equal or higher than 10^{-6} *M*. At MTX serum

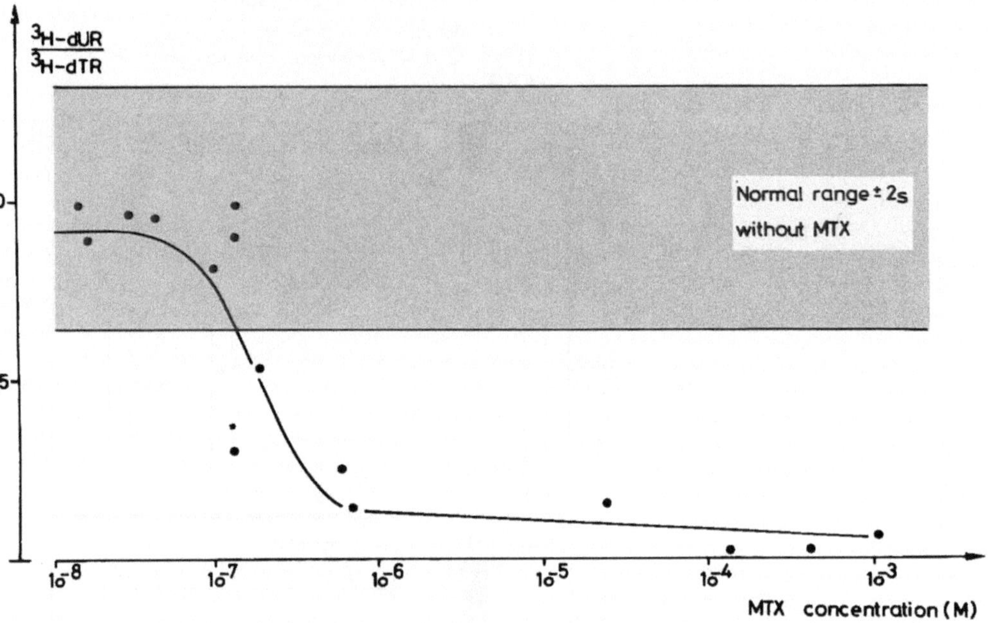

Fig. 7. Relation between MTX serum concentration and ^{3}H-dUR/^{3}H-dTR ratio in bone marrow cells under treatment with HDMTX/CF

concentrations of 10^{-7} *M*, CF is effective at doses which can be controlled by the normalization of the dUR/dTR ratio. According to these results, early CF application is ineffective and seems to be of no benefit, although it is demanded in most of the published schedules for HDMTX/CF therapy. Recently, Camitta and Holcenberg [4] proposed a delayed Leucovorin rescue 24 h after HDMTX therapy as therapeutic regimen and showed it to be as safe as the conventional rescue.

When MTX elimination is retarded and MTX serum levels remain above 10^{-6} *M* after 48 h or at about 10^{-7} *M* after 72 h, the CF rescue with "normal" doses is ineffective, since both MTX and CF enter the cell by the same active transport mechanism and inhibit each other competitively [9]. Thus, high MTX concentrations almost totally prevent the transport of low CF doses into the cell.

To save these patients from perhaps lethal complication, massive doses of Leucovorin are necessary [6]. On the assumption that Leucovorin as well as methotrexate is distributed in 76% of the body volume [7], the Leucovorin doses for a rescue effect can be calculated according to the formula

$$\text{Leucovorin (mg)} = 10 \times \text{MTX (mg/l)} \times 0.76 \times \text{body weight (kg)}.$$

Thus, the Leucovorin dose for a 70-kg patient would be 266 mg every 6 h at an MTX serum concentration of 10^{-6} *M* 48 h after the MTX infusion. After four consecutive applications of this dose, further Leucovorin treatment is adapted to the MTX serum level. This calculation is important as the MTX clearance can be delayed independent of the renal function, in rare cases [3, 12]. Recently, Stoller and co-workers [13] proposed a similar therapeutic regimen. Moreover, in critical cases the monitoring of the DNA metabolism in the bone marrow cells by means of the dUR/dTR ratio can determine whether the Leucovorin dose is enough to prompt the desired rescue effect.

References

1 Bertino JR (1977) "Rescue" techniques in cancer chemotherapy: Use of Leucovorin and other rescue agents after methotrexate treatment. Semin Oncol 4:203–216

2 Bleyer WA (1977) Methotrexate: Clinical pharmacology, current status and therapeutic guidelines. Cancer Treat Rev 4:87–101

3 Bleyer WA (1978) The clinical pharmacology of methotrexate. Cancer 41:36–51

4 Camitta BM, Holcenberg JS (1978) Safety of delayed Leucovorin "rescue" following high-dose methotrexate in children. Med Pediatr Oncol 5:55–59

5 Djerassi I (1975) High-dose methotrexate (NSC-104) and citrovorum factor (NSC-3590) rescue: Background and rationale. Cancer Chemother Rep 6:3–6

6 Djerassi I, Kim JS, Nayak N, Ohanissian H, Adler S, Hesieh S (1977) New "rescue" with massive dose of citrovorum factor for potentially lethal methotrexate toxicity. Cancer Treat Rep 61:749–750

7 Goldmann ID (1975) Membrane transport of methotrexate (NSC-740) and other folate compounds: Relevance to rescue protocols. Cancer Chemother Rep 6:63–72

8 Sauer H, Jaenicke L (1974) Zur Aufhebung des zytostatischen Effekts von Amethopterin (Methotrexat) durch Methyl-Tetrahydrofolsäure. Blut 28:321–326

9 Sauer H, Schalhorn A, Wilmanns W (1978) Zum biochemischen Mechanismus des Citrovorum-Faktor-Schutzes nach hochdosierter Methotrexat-Behandlung maligner Tumoren. Therapiewoche 28:7809–7814

10 Sauer H, Schalhorn A, Wilmanns W (1979) Biochemical control of the folinic acid rescue effect after high-dose methotrexate (MTX) therapy. In: Kislink RL, Brown GM (eds) Chemistry and biology of pteridines. Elsevier/North-Holland, New York Amsterdam Oxford, pp 683–688

11 Sauer H, Schalhorn A, Wilmanns W (1979) The biochemistry of the citrovorum factor rescue effect in normal bone marrow cells after high-dose methotrexate treatment. Eur J Cancer 10:1203–1209

12 Stoller RG, Hande KR, Jacobs SA, Rosenberg SA, Chabner BA (1977) Use of plasma pharmacokinetics to predict and prevent methotrexate toxicity. N Engl J Med 297:630–633

13 Stoller RG, Kaplan HG, Cummings FJ, Calabresi P (1979) A clinical and pharmacological study of high-dose methotrexate with minimal Leucovorin rescue. Cancer Res 39:908–912

14 Wilmanns W, Kehr D (1970) DNS-Synthese in Leukämiezellen unter der Einwirkung von Methotrexat, 5-Fluoro-Uracil und Cytosin-Arabinosid in vitro. Pharmacol Clin 2:161–167

15 Wilmanns W, Sauer H (1979) Rational use of antimetabolites in cancer chemotherapy with special reference to high-dose methotrexate/citrovorum factor rescue therapy. In: Skoda J, Langen P (eds) Antimetabolites in biochemistry, biology and medicine. Pergamon, Oxford New York, pp 233–245

High-Dose Methotrexate in Combination Chemotherapy for Small Cell Lung Cancer

F. A. Greco, K. R. Hande, R. L. Richardson, and R. K. Oldham*

Summary

High-dose methotrexate and Leucovorin (calcium folinate) rescue was evaluated as induction chemotherapy in combination with cyclophosphamide, doxorubicin, and vincristine in 21 patients with extensive-stage small cell lung cancer. Nine (42%) of 21 had a complete remission. The median duration of remission has been short (5 months), and attempts are now under way to improve consolidation chemotherapy. In general, the degree of myelotoxicity was not increased by the high-dose methotrexate, although the antitumor activity of the combination appears enhanced. Attempts at further increasing the intensity of this regimen or comparative trials with other therapy appears warranted.

Introduction

Chemotherapy for patients with small cell carcinoma of the lung has improved over the past few years [3, 4, 6, 8]. The two most important disease-related factors are *stage of disease* and *performance status* in determining prognosis and the outcome of many combination chemotherapy regimens. Patients with limited-stage disease (no demonstrable metastases outside the chest) have a better prognosis than patients with extensive-stage disease [8] (demonstrable extrathoracic metastasis). Multiple combinations of drugs and various schedules are currently being tested. Patients with extensive-stage disease are rarely cured with any chemotherapeutic regimen. Therefore, aggressive investigation in this group of patients appears particularly warranted to identify more effective combination chemotherapeutic approaches. The combination of the three active drugs cyclophosphamide, doxorubicin (adriamycin), and vincristine, or CAV, is one of several combinations which has been shown to be effective in producing responses and increasing survival in patients with extensive-stage small cell carcinoma of the lung [2, 9]. There appears to be a dose-response curve for CAV and for other forms of combination chemotherapy. A greater number of complete remissions occur with more intensive induction therapy [5, 10], but there is usually more serious toxicity with the more aggressive approaches [7, 11].
One method of increasing the intensity of induction chemotherapy without necessarily increasing severe toxicity involves the use of an additional active drug in combination

* This research was supported in part by JFCF, ACS 394; PHSG 5M01 RR-95; Division of Cancer Treatment of the National Cancer Institute

which does not possess major overlapping toxicity with the other drugs. This represents one principle in the classic combination chemotherapy approach. High-dose methotrexate followed by Leucovorin (calcium folinate) rescue is a theoretically attractive component of combination chemotherapy for small cell lung carcinoma. If patients are selected carefully and urine volume and alkalinization are maintained, methotrexate (3–10 mg/m^2) intravenously (IV) followed by rescue is usually not associated with myelosuppression (less than 5%, of courses) [12, 15]. In addition, pharmacologic monitoring of drug levels enables one to adjust Leucovorin dosage if necessary. High-dose methotrexate is an active single drug in small cell carcinoma patients, as has been noted by PITMAN and FREI [12], SKARIN et al. [14], and GRECO et al. [7] (overall response rate 35%).

High-dose methotrexate with Leucovorin rescue can be given with a myelotoxic combination without necessarily increasing myelotoxicity, as has been demonstrated in patients with diffuse histiocytic lymphoma [13]. We have also completed a pilot study at Vanderbilt University Hospital in selected ambulatory extensive-stage patients with small cell carcinoma of the lung. We initially employed the effective induction combination of CAV with the addition of high-dose methotrexate with Leucovorin rescue given *every 3 weeks* for a total of two courses. The schedule was concurrent administration of all chemotherapy in an attempt to intensify induction without increasing toxicity. No maintenance therapy was given to these patients after a total of six cycles of chemotherapy.

After assessing the toxicity, response rate, and response durations of the patients in our initial study, a second study was begun using *weekly* administration of high-dose methotrexate with rescue as part of induction therapy in combination with CAV. The rationale for weekly high-dose methotrexate with rescue was to provide additional nonmyelosuppressive antitumor activity during the period of pancytopenia induced by the previously administered cyclophosphamide and doxorubicin. Theoretically, the methotrexate followed by Leucovorin rescue would spare the bone marrow and increase the therapeutic index. Furthermore, the weekly schedule of high-dose methotrexate with rescue may be more effective than the every 3 week schedule, as has been reported in osteogenic sarcoma. In an attempt to avoid drug resistance and early relapse, intensive non-cross-resistant consolidation chemotherapy with VP-16-213 (epipodophyllotoxin) and hexamethylmelamine was given following induction therapy and subsequently alternated with CAV. We report here the preliminary results of these investigations.

Materials and Methods

Twenty-one patients with extensive-stage small cell lung cancer were treated. None of the patients had received prior radiotherapy or chemotherapy. There were 18 male and three female patients, their ages ranging from 41–65 years. All patients had a functional status of above 40 on the Karnofsky scale. To define the extent of disease, the investigation of most patients included history, physical examination, chest X-ray, bronchoscopy, CBC, liver functions (SGOT, SGPT, bilirubin, alkaline phosphatase), calcium, BUN, creatinine, radionuclide liver and bone scan, bone marrow aspiration and biopsy, and computerized axial tomographic X-rays of the brain. The extent of metastatic involvement in the 21 patients is shown in Table 1. All Patients had 24-h

Table 1. Initial staging: Extensive-stage small cell lung cancer

Test	Abnormal (%)
Chest X-ray	21/21 (100)
Bronchoscopy	11/18 (61)
Liver scan	11/21 (52)
Bone marrow biopsy	8/19 (42)
Brain scan	4/17 (23)

Table 2. High-dose methotrexate every 3 weeks in combination chemotherapy

1) Cyclophosphamide 1,000 mg/m^2 IV push
2) Adriamycin 40 mg/m^2 IV push
3) Vincristine 1 mg/m^2 IV push
4) Methotrexate (MTX) 6,000 mg/m^2 IV infusion over 6 h
5) Leucovorin 15 mg/m^2 IM beginning 2 h after MTX infused and continuing q 6 h × 12 doses
6) Urinary volume (100 cm^3/h) and alkalinization (pH 7 or greater); 48-h MTX level
7) Above repeated q 3 weeks × 2; then evaluation of response
8) Continue CAV with methotrexate (500 mg/m^2 PO followed by Leucovorin PO) q 3 weeks × 2 courses, then CAV alone × 2 courses q 3 weeks

creatinine clearances of above 50 ml/min, and patients were excluded from this therapy if they had large effusions.

Patients were treated at the Clinical Research Center at Vanderbilt University Hospital. The first nine patients received CAV and high-dose methotrexate followed by Leucovorin rescue every *3 weeks* for two courses as outlined in Table 2. An additional two courses of CAV plus oral methotrexate (500 mg/m^2) and Leucovorin were given followed by two courses of CAV. All therapy was then stopped. The pretreatment functional status of these first nine patients was particularly good (mean of 80 on the Karnofsky scale).

The next 12 patients received induction therapy with CAV plus *weekly* high-dose methotrexate and Leucovorin rescue as outlined in Table 3. We were less selective in placing patients on this therapy and the mean functional status was 60 on the Karnofsky scale. Following the first 4 weeks of induction chemotherapy, they also received VP-16-213, hexamethylmelamine, and vincristine alternating with CAV. All patients received prophylactic cranial radiotherapy (3,000 rads over 2 weeks).

Methotrexate plasma levels were measured by means of a competitive bindings assay. If 48-h postinfusion levels were less than 5×10^{-7} *M*, Leucovorin was discontinued after 12 doses.

Response was evaluated completely after 16 weeks of therapy, repeating each test which was initially abnormal. A complete remission was defined as complete disappearance of all evidence of neoplastic disease. Partial remission represented a 50% or greater decrease in the perpendicular diameter of measurable lesions or a clear reduction in evaluable lesions. Response durations and survival were measured from the time of first therapy.

Table 3. High-dose methotrexate weekly in combination chemotherapy

Week	1	2	3	4	5	6	7	8	9	10	11	12	13	14	15	16
Treatment	C A V M	M	M	C A V M			H VP V*			C A V			H VP V*			C A V

C, Cyclophosphamide 1,000 mg/m² IV; A, adriamycin 40 mg/m² IV; V, vincristine 1 mg/m² IV; M, methotrexate 6 g/m² IV over 6 h followed by Leucovorin 15 mg/m² IV q 6 h × 12 doses; H, hexamethylmelamine 8 mg/kg PO × 7 days; VP, VP-16 180 mg/m² IV × 3 doses; V, vincristine 1 mg IV × 3 doses

Results

Twenty patients were evaluable for response and there was one early death. All 20 patients had an objective and subjective response to therapy. After 16 weeks of therapy, nine (42%) of 21 patients experienced a complete remission and 11 (51%) of 21 a partial remission. As judged by chest X-ray alone, eight of the nine complete remissions occurred by 8–10 weeks. Of the nine patients receiving high-dose methotrexate every 3 weeks, six had complete remission. Three of 12 patients receiving weekly high-dose methotrexate had a complete remission. Five of the patients with partial remissions in this group had rather remarkable tumor shrinkage, but slight abnormalities remained on bone or liver scans.

The mean duration of remission for the entire group is 8+ months (range 3–13+ months). The median duration of complete remission is 5 months. The median survival of the group is 12 months (range 1–17+ months). Of the nine complete remissions, four remain alive at 6+, 7+, 11+, and 15+ months. Six of 11 partial remissions are alive at 6+, 6+, 9+, 9+, 9+, and 17+ months. Two of the first nine patients who received the methotrexate every 3 weeks are alive (15+, 17+ months). Eight of the 12 patients are currently alive who received weekly methotrexate (6+, 6+, 6+, 7+, 9+, 9+, 9+, and 11+ months).

One patient died as a result of severe myelosuppression with sepsis. He developed acute renal failure and methotrexate toxicity after the first dose despite increased Leucovorin administration. He was the only drug-related death, and the only patient to experience definate severe myelosuppression from methotrexate. The mean white blood cell nadir for all patients was 1,500/mm³ (range 500–2,900) and platelet nadir 110,000/mm³ (range 350–225,000). A detailed evaluation of hematologic toxicity following CAV plus high-dose methotrexate is presented in Table 4. There were no significant differences in hematologic toxicity when the weekly methotrexate schedule was compared with the every 3 week schedule. Except for the one drug-related death, the myelotoxicity did not appear substantially increased over that expected with CAV alone. The myelotoxicity following VP-16-213 and hexamethylmelamine was generally less severe than the induction regimen.

Neurotoxicity was an important problem. All patients developed signs of mild to moderate peripheral neuropathy. One patient had severe weakness from neuromyopathy, and the vincristine, VP-16-213, and hexamethylmelamine were discontinued. Four other patients developed orthostatic hypotension late in their treatment course

Table 4. Drug toxicity following induction chemotherapy

WBC nadir/mm^3	Number of patients
>3,000	4
2,000–3,000	5
1,000–2,000	7
<1,000	5
Platelet nadir/mm^3	
>100,000	15
50,000–100,000	5
< 50,000	1

which was attributed to the combination of neurotoxic drugs. Each recovered when the drugs were discontinued.

Plasma methotrexate levels were not significantly different when methotrexate was given with CAV (mean 2.2×10^{-7} *M*) or alone (mean 4.6×10^{-7} *M*).

Discussion

The use of high-dose methotrexate followed by Leucovorin rescue in combination with CAV represents an attempt to increase the intensity and efficiency and not the toxicity of induction therapy for patients with small cell lung cancer. The toxicity in our phase II investigations has not been severe. In general, the hematologic toxicity of the every 3 week and the weekly high-dose methotrexate plus CAV was no greater than expected from CAV plus chest radiotherapy [9].

The complete remission rate to the induction chemotherapy was approximately 40%. These patients were reevaluated rather vigorously and this complete remission rate is equal to or greater than the other intensive therapies [1, 4, 5, 10]. However, our patients were selected for good performance status and renal function and this may partially explain the high complete remission rate. The duration of complete remission in the unmaintained patients was short (median 5 months).

This fact was responsible for the subsequent use of the non-cross-resistant combination of VP-16-213 and hexamethylmelamine following induction therapy in hopes of killing resistant tumor cells and extending the duration of remission. It is too early to adequately evaluate the effect on remission duration and survival. However, the median survival of these extensive-stage patients was 12 months. We have been impressed by the relatively long survival of patients with partial responses, and believe the kinetic activity of the tumor has been altered by therapy.

The lack of severe toxicity and the relative efficacy of weekly high-dose methotrexate when combined with CAV suggests that investigation should continue in order to determine whether other drugs might be combined with this regimen to further increase the intensity and perhaps the efficacy of induction therapy.

References

1 Abeloff MD, Ettinger DS, Khouri N (1970) Intensive induction therapy for small cell carcinoma of the lung (SCC). Proc Am Soc Clin Oncol 20:328
2 Brereton HD, Kent CA, Johnson RE (1977) Chemotherapy and radiotherapy for small cell lung cancer: A remedy for past therapeutic failure. Proc Am Soc Clin Oncol 18:275
3 Broder LE, Cohen MH, Selawry OS (1977) Treatment of bronchogenic carcinoma II. Small cell lung cancer. Cancer Treat Rev 4:219–260
4 Bunn PA, Cohen MH, Ihde DC, Fossieck BE, Matthews MJ, Minna JD (1977) Advances in small cell bronchogenic carcinoma. Cancer Treat Rep 61:333–342
5 Cohen MH, Creaven PJ (1977) Intensive chemotherapy of small cell bronchogenic carcinoma. Cancer Treat Rep 61:349–354
6 Einhorn LH, Bond WH, Hornback N, Tekjoe B (1978) Long-term results in combined modality treatment of small cell carcinoma of the lung. Semin Oncol 5:309–313
7 Greco FA, Brereton HD, Zimbler H, Merrill JM, Johnson RE (1976) Adriamycin and enhanced radiation reaction in normal esophagus and skin. Ann Intern Med 85:294–298
8 Greco FA, Einhorn LH, Richardson RL, Oldham RK (1978) Small cell lung cancer: Progress and perspectives. Semin Oncol 5:323–335
9 Greco FA, Richardson RL, Stroup SL, Shulman S, Oldham RK (1978) Therapy of oat-cell carcinoma of the lung: Complete remissions, acceptable complications and improved survival. Br Med J 2:10–11
10 Kent CH, Brereton HD, Johnson RE (1977) "Total" therapy for oat cell carcinoma of the lung. Int J Radiat Oncol Biol Phys 2:427–432
11 Merrill JM, Brereton HD, Kent CH, Johnson RE (1976) Anorectal disease in patients with non-hematological malignancy. Lancet 1:1105–1107
12 Pitman E, Frei E (1977) Weekly methotrexate citrovorum (MTX-CF) with alkalinization: Tumor response in pase II study. Proc Am Assoc Cancer Res 18:124
13 Skarin A, Canellos G, Frei E (1978) Therapy of unfavorable histology non-Hodgkin's lymphoma with high dose methotrexate and citovorum rescue, bleomycin, adriamycin, cyclophosphamide, Oncovin, and Decadron. Proc Am Soc Clin Oncol 19:400
14 Skarin A, Greene H, Canellos G, Takovrin R, Frei E (1979) High dose methotrexate with citrovorum factor rescue alternating with combination chemotherapy in small cell lung cancer. Proc Am Soc Clin Oncol 20:238
15 Stoller RG, Hande KR, Jacobs S, Chabner B (1977) Use of plasma pharmacokinetics to predict and prevent methotrexate toxicity. N Engl J Med 297:630–633

Clinical and Laboratory Reevalution of Dichloromethotrexate

B. Fernbach, I. Takahashi, T. Ohnuma, and J. F. Holland

Summary

Clinical and pharmacologic effects of dichloromethotrexate (DCM) were reevaluated by an intermittent intravenous large dose schedule in patients with advanced malignancies. DCM was tolerated without Leucovorin (calcium folinate) in man, even when the initial immunoassayable DCM level approached 10^{-3} *M*. Hepatic dysfunction occurred more frequently at high doses. Hematologic toxicity was not dose-limiting. Plasma decay of DCM was comparable to that of methotrexate (MTX). Of 50 patients treated, five including two with hepatic metastasis from colon carcinoma, responded with more than 50% regression of tumor.
In vitro comparison of DCM and MTX in Molt 3 cells revealed that DCM was slightly more inhibitory than MTX on an equimolar basis. In the presence of 2.5 g/dl of human serum albumin (HA), however, inhibitory effects of DCM decreased markedly. The decreased biologic effects of DCM compared to those of MTX are due to much higher binding to HA by DCM. This phenomenon appears to explain all of the clinical and pharmacologic characteristics of DCM.

Introduction

Dichloromethotrexate (DCM) given at optimal doses prolonged the survival of mice bearing L1210 leukemia more than fourfold longer than methotrexate (MTX) [8] and inhibited 6C3HED lymphoma more than 11-fold[1]. By comparison, DCM was about tenfold less toxic than MTX in dogs when given daily parenterally. A recent study showed that renal precipitation of the drug was the dose-limiting toxicity of intravenous (IV) administration of DCM in monkeys which were not hydrated and alkalinized (D. A. Cooney, personal communication).
The initial clinical studies carried out 15 years ago on DCM [7] compared the drug with MTX at both daily oral (PO) and twice weekly intramuscular (IM) schedules in patients with lymphoma. It was shown that there was no difference in antitumor activity at equitoxic doses between the two agents. Five times more DCM than MTX was tolerated in man. A randomized comparison of DCM given twice weekly IM vs three times weekly IM in patients with lung cancer revealed no significant differences

1 Dichloromethotrexate, NSC-29630, IND-3168, Annual Report to the Food and Drug Administration, 1976, Investigational Drug Branch, Cancer Therapy Evaluation Program, Division of Cancer Treatment, NCI

in antitumor effects, toxicity, or survival time [1]. DCM produced a small number of responses in patients with hepatocellular carcinoma [16].

Clinical pharmacologic studies using DCM-CL^{36} indicated that, in contrast to MTX, as much as half the IV-administered DCM was excreted in the feces; 30%–40% of the DCM appeared in the urine within 2 days and the rest was excreted in the stool, starting 2–3 days after the administration of the drug. One-third of the inactivated form of DCM, 7-hydroxy-DCM, was recovered from 24-h urine [4].

Intermittent administration of large doses of MTX followed by Leucovorin (LV) (calcium folinate) was effective in protecting the host and in improving the therapeutic efficacy of the drug in animals [9] and in man [5, 11, 12]. Increase in dihydrofolate reductase and decrease in the transport of MTX have been regarded to be the major mechanisms of resistance [2] and constitute a rationale for using MTX at the large dose. The dose-limiting toxicity of large-dose MTX is nephrotoxicity [3, 11]. Inadequate renal clearance of MTX is accompanied by sustained high levels of plasma MTX and this results in the manifestation of other toxicities such as myelosuppression, stomatitis and other gastrointestinal toxicities, and cutaneous eruption. Protocols have been evolved for the precise sequence of hydration, measurement of creatinine clearance, alkalinization of urine, and MTX blood level determination in order to minimize this complication.

We began clinical and laboratory reevaluation of DCM [6, 15] because (a) DCM is highly active in murine systems, (b) the major excretion route of DCM is through the bile rather than the kidney, which should help avoid nephrotoxicity, and (c) large intermittent IV doses of DCM plus LV have not been studied.

Materials and Methods

DCM was supplied by the National Cancer Institute, Bethesda, Maryland, in a 20-ml vial containing lyophilized DCM 250 mg and soidum hydroxide to adjust the pH to 7.5–8.0.

Clinical Studies

Fifty patients (19 men and 31 women) with advanced malignant neoplasms were included in the study. Their ages ranged from 28 to 77 years with a mean of 51 years. All patients had cancer or leukemia which had been microscopically confirmed and which was not considered amenable to conventional therapy. Table 1 lists the disease categories.

Base-line studies included physical examination, body weight and height, complete blood counts and complete automated chemical profile (SMA 6 and 12), urinalysis, chest X-ray, and measurements of tumor lesions. Bone marrow examinations were carried out in all leukemic patients.

Prior to administration of DCM, all patients were hydrated with 5% dextrose in water or 5% dextrose in 0.45% saline to assure urine output of more than 200 ml/h and alkalinization with sodium bicarbonate PO or IV, and, if necessary, acetazolamide IV, to assure urine pH of more than 7.0. Patients with creatinine clearance of less than 60 ml/min were excluded from the study.

Table 1. Disease categories

Diagnosis	Number
Colon cancer	16
Breast cancer	8
Lung cancer, AML, lymphoma, ovarian cancer	3 each
Sarcoma, melanoma, head and neck cancer	2 each
Gall bladder cancer, gastric cancer, esophageal cancer, Hodgkin's disease, chordoma, glioblastoma, ependymoma	1 each
Total	50

A cohort of three patients was entered sequentially at each dose level with an interval of not less than 1 week for the first and next two patients. The initial dose of DCM was 125 mg/m^2 IV given as a 30-min infusion. This dose corresponded to approximately one-fourth the cumulative minimal toxic dose of DCM, 1.0 mg/kg/day by a 14-day IM schedule [6], or one-fourth the cumulative weekly dose of DCM, 200 mg/m^2 given twice weekly IM [1]. This also corresponded to the cumulative minimal toxic dose of 12 mg/m^2/day (4-h infusion) × 10 days studied in hepatoma patients [16].
Subsequent patients were entered at higher dose levels according to a geometric progression if no dose-limiting toxicity had occurred at the preceding dose levels. We adopted the rapid escalation in anticipation that very high doses of DCM would be tolerated with LV rescue. The dose was repeated every 3 weeks or as often as tolerated, as long as therapeutic effects were observed.
Clinical toxicity and therapeutic effects were evaluated according to criteria adopted by the Cancer and Leukemia Group B [14].

Laboratory Studies

For the determination of DCM serum levels, blood was drawn at timed intervals after the short DCM infusion. Immunoreactive DCM blood levels were measured by using a commercially available radioimmunoassay (RIA) kit (Diagnostic Biochemistry, Inc., San Diego, California). Some serum samples were also subjected to competitive enzyme binding assay using L. casei dihydrofolate reductase (New England Enzyme Center, Boston, Massachusetts).
Human acute lymphocytic leukemia cell line Molt 3 [13] was used for in vitro comparison of MTX and DCM. Cells were maintained in suspension in culture flasks containing RPMI medium 1640 with 10% (v/v) heat-inactivated fetal, calf serum (FCS), penicillin and streptomycin, and fed with fresh medium three times per week. Cells in stock culture were counted daily and used when they were in an exponential growth phase.
To determine the effects of DCM and MTX on cell growth, the initial cell number in individual culture tubes was adjusted to 1.5×10^5/ml; $^1/_{10}$ ml of each drug solution at different concentrations was added to 10 ml of the cell suspension in individual culture tubes on day 0. Cells were not fed during the period of the experiments. Viable cells were determined by the trypan blue dye exclusion method, and dose-response curves were obtained by calculating the percentage of viable cells on day 3 as compared to those in the control tubes containing no drug.

The binding of both drugs to human serum albumin (HA) was determined by the degree to which cell growth was inhibited by the ultrafiltrates. Equimolar concentrations (5×10^{-6} *M*) of DCM and MTX were incubated at 37° C from day −1 to day 0 in 10 ml of RPMI medium 1640 containing HA (2.5 g/dl). On day 0, 5 ml of each sample were transferred into Centriflo type 50A membrane cones (Amicon Corp., Lexington, Massachusetts) and centrifuged at 1000 *g* for 30 min. The ultrafiltrate and the parent medium were sterilized by passage through a 0.45-µm Millipore-filter membrane, and 0.1 ml of each material was added to each culture tube containing 10 ml of HA-free culture medium and cells. Drug solutions which contained no HA were processed similarly and used as controls. The percentage of viable cells on day 3 was determined, and the biologically active molar concentration of each drug was calculated from the dose-response curve in HA-free culture medium. The percentage of drug binding to HA was determined by the following formula:

$$\% \text{ binding} = \frac{X - Y}{X} \times 100$$

where *X* is the biologically active molar concentration of ultrafiltrate obtained after incubation without HA and *Y* is the biologically active molar concentration of ultrafiltrate obtained after incubation with HA.

The effects of DCM and MTX on cells pretreated with HA were determined as follows. Cells (1.5×10^5/ml) were grown in RPMI medium 1640 containing 10% FCS and antibiotics with or without HA (2.5 g/dl; 3.78×10^{-4} *M*) at 37° C from day −1 to day 0. After three washings with fresh culture medium, the cells were reincubated in culture medium containing equimolar concentrations (5×10^{-8} *M*) of DCM or MTX. The percentage of viable cells was determined on day 3.

To minimize differences in the condition of the cells, DCM and MTX were used simultaneously in each of the comparative experiments. All experiments were carried out in triplicate and repeated at least twice.

Results

Toxic and Therapeutic Effects of DCM in Man

The dose escalation of DCM, numbers of patients and courses entered to each dose level, and attendant toxicity are listed in Table 2. The geometric escalation of this drug resulted in development of severe leukopenia and thrombocytopenia in one patient at 1,000 mg/m^2. For this reason, an intermediary dose of 750 mg/m^2 was tested. After confirmation that no further severe toxicity occurred in 25 additional courses at 750 mg/m^2 and 1,000 mg/m^2, the doses were cautiously escalated to 2,500 mg/m^2.

A 50% or greater increase in creatinine occurred in ten patients. In eight patients, the range was 1.5–2.6 mg%. In one patient, creatinine increased to 9.4 mg%. The patient required dialysis for 2 weeks and then recovered normal renal function. A second patient had a creatinine elevation to 6.5 mg%, did not require dialysis, and creatinine returned to normal.

No patient developed significant bone marrow suppression (WBC < 4,000/µl, platelets < 100,000/µl) without a 50% or more increase in creatinine. Two early patients with increased creatinine levels had leukocyte nadirs of 200 and 650/µl, and

Table 2. Dose escalation of dichloromethotrexate and clinical toxicities

Dose (mg/m^2)	Patients	Courses	WBC < 4000/µl	Platelets < 100,000/µl	Hepatic	Renal	Stomatitis
125	3	3	0	0	0	0	0
250	4	4	0	0	0	0	0
500	10	0	0	0	0	0	0
750	6	8	1	1	1	1	1
1,000	11	18	2	2	0	2	2
1,250	5	6	0	0	2	0	0
1,500	6	9	0	0	2	2	0
1,750	2	3	0	0	1	0	0
2,000	13	18	2	0	0	4	2
2,250	4	7	0	0	1	0	0
2,500	3	6	0	0	3	1	1

platelet nadirs of 20,000 and 26,000/µl, respectively. With the emergence of this pattern, it was decided to utilize LV rescue when there was a 50% increase in creatinine at 24 h. Rescue consisted of 25 mg of LV every 6 h until the creatinine returned to normal and the DCM levels were $< 10^{-7}$ *M*. Six patients received LV rescue, four had no bone marrow toxicity, and two had leukopenia with nadirs of 2,900/µl and 500/µl, respectively. Five patients had 50% or greater increases in bilirubin (range 1.3–3.6 mg%) and seven had 50% or greater increases in SGOT or SGPT (range 75–409 mg/ml). These changes occurred within the first week after treatment and disappeared within 3 weeks. Six patients had stomatitis. Isolated oral ulcers occurred in mild cases and more generalized inflammation in severe cases.

Risk factors for toxicity included mild ascites and edema ($n = 1$), poor performance status ($n = 3$), and advanced age ($n = 1$). Two patients had no apparent risk factors. Although toxicity was generally erratic and unpredictable, at high doses of DCM, transient deterioration of hepatic functions was common and renal toxicity appeared frequently. No further escalation seemed indicated after 2,500 mg/m^2, because DCM blood levels were approaching 10^{-3} *M* and therapeutic effects had begun to appear at lower doses.

Therapeutic effects of DCM are shown in Table 3. Five of 36 evaluable patients had partial response (PR), tumor regression to less than 50% of their pretreatment areas, lasting 1–5 months. It is noteworthy that the two PR occurred in patients with colon carcinoma metastatic to the liver.

Pharmacokinetic and Cellular Pharmacologic Effects of DCM

Serum DCM levels of four patients who received 2,000 mg/m^2 of the drug are shown in Fig. 1. The serum decay of immunoreactive DCM was essentially comparable to that reported for high doses of MTX [10], except that at later hours a more flattened decay curve suggested a triphasic decay. Ten serum samples measured by both RIA and competitive enzyme binding assay revealed comparable serum DCM concentrations, indicating that serum RIA measured no inactive metabolite(s).

Table 3. Responses to dichloromethotrexate (months)

	Patients	Partial response	Minor response	Stabilization
Colon cancer	16	2 (5, 1)	2 (1)	–
Breast cancer	8	1 (1)	–	–
Mycoses fungoides	1	1 (1)	–	–
Chordoma	1	1 (2)	–	–
AML	3		1 (1/2)	–
Head and neck cancer	2	–	1 (1)	–
Hodgkin's disease	1	–	1 (1)	–
Ovarian cancer	3	–	–	1 (3)
Gall bladder cancer	1	–	–	1 (4)

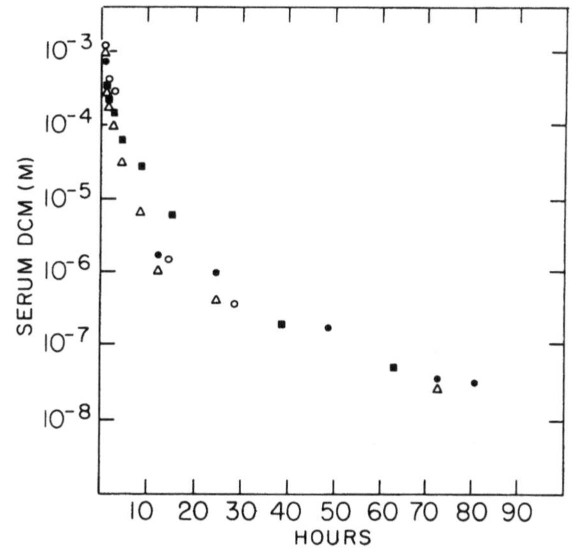

Fig. 1. Serum dichloromethotrexate levels of four patients (shown in four symbols) who received 2,000 mg/m² of the drug as a 30-min infusion

The inhibitory effects of DCM and MTX on Molt cells were compared and the results are shown in Fig. 2. On an equimolar basis, the inhibitory effect of DCM was, if anything, slightly more pronounced than that of MTX.

The data on pharmacokinetic effects of DCM in man provided essentially similar concentration · time (C×t) values for MTX. The comparable inhibitory effects of DCM and MTX in vitro posed the paradox of why much larger doses of DCM were tolerated in man without LV. This paradox was solved by the following experiments. When DCM and MTX were compared in vitro in the presence of 2.5 g/dl of HA, the inhibitory effects of DCM were markedly decreased (Fig. 3). Thus, at the ID_{90}, a fivefold increase in DCM concentration was required in the presence of HA to produce the same degree of inhibition as without HA, while the equitoxic concentration of MTX in the presence of HA increased only twofold. Preincubation of Molt cells with HA did not influence the inhibitory effects of DCM and MTX. The results of the experiments on binding are shown in Table 4. When 0.1 ml of the ultrafiltrates obtained from an incubation mixture of DCM (5×10^{-6} *M*) and HA (2.5

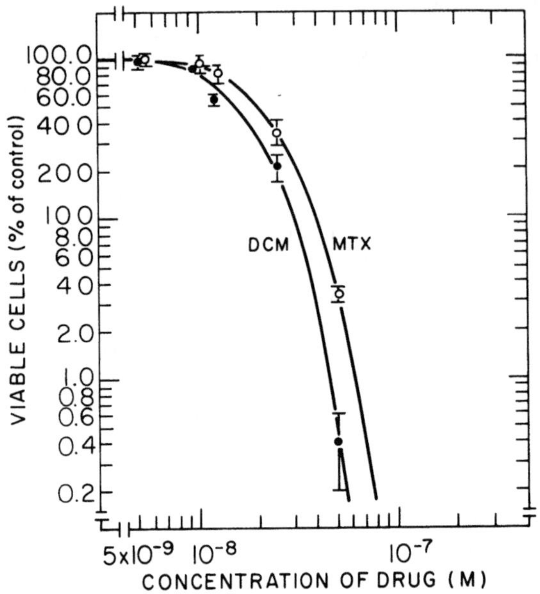

Fig. 2. Inhibitory effects of dichloromethotrexate and methotrexate on Molt cell growth in RPMI medium 1640 on the 10% fetal calf serum and antibiotics

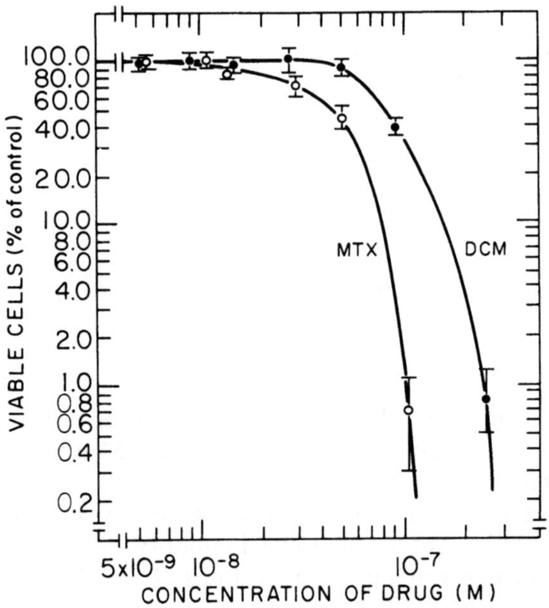

Fig. 3. Inhibitory effects of dichloromethotrexate and methotrexate on Molt cell growth in RPMI medium 1640 with 10% fetal calf serum, antibiotics, and 2.5 g/dl of human serum albumin

g/dl) were added to individual culture flasks, the viable cells on day 3 were 91% of the control. The binding of DCM to HA was calculated to be approximately 83.5%. In a similar study with equimolar MTX, viable cells were 9% of control, and the binding to HA was 49%. These results demonstrated clearly that DCM binds more extensively to HA than does MTX, and that this binding appears to determine biologic activity.

Table 4. Binding of dichloromethotrexate and methotrexate to human albumin in vitro[a]

	Viable cells ($\times 10^5$/ml)	% Viable cells	% Binding
Control	7.53	100.0	
DCM			
Incubated with HA	6.90	91.0	83.5
Incubated without HA	0.07	0.08	
MTX			
Incubated with HA	0.68	9.0	49.0
Incubated without HA	0.03	0.4	

[a] From Takahashi et al. [15]

Discussion

The present study revealed that large doses of DCM were tolerated in man without LV rescue when given on an intermittent IV schedule. Hematologic toxicity was erratic, unpredictable, and not dose-limiting. Renal toxicity from tubular precipitation of large doses of DCM, reported in animals, appears to have been avoided in man by hydration and alkalinization. Radioimmunoassay of serum DCM revealed that serum decay of DCM was essentially similar to that seen after large doses of MTX, giving $C \times t$ values essentially similar to MTX on an equimolar basis. DCM and MTX had similar inhibitory effects in vitro.

The apparent paradox of man's ability to tolerate higher doses of DCM without LV was explained, at least in part, by our demonstration in vitro that DCM binds more extensively to HA than does MTX. The bound drug is biologically inactive and the concentration of free, biologically active drug in circulation is thus much smaller than was identified by RIA. Since glomerular filtration is usually limited by the extent of binding to HA, the relatively less urinary excretion of DCM than MTX might be explained by the high binding of the drug to HA. In addition, albumin, which is known to be catabolized by the liver, might serve as a carrier to transport DCM to the hepatic cells where it may undergo metabolic transportation and eventual biliary excretion. The greater frequency of hepatic dysfunction at high doses of DCM compared to MTX should be considered from this viewpoint.

Only free, unbound drug filters through the capillary wall to the interstitial fluid, then to the cell wall for transport, and eventually to the intracellular target enzymes, thus exerting its biologic activities. High binding of DCM to HA would virtually preclude exit from the capillaries. Lack of dose-limiting hematologic effects of DCM may be explained on this basis.

The dose of MTX tolerated in man without LV rescue when given by 30-min infusion is not known. However, an earlier observation that five times more DCM than MTX was tolerated in man is consistent with the ratio of unbound drug concentrations obtained in vitro (free DCM: 16.5%, and free MTX: 51%; see Table 4).

It appears, therefore, that the unique clinical characteristics of DCM compared to MTX may be explained on the basis of more extensive binding of DCM to albumin. We have currently embarked on studies to exploit this therapeutically. Albumin binding should be considered an important biologic characteristic governing the pharmacologic and clinical effects of antineoplastic agents.

Acknowledgments. The authors thank SANDRA BROOKS, R. N., and SUSAN SATTLER, R. N., for skillful oncologic nursing participation during the clinical study. This work was supported in part by contract N01-CM-53837 from the Division of Cancer Treatment, National Cancer Institute, National Institutes of Health, Bethesda, Maryland; by USPHS research grant CA 15390; by the United Leukemia Fund, Inc., New York, New York; and by the Chemotherapy Foundation, Inc., New York, New York.

References

1 Band PR, Ross CA, Holland JF (1973) Comparison of two dose schedules of dichloromethotrexate (NSC-29630) in lung cancer. Cancer Chemother Rep 57: 79–82
2 Brockman RW (1974) Mechanism of resistance. In: Sartorelli AC, Johns DG (eds) Antineoplastic and immunosuppressive agents. Springer, New York, pp 352–410
3 Condit PT, Chanes RE, Joel W (1969) Renal toxicity of methotrexate. Cancer 23: 126–131
4 Davidson JD, Oliverio VT (1963) The physiologic disposition of dichloromethotrexate-Cl^{36} in man. Clin Pharmacol Ther 6: 321–323
5 Djerassi I, Rominger J, Kim JS, Turchi J, Suvansri U, Hughes D (1972) Phase I study of high doses of methotrexate with citrovorum factor in patients with lung cancer. Cancer 30: 22–30
6 Fernbach B, Ohnuma T, Takahashi I, Greenspan EM, Holland JF (1979) Reevaluation of dichloromethotrexate. Proc Am Assoc Cancer Res and Am Soc Clin Oncol 20: 163
7 Frei E III, Spurr CL, Brindley CO, Selawry O, Holland JF, Rall DR, Wasserman LR, Hoogstraten B, Shnider BI, McIntyre OR, Matthews LB Jr, Miller SP (1965) Clinical studies of dichloromethotrexate (NSC 29630). Clin Pharmacol Ther 6: 160–171
8 Goldin A, Humphreys SR, Venditti JM, Mantel N (1959) Prolongation of life span of mice with advanced leukemia (L1210) by treatment with halogenated derivatives of amethopterin. J Natl Cancer Inst 22: 811–823
9 Goldin A, Venditti JM, Klein I, Mantel N (1966) Eradication of leukemic cells L1210 by methotrexate and methotrexate plus citrovorum factor. Nature 212: 1548
10 Isacoff WH, Morrison PF, Aroesty J, Willis KL, Block JB, Lincoln TL (1977) Pharmacokinetics of high dose methotrexate with citrovorum factor rescue. Cancer Treat Rep 61: 1665–1674
11 Jaffe N, Frei E III, Traggis D, Bishop Y (1974) Adjuvant methotrexate and citrovorum factor treatment of osteogenic sarcoma. N Engl J Med 291: 994–997
12 Levitt M, Mosher MB, DeConti RC, Farber LR, Skeel RT, Marsh JC, Mitchell MS, Papac RJ, Thomas ED, Bertino JR (1973) Improved therapeutic index of methotrexate with "Leucovorin rescue." Cancer Res 33: 1792–1734
13 Ohnuma T, Arkin H, Minowada J, Holland JF (1978) Differential chemotherapeutic susceptibility of human T-lymphocytes and B-lymphocytes in culture. J Natl Cancer Inst 60: 749–752
14 Ohnuma T, Nogeire C, Cuttner J, Holland JF (1978) Phase I study with neocarzinostatin: Tolerance to two hour infusion and continuous infusion. Cancer 42: 1670–1679
15 Takahashi I, Ohnuma T, Holland JF (1979) A comparison of the biological effects of dichloromethotrexate and methotrexate on human leukemic cells in culture. Cancer Res 39: 1264–1268
16 Vogel Cl, Adamson RH, DeVita VT, Johns DG, Kyalwazi SK (1972) Preliminary clinical trials of dichloromethotrexate (NSC-29630) in hepatocellular carcinoma. Cancer Chemother Rep 56: 249–258

An Overview of the Clinical Pharmacology of N-Phosphonacetyl-L-Aspartate (PALA), a New Antimetabolite

C. Erlichman

N-Phosphonacetyl-L-aspartic acid (PALA) is a new synthetic antimetabolite which inhibits de novo pyrimidine biosynthesis. Its significant activity against Lewis lung carcinoma, B16 melanoma, and glioma 26 suggested that it might be useful in the treatment of human solid tumors. Phase I trials revealed that dose-limiting toxicity included skin reactions, diarrhea, and stomatitis. Pharmacologic studies demonstrated rapid renal excretion of more than 70% of the unmetabolized drug in 24 h. Peak plasma levels correlated with dose of PALA administered. Partial responses to PALA were seen in one patient with melanoma, one with chondrosarcoma, and one with colon carcinoma. The potential for PALA's use in combination chemotherapy, particularly with 5-fluorouracil, is discussed.

Introduction

N-Phosphonacetyl-L-aspartic acid (PALA) was synthesized by Collins and Stark [2] as an analogue of the transition state intermediate of the reaction catalyzed by aspartate transcarbamylase (ATC). This reaction, whereby carbamyl phosphate and aspartate combine to form carbamylaspartate, is the second step in de novo pyrimidine biosynthesis (Fig. 1). PALA competitively inhibits the binding of carbamyl phosphate to ATC with a K_i of approximately 10^{-8} *M*. In *Escherichia coli*, ATC is a key enzyme in de novo pyrimidine biosynthesis. Thus, inhibition of this enzyme by PALA significantly diminished pyrimidine biosynthesis. However, carbamyl synthetase, and not ATC, is the rate-limiting enzyme in the de novo pathway of pyrimidine biosynthesis in mammalian cells [11]. Furthermore, a "salvage pathway" for pyrimidine nucleotide biosynthesis potentially exists in mammalian cells which could supply the necessary precursors either preferentially or in the case of inhibition of the de novo pathway. Despite these two potential biochemical drawbacks, PALA has demonstrated interesting antineoplastic activity in murine systems. On this basis and its predictable, tolerable, and reversible toxicity in animals, PALA has undergone phase I trial in the United States in the past year. This paper presents some of the pertinent preclinical data and a summary of the phase I results and discusses possible future roles for PALA as a new antimetabolite in the study and therapy of cancer.

Preclinical Studies of PALA

PALA was screened in a variety of murine tumors and demonstrated an unusual spectrum of activity. It had significant activity against Lewis lung carcinoma, B16

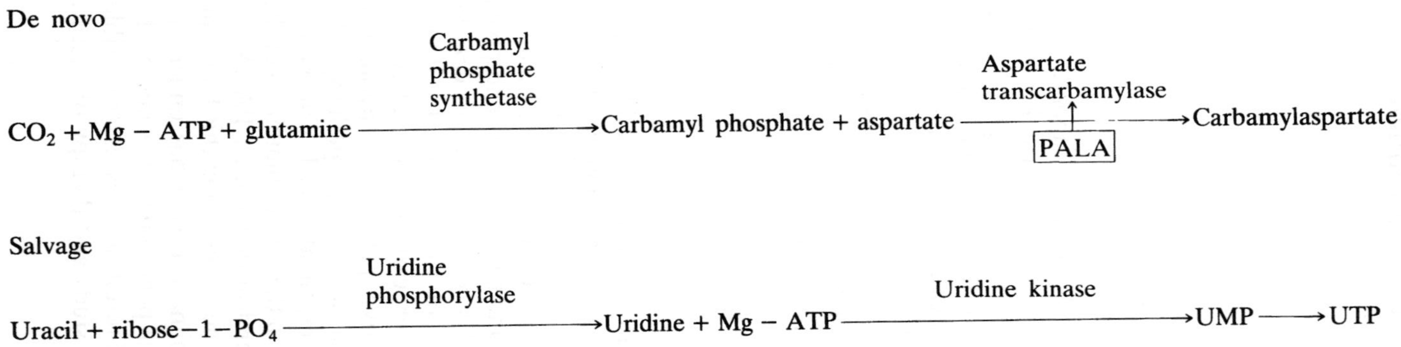

Fig. 1. Pathways for pyrimidine biosynthesis. Mg, Magnesium; ATP, adenosine triphosphate; UMP, uridine monophosphate; UTP, uridine triphosphate

melanoma, and glioma 26, moderate activity against a subline of P388 leukemia, but no activity against L1210 leukemia [8]. This significant activity in murine solid tumors suggested that PALA might have activity in human solid tumors, whereas efficacy in hematologic malignancies was not expected.

Studies of PALA biochemical pharmacology were performed in vitro and in vivo to elucidate some of the parameters which might be important in therapy with this agent. PALA significantly inhibited the de novo synthesis of pyrimidines in one human colon cancer cell line [15]. This persisted for long periods of time and was associated with inhibition of growth. Mutant cells, resistant to PALA, were developed and showed increased ATC levels in comparison to the original PALA-sensitive cells [9]. PALA-treated animals and cells could be "rescued" by the administration of carbamylaspartate or uridine [7]. Presumably, carbamylaspartate bypasses the metabolic block created by PALA whereas uridine is utilized through the "salvage pathway" to supply the necessary pyrimidine nucleotide precursors. PALA intracellular uptake has been examined in vitro and was found to be slower in resistant cell lines [6]. However, it is not sufficiently clear at this time whether changes in uptake play a significant role in sensitivity to PALA. The potential importance of the salvage pathway in the sensitivity of tumors to PALA has been mentioned previously. Although the salvage pathway may play an important role in resistance to PALA in certain tumors, crucial experiments addressing this question have not as yet been reported. The flux across the de novo pathway using $^{14}CO_2$ or ^{14}C-aspartate in PALA-sensitive and PALA-resistant cells relative to the flow of pyrimidine bases or nucleosides through the salvage pathway in the same cells may provide insight into the importance of salvage. Furthermore, an understanding of the relative importance of these two pathways in normal and malignant cells might suggest that rescue with exogenous pyrimidine nucleosides such as uridine would increase the therapeutic index for PALA.

Preclinical toxicology and disposition studies were carried out in mice, dogs, and monkeys. The major toxicities were: (a) gastrointestinal, manifested by diarrhea, emesis, hematemesis, and hematochezia; and (b) neurologic with sedation and seizures. The toxicity was dose-dependent, reversible, and did not appear to be cumulative. No significant hematopoietic or renal toxicity was observed. Drug disposition studies in animals revealed that there was significant uptake of PALA in bone and kidney and that most of the PALA was excreted in the urine unchanged in the first 24 h [1]. These preclinical studies suggested that PALA would be suitable for phase I trials in man. The results of these trials are summarized in the following section.

Clinical Studies of PALA

PALA has undergone phase I trials in several centers in the USA using different dose schedules (Table 1) [3–5, 14, 16]. Toxicity did not appear to be schedule-dependent. Dose-limiting toxicity was due to skin and/or gastrointestinal reactions. No significant hematopoietic, hepatic, or renal toxicities were noted.

In the National Cancer Institute (NCI) phase I trial of PALA, given as a daily bolus for 5 days, the skin toxicity was manifested by a macular, erythematous, and occasionally pruritic eruption which was most common in the head and neck regions and intertriginous areas. Although the rash was usually localized to these areas it did

Table 1. Phase I PALA studies

Institute	Schedule	Maximum dose	Recommended dose	Reference
Memorial S.K.I	IV q week × 3	6.75 $g/m^2/day$	4.5 $g/m^2/day$ (PS > 60)	[5]
	IV q week × 3		$3.75^a/m^2/day$ (PS ≤ 60)	
M. D. Anderson	IV q 2 weeks	6 $g/m^2/day$	5 $g/m^2/day$	[16]
DCT/NCI	IV q d × 5 q 3 weeks	2 $g/m^2/day$	1.5 $g/m^2/day$	[3]
Mount Sinai	IV 24-h infusion	10.5 $g/m^2/day$	8.7 $g/m^2/day$	[14]
Sidney Farber	IV 4-day infusion	2 $g/m^2/day$	1.5–1.8 $g/m^2/day$	[4]
Mayo Clinic	IV q d × 5 q 6 weeks	1.25 $g/m^2/day$	1.25 $g/m^2/day$	

P.S. performance status (Karnofsky Scale)

become generalized at the higher doses. At the maximum dose level achieved (2 $g/m^2/day$), four of five patients experienced severe, extensive skin toxicity. Although no significant exfoliation was seen in the NCI trial, this has been reported by other centers. The rash usually began days 5–8 of a 21-day cycle and resolved by day 14 in most cases. There was no correlation with age, sex, diagnosis, or previous radiotherapy or chemotherapy. At all centers the rash was dose-related and reversible but not cumulative.

Gastrointestinal toxicity was manifested as nausea and/or vomiting which was mild, stomatitis (which occurred in association with diarrhea), and hematochezia. Diarrhea, which was the major gastrointestinal toxicity, usually began on days 3–7 of a cycle and resolved in 1 week. No episode of hematochezia was associated with significant blood loss. Gastrointestinal toxicity usually occurred during courses associated with the skin toxicity and was also dose-dependent, reversible, but not cumulative.

There was some suggestion of neurotoxicity in several of the phase I trials. This neurotoxicity ranged from paresthesias to sedation and seizures. The seizures were grand mal in nature and usually occurred late in a cycle. Five patients have had seizures. Three of these had structural lesions. Seizures occurred after at least two cycles in all cases. It is not clear at this time whether these seizures are a manifestation of chronic PALA toxicity, but, in view of these reported cases, it would be advisable to exclude patients with evidence of central nervous system lesions from PALA therapy.

In the phase I studies no complete responses have been observed. Partial responses were observed in one case each of melanoma, chondrosarcoma, and colon carcinoma. Stable disease was documented in four patients with melanoma, seven patients with colon carcinoma, five patients with carcinoma of the lung, two patients with carcinoma of the bladder, three patients with sarcoma, two patients with hypernephroma, and one each with carcinoid and ovarian carcinoma.

Pharmacokinetic studies of PALA using various of the available assay methods were carried out in some of the patients treated in the phase I studies. There was general agreement among the centers reporting these results as follows: (a) PALA plasma levels decreased biexponentially with a $t_{1/2}\beta$ which averaged between 5 and 8 h at different centers, (b) the $t_{1/2}\beta$ reflected renal excretion which was the main route of elimination, (c) the majority of the drug accumulated in the urine within the first 24 h, (d) no metabolites were detected in the patients studied, and (e) peak plasma levels were linear with dose.

In an attempt to establish biochemical correlates of toxicity or therapeutic response, levels of ATC were examined in tumor tissue and circulating leukocytes [10, 12]. In the leukocytes, the inhibition of ATC was rapid and persistent with levels of activity returning to 50% of pretreatment levels by day 10 on a daily × 5 schedule of PALA therapy. However, it is not clear whether this reflects a similar inhibition of ATC activity in tumor tissues. Pretreatment analysis of ATC in tumor specimens did not shown any correlation between enzyme activity and tumor type. Levels of ATC activity in skin and gastrointestinal mucosa were lower than in circulating leukocytes. This suggests a correlation of toxicity seen in the phase I trials with low levels of ATC activity. All these results are preliminary and further serial specimens will need to be analyzed in order that sound conclusions may be reached.

Discussion

At this point, the role of PALA in future cancer therapy is unclear. The predictable, reversible, and tolerable toxicity observed in the phase I trials makes phase II studies feasible. These are under way at present and results should be forthcoming on PALA's single-agent activity in the near future.

The results of the phase I studies do not suggest that any specific schedule has an advantage over another. However, using information available from preclinical studies and from pharmacokinetics in the phase I trials, we may be able to suggest schedules which might give an optimal chance for therapeutic effect. Growth inhibition of various cell lines in culture by PALA required continuous exposure to relatively high levels ($> 10^{-5}$ M) for prolonged periods of time. As previously mentioned, the uptake of PALA may be a limiting factor in its therapeutic efficacy. If so, prolonged exposure to PALA and/or high concentrations should result in greater intracellular uptake. Animal studies showed that optimal activity of PALA was achieved in multidose schedules. Phase I pharmacokinetics revealed that high plasma levels are achieved by rapid infusion, but these levels are quickly dissipated due to rapid renal excretion of PALA. On the basis of these four points, it would appear that a prolonged continuous infusion or a multidose schedule could achieve an optimal effect of PALA therapy.

Combination therapy with PALA is a promising area of exploration in view of its spectrum of toxicity and its biochemical action. The lack of myelosuppression makes it an attractive partner in combination with myelosuppressive agents. The biochemical rationale for combining PALA with 5-fluorouracil (5-FU) is particularly appealing. PALA inhibition of the de novo pathway could conceivably increase utilization of preformed pyrimidines through the salvage pathway. If 5-FU were administered, there might be increased incorporation of the 5-FU into the nucleotide pools with enhanced thymidylate synthetase inhibition and/or increased incorporation into RNA. In fact, there is some evidence that PALA does cause increased incorporation of 5-FU into RNA in some tumor systems [13]. Another proposed mechanism by which PALA and 5-FU may be synergistic involves the presumed increase in intracellular phosphoribosylpyrophosphate (PRPP) pools which would become available for 5-FU activation when PALA blocks de novo pyrimidine biosynthesis. This has been suggested as a mechanism for methotrexate – 5-FU synergism in some cell lines. Similar biochemical mechanisms can be hypothesized for PALA and cytosine arabinoside combinations. Finally, the possibility of uridine rescue of normal tissue in preference to tumor tissue, as mentioned earlier, needs further examination.

Thus, the role of PALA in cancer chemotherapy is yet to be defined. The studies ongoing at this time will hopefully clarify its usefulness.

References

1 Chadwick M, Silveira DM, MacGregor JA, Branfman AR, Liss RH, Yesair DW (1978) Physiological disposition of PALA in several species. Proc Am Assoc Cancer Res 19: 182

2 Collins KD, Stark GR (1971) Aspartate transcarbamylase, interaction with the transition state analogue *N*-(phosphonacetyl)-L-aspartate. J Biol Chem 246: 6599–6605

3 Erlichman C, Strong J, Wiernik P, Edwards L, Cohen M, Levine A, Hubbard S, Chabner B (1979) Phase I trial of PALA (*N*-phosphonacetyl-L-aspartate). Proc Am Soc Clin Oncol 20: 314

4 Ervin TJ, Blum RH, Canellos GP (1979) *N*-Phosphonacetyl-L-aspartate (PALA), phase I trial. Proc Am Assoc Cancer Res 20: 200

5 Gralla RJ, Casper ES, Golbey RB, Young CW (1979) Phase I and preliminary phase II studies with *N*-(phosphonacetyl)-L-aspartic acid (PALA). Proc Am Assoc Cancer Res 20: 115

6 Jayaram HN, Cooney DA, Vistica DT, Kariya S, Johnson RK (1979) Mechanisms of sensitivity or resistance of murine tumors to *N*-(phosphonacetyl)-L-aspartate. Cancer Treat Rep 63: 1291

7 Johnson RK (1977) Reversal of toxicity and antitumor activity of *N*-(phosphonacetyl)-L-aspartate by uridine or carbamyl-DL-aspartate in vivo. Biochem Pharmacol 26: 81–84
8 Johnson RK, Inouye T, Goldin A, Stark GR (1976) Antitumor activity of *N*-(phosphonacetyl)-L-aspartic acid, a transition state inhibitor of aspartate transcarbamylase. Cancer Res 36: 2720–2725
9 Kempe TD, Swyryd EA, Bruist M, Stark GR (1976) Stable mutants of mammalian cells that overproduce the first three enzymes of pyrimidine nucleotide biosynthesis. Cell 9: 541–550
10 Kensler TW, Jayaram HN, Cooney DA, Petrucci PE (1979) Inhibition of L-aspartate transcarbamylase (ATCase) in human leucocytes by *N*-(phosphonacetyl)-L-aspartic acid (PALA): Use of peripheral white blood cells as enzymic indicators. Proc Am Assoc Cancer Res 20: 243
11 Levine RL, Hoogenraad NJ, Kretchmer N (1974) A review: Biological and clinical aspects of pyrimidine metabolism. Pediatrics 8: 724–734
12 Moore EC, Friedman J, Valdievieso M, Marti JR, Russ J, Loo TL (1979) *N*-(Phosphonacetyl)-L-aspartate (PALA) concentration and aspartate carbamoyl-transferase (ATCase) activity in biopsy specimens of patients treated with PALA. Proc Am Assoc Cancer Res 20: 221
13 Nayak R, Martin D, Stolfi R, Furth J, Spiegelman S (1978) Pyrimidine nucleosides enhance the anti-cancer activity of FU and augment its incorporation into nuclear RNA. Proc Am Assoc Cancer Res 19: 63
14 Ohnuma T, Hart R, Roboz J, Andrejczuk A, Holland JF 1979) Clinical and pharmacological studies with phosphonacetyl-L-aspartate (PALA). Proc Am Soc Clin Oncol 20: 344
15 Tsuboi KK, Edmunds HN, Kwong LK (1977) Selective inhibition of pyrimidine biosynthesis and effect on proliferative growth of colonic cancer cells. Cancer Res 37: 3080–3087
16 Valdivieso M, Moore EC, Loo TL, Bodey GP, Freireich EJ (1979) Phase I clinical study of *N*-(phosphonacetyl)-L-aspartate (PALA, NSC 224131). Proc Am Assoc Cancer Res 20: 187

N-(Phosphonacetyl)-L-Aspartate (PALA): Current Status

M. Rozencweig*, R. Abele, M. Piccart, D. D. Von Hoff, and F. M. Muggia

Summary

N-(Phosphonoacetyl)-L-aspartate (PALA) is a synthetic antimetabolite exhibiting striking oncolytic properties against a wide variety of experimental solid tumors. The clinical dose-limiting factor is mucocutaneous toxicity which is reversible and dose-related. Delineation of the single-agent activity of PALA in human cancer must still await results of recently activated trials.

Introduction

N-(Phosphonoacetyl)-L-aspartate (PALA) is a new anticancer agent which was synthesized by COLLINS and STARK [3] as an analogue of the transition state for the reaction catalyzed by aspartate transcarbamylase. The chemical structure of this antimetabolite is depicted in Fig. 1.

The drug exhibits excellent antitumor effect against various mouse solid tumors, whereas little or no activity has been detected in commonly sensitive murine leukemias. These striking observations led to the prompt introduction of this compound into clinical trials. A large number of phase II studies have been recently activated and should rapidly delineate the role of PALA as a single agent in the treatment of human cancer. This overview summarizes the current status of this new agent, complementing the biochemical pharmacology described above.

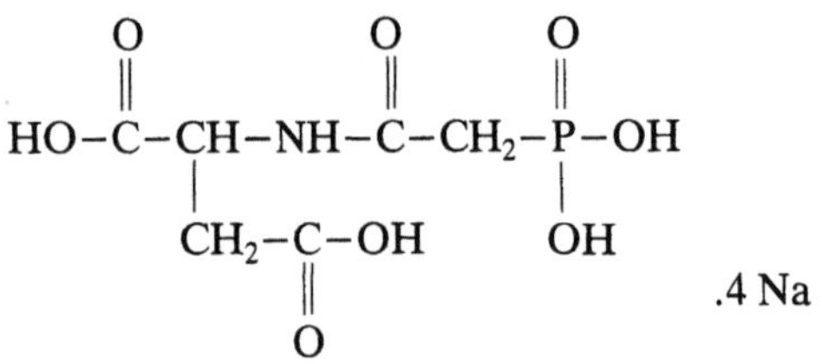

PALA
NSC-224131

Fig. 1

* The authors acknowledge the help of Ms. GENEVIÈVE DECOSTER in the preparation of this manuscript. This work was supported by grant 3.4535.79 from the "Fonds de la Recherche Scientifique Médicale" (FRSM, Belgium), and by contract NIH NO1/CM53840 from the National Cancer Institute, Bethesda, Maryland, USA

Pharmaceutical Data

For clinical use, PALA is available only to qualified investigators through the Investigational Drug Branch of the National Cancer Institute. The compound is very stable as the bulk drug or in aqueous solution. It is supplied for intravenous (IV) injection in 10-ml ampules containing 100 mg/ml of PALA, sodium hydroxide to adjust to pH 6.5–7.5, and water for injection USP. The intact ampules should be stored at 2°–8° C.

Preclinical Information

Biologic Properties

PALA is a potent inhibitor of aspartate transcarbamylase, a key enzyme in the de novo biosynthesis of pyrimidine nucleotides [3]. This inhibition results in cytotoxic effects which may be reversed in vivo by uridine and carbamyl-DL-aspartate [12]. PALA has been shown to enhance the entry of 5-fluorouracil into nuclear RNA [8]. It does not appear to impair cell-mediated immune response as measured by the rejection rate of a tumor allograft in mice [13].

Animal Tumor Data

PALA is curative without clear schedule dependency in the usually refractory Lewis lung carcinoma [21]. The drug is also active against a variety of other mouse solid tumors including $CD8F_1$ mammary carcinoma, glioma 26, B16 melanoma, colon carcinoma 26, C3H mammary carcinoma, and mammary xenograft MX-1 [9, 13]. In contrast, L1210 and P388 murine leukemias are relatively or completely resistant to PALA, whereas these tumor models exhibit sensitivity to the vast majority of standard chemotherapeutic agents. Of note, collateral sensitivity to PALA has been described in P388 cell lines resistant to cytosine arabinoside and 5-fluorouracil [16]. No antitumor activity has been observed with oral PALA in experimental murine tumors.

The unusual spectrum of activity of PALA has been related to a direct relationship between natural or acquired drug resistance, cellular levels of aspartate transcarbamylase, and cell proliferation rate [13, 14]. Thus, higher enzyme activity and faster cell proliferation characterize the L1210 leukemia relative to Lewis lung carcinoma. Cellular uptake mechanisms and pyrimidine salvage pathways might also interfere with the cytotoxic properties of the drug [11].

Animal Toxicology

In the mouse, acute toxicity studies indicated an LD_{10} of 3.2 g/m^2. Histopathologic evaluation after the administration of a lethal dose did not reveal any pathologic changes except in the liver, where PALA produced a dose-dependent and dose-limiting toxicity [13].

In the dog, the toxic low dose was 2.4 g/m^2 for the single-dose study, and between 0.3 and 0.6 g/m^2/day for the daily administration for 5 consecutive days. Dose-limiting toxicity resulted from toxic effects in the gastrointestinal tract and the central nervous system (CNS). Gastrointestinal toxicity was dose-related and reversible at sublethal doses. It consisted of vomiting, hematemesis, diarrhea, and melena. Histologic examination revealed hemorrhagic and suppurative atrophy of the intestinal mucosa. CNS effects at sublethal doses were essentially apparent with the single-dose schedule and included seizures, loss of corneal reflex, and ataxia. No histologic lesions could be identified to account for these CNS manifestations. Finally, sporadic and transient shifts in serum enzymes and electrolytes were also encountered, but could not be clearly related to specific target organ impairment. These toxicology studies also pointed to the lack of drug-induced myelosuppression.

Experimental Pharmacology

Various analytic methods have been developed for quantitating PALA [1, 4, 5, 8 , 19, 22], but limited pharmacokinetic data are presently available. The drug is poorly absorbed when given orally [1]. After IV administration of the radiolabeled compound to mice [1, 2], the drug is eliminated from plasma and tissues with an initial half-life of about 1 h and a secondary half-time of from 1–1.25 days. Radioactivity may be detected in the brain shortly after treatment. Whole-body radioautographic techniques indicate that PALA is deposited and retained in bones. The drug is rapidly excreted in the urine, where more than 80% of the administered dose may be recovered.

Clinical Studies

Toxic Effects

Clinical information presently available on PALA is essentially based on currently completed phase I trials (Table 1). In these trials, mucocutaneous toxicity was consistently found to be dose-related and dose-limiting. Low performance status [10], hepatic dysfunction, and increase of third space [19] appeared to enhance the risk and the severity of toxic manifestations.

Skin toxicity was most frequently encountered and consisted of an exfoliative dermatitis starting as an erythematous macular rash involving skin-fold surfaces, the

Table 1. Phase I trials with PALA

Schedule (reference)	Dose/g/m^2/day	
	Recommended	Tested
Single dose every 2 weeks [23]	5	0.8 –15.0
Every day for 5 days every 3 weeks [6]	1.5	0.1 – 2.0
Weekly for 3 weeks [10]	4.5	0.9 – 6.75
Continuous infusion for 24 h every 3 weeks [19]	8.7	0.5 –10.5
Continuous infusion for 5 days every 3 weeks [7]	1.8	0.15– 2.0
Continuous infusion for 5 days every 3 weeks [19]	–	0.8 – 1.74

trunk, and the face. Skin biopsies have revealed toxic necrolysis of the basement membrane [8].
Mild to moderate stomatitis often accompanied skin toxicity [10]. Diarrhea became uniformly prominent at high doses of the drug. Anorexia, nausea, and vomiting have also been described.
Other toxic effects were rarely observed and included transient neurologic symptoms with lethargy, weakness, paresthesias of lips and extremities, SGOT elevations, phlebitis, fever, and negligible myelosuppression.

Antitumor Activity

Antitumor effect of PALA has been detected in phase I trials in sarcoma [7, 19, 23], colon cancer [6, 7], melanoma, and ovarian cancer [23]. The single-agent activity of PALA is presently investigated in a large number of tumor types. Phase II experience with this agent remains limited at this point. Minor responses have been achieved in three of 21 patients with non-small cell lung cancer and in two of ten patients with bladder cancer [10].

Clinical Pharmacology

The specific activity of aspartate transcarbamylase in human leukocytes is relatively high as compared with that found in the skin and the colonic mucosa [15]. In patients given oncostatic infusions of PALA, this leukocytic enzyme is rapidly and strongly inhibited; restitution of enzyme activity is slow after cessation of therapy with a half-maximal restoration time of about 280 h [15].
The activity of aspartate transcarbamylase was considerably lower in PALA-resistant human tumors as compared with PALA-sensitive murine tumors [17]. In man, the enzymatic activity could be reduced to 0–10% of the pretreatment values within 1.5–6 h after the administration of a single dose. Enzymatic inhibition was correlated with tumor concentrations of PALA and was still apparent after 6 days [17].
Pharmacokinetic data are still very preliminary [6, 8, 19]. Ohnuma et al. [19] reported a median serum concentration of 250 μM (range: 137–400 μM) at the end of a 24-h infusion of 4 g/m^2 of PALA. Serum drug levels decreased biexponentially with an initial half-life of 100 min and a secondary half-life of 8 h. Most of the drug was recovered in the urine within 30 h. The drug was primarily excreted unmetabolized [6].

Discussion

PALA is a new antimetabolite that differs strikingly from other antimetabolites in terms of experimental antitumor activity. In addition, cell lines resistant to cytosine arabinoside or 5-fluorouracil have shown collateral sensitivity to PALA [16].
The currently available phase I reports suggest that the mode of administration does not markedly affect the pattern of toxic effects induced by PALA. Of possible relevance, no clear schedule dependency had been found for the antitumor activity in the mouse, and pharmacokinetics is essentially similar in mouse and man.
At doses recommended for phase II studies, mucocutaneous toxicity is usually well tolerated, but may become occasionally severe. Whether PALA-induced toxic effects

are cumulative has not yet been properly estimated. There are no data correlating drug toxicity and renal function. However, pharmacokinetic studies call for the greatest care if PALA is to be administered to patients with renal impairment.

Uridine and carbamyl-DL-aspartate have been used experimentally to reverse the PALA-induced inhibition of aspartate transcarbamylase [12]. A possible tissue selectivity of this reversibility should be explored to determine whether rescue measures might be of therapeutic benefit. The lack of significant myelosuppression in patients treated with PALA is consistent with its lack of activity in the L1210 system [20]. This attractive property might become an important consideration for future combination chemotherapy regimens. At present, there is no published information on synergistic combinations in animal tumor systems.

The remarkable sensitivity of some usually refractory solid tumors in mice has been ascribed to low levels of aspartate transcarbamylase [13, 14]. The clinical relevance of these findings remains to be established. In humans, the specific activity of the enzyme was reported to be much higher in leukocytes than in the skin or colonic mucosa, which both are prime targets of drug toxicity [15]. On the other hand, it would appear that low tumoral enzyme activities and at least transient total blockade of aspartate transcarbamylase are not sufficient requirements to observe anticancer effects in man [17]. These determinations should undoubtedly be repeated in phase II trials using more homogenous samples of patients with better prognosis and more prolonged treatments.

The clinical spectrum of antitumor activity is being actively investigated. Disease-oriented studies in colon cancer, melanoma, and sarcoma deserve particular attention in view of the phase I experience. Positive results achieved in various murine mammary tumors including the human xenograft make breast cancer an important candidate for clinical testing. Of note, PALA was found to cross the so-called "blood-brain barrier" and to exert marked activity against glioma 26. Its neurologic toxicity further suggests a possible role in the treatment of malignancies of the central nervous system. Retention of PALA in mouse bone also warrants its investigation in osseous tumors.

In conclusion, PALA is an investigational anticancer agent with very attractive experimental characteristics. It is still premature to assess its therapeutic usefulness, but this should be rapidly clarified with currently expanding clinical experience.

References

1 Chadwick M, Silveira DM, MacGregor JA, Branfman AR, Liss RH, Yesair DW (1978) Physiological disposition of PALA in several species. Proc Am Assoc Cancer Res and Am Soc Clin Oncol 19: 182

2 Chadwick M, Silveira DM, McGarrigle PL, Liss RH, Schepis PJ (1979) Distribution of PALA in tissues and tumors of mice after intravenous administration. Proc Am Assoc Cancer Res and Am Soc Clin Oncol 20: 241

3 Collins KD, Stark GR (1971) Aspartate transcarbamylase. Interaction with the transition state analogue N-(phosphonacetyl)-L-aspartate. J Biol Chem 246: 6599-6605

4 Cooney DA, Karlowicz MG, Cubillan J, Roettger M, Jayaram HN (1978) An enzymatic technique for measuring N-phosphonacetyl-L-aspartic acid in tissues. Cancer Treat Rep 62: 1503–1507

5 Erlichman C, Chabner BA (1979) A competitive protein binding assay for N-phosphonacetyl-L-aspartate (PALA). Proc Am Assoc Cancer Res and Am Soc Clin Oncol 20: 185

6 Erlichman C, Strong, J, Wiernick P, Edwards L, Cohen M, Levine A, Hubbard S, Chabner B (1979) Phase I trial of PALA (N-phosphonacetyl-L-aspartate). Proc Am Assoc Cancer Res and Am Soc Clin Oncol 20: 314
7 Ervin, TJ, Blum RH, Canellos GP (1979) N-Phosphonacetyl-L-aspartate (PALA), phase I trial. Proc Am Assoc Cancer Res and Am Soc Clin Oncol 20: 200
8 Friedman J, Moore EC, Hall SW, Loo TL (1979) Enzymatic assay for the antitumor agent N-(phosphonacetyl)-L-aspartic acid (PALA). Cancer Treat Rep 63: 85–88
9 Goldin A, Venditti JM, Muggia FM, Rozencweig M, De Vita VT (1979) New animal models in cancer chemotherapy. In: Fox BW (ed.) Advances in Medical Oncology, Research and Eduction, vol. 5, Basis for Cancer Therapy 1. Pergamon Press, Oxford, pp 113–122
10 Gralla RJ, Casper ES, Golbey RB, Young CW (1979) Phase I and preliminary phase II studies with N-(phosphonacetyl)-L-aspartic acid (PALA). Proc Am Assoc Cancer Res and Am Soc Clin Oncol 20: 115
11 Jayaram HN, Cooney DA, Vistica DT, Kariya S, Johnson RK (1979) Mechanisms of sensitivity or resistance of murine tumors to N-(phosphonacetyl)-L-aspartate. Cancer Treat Rep 63: 1291–1302
12 Johnson RK (1977) Reversal of toxicity and antitumor activity of *N*-(phosphonacetyl)-L-aspartate by uridine or carbamyl-DL-aspartate in vivo. Biochem Pharmacol 26: 81–84
13 Johnson RK, Swyryd EA, Stark GR (1978) Effects of N-(phosphonacetyl)-L-aspartate on murine tumors and normal tissues in vivo and in vitro and the relationship of sensitivity to rate of proliferation and level of aspartate transcarbamylase. Cancer Res 38: 371–377
14 Kempe TD, Swyryd EA, Bruist M, Stark GR (1976) Stable mutants of mammalian cells that overproduce the first three enzymes of pyrimidine nucleotide biosynthesis. Cell 9: 541–550
15 Kensler TW, Jayaram HN, Cooney DA, Petrucci PE (1979) Inhibition of L-aspartate transcarbamylase (ATCase) in human leucocytes by N-(phosphonacetyl)-L-aspartic acid (PALA): Use of peripheral white blood cells as enzymic indicators. Proc Am Assoc Cancer Res and Am Soc Clin Oncol 20: 243
16 Laster WR Jr, Schabel FM Jr (1979) Collateral sensitivity of P388/Ara-C and P388/5-FU to N-(phosphonacetyl)-L-aspartate (PALA). Proc Am Assoc Cancer Res and Am Soc Clin Oncol 20: 95
17 Moore EC, Friedman J, Valdivieso M, Marti JR, Russ J, Loo TL (1979) N-(Phosphonoacetyl)-L-aspartate (PALA) concentration and aspartate carbamoyltransferase (ACTase) activity in biopsy specimens of patients treated with PALA. Proc Am Assoc Cancer Res and Am Soc Clin Oncol 20: 221
18 Nayak R, Martin D, Stolfi R, Furth J, Spiegelman S (1978) Pyrimidine nucleosides enhance the anti-cancer activity of FU and augment its incorporation into nuclear RNA. Proc Am Assoc Cancer Res and Am Soc Clin Oncol 19: 63
19 Ohnuma T, Hart R, Roboz J, Andrejczuk A, Holland JF (1979) Clinical and pharmacological studies with phosphonoacetyl-L-aspartate (PALA). Proc Am Assoc Cancer Res and Am Soc Clin Oncol 20: 344
20 Rozencweig M, Von Hoff DD, Venditti JM, Muggia FM (1976) Correlation between experimental activity of anticancer agents and their hematologic toxicity in man. Blood 48: 984
21 Schabel FM Jr, Laster WR Jr, Rose WC (1979) The role of experimental tumor systems. In: Muggia FM, Rozencweig M (eds) Lung cancer: Progress in therapeutic research. Raven, New York, pp 15–35
22 Strong JM, Kinney YE, Branfman AR, Cysyk RL (1979) Determination of N-(phosphonacetyl)-L-aspartic acid (PALA) in dog serum and urine by gas chromatography and selected ion monitoring. Cancer Treat Rep 63: 775–780
23 Valdivieso M, Moore EC, Loo TL, Bodey GP, Freireich EJ (1979) Phase I clinical study of N-(phosphonoacetyl)-L-aspartate (PALA, NSC 224131). Proc Am Assoc Cancer Res and Am Soc Clin Oncol 20: 187

Synthesis, Biologic Effects, and Biochemical Properties of Some 2′-Azido- and 2′-Amino-2′-Deoxyarabinofuranosyl Pyrimidines and Purines

M. Bobek, Y.-C. Cheng, E. Mihich, and A. Bloch

Summary

Various 2′-azido- and 2′-aminoarabinofuranosyl purine and pyrimidine nucleosides have been synthesized. Among these, the derivatives of cytosine and of adenine inhibit the growth of some tumor cell lines in vitro and in vivo. 2′-Azidoarabinofuranosyl cytosine also interferes with the replication of herpes simplex virus types I and II. Whereas 2′-azidoara-C is resistant to deamination by a partially purified CdR deaminase from KB cells, the adenine derivatives are substrates for aminohydrolases partially purified from calf and mouse intestines. Both azido- and aminoara-C are phosphorylated by partially purified CdR kinases from leukemia L1210 and from human AML blast cells. The accumulated data encourage exploration of the clinical utility of the more potent of these analogues.

Introduction

The arabinofuranosyl derivatives of cytosine (ara-C) and of adenine (ara-A) possess significant antitumor and antiviral activity, particularly when their susceptibility to enzymatic deamination is moderated by the use of deaminase inhibitors [7, 8]. Since replacement of the 2′-hydroxyl group with other functions entailed the potential of increased antitumor and antiviral action simultaneous with decreased susceptibility to deamination, we embarked upon the synthesis of 2′-amino- and 2′-azido-2′-deoxyarabinofuranosyl cytosine and adenine, and evaluated the biologic and biochemical properties of these compounds. Analogous derivatives of uracil, thymine, guanine, and hypoxanthine were also prepared and tested. This communication reports the results of this investigation.

Materials and Methods

Synthetic Procedures

The compounds were synthesized by the general methods outlined in Figs. 1 and 2. The key sugar intermediate 1-chloro-3-*O*-acetyl-5-*O*-benzoyl-2-azido-2-deoxyarabinofuranose was prepared from diisopropylidene allose (Fig. 1). Displacement of the sulfonyl group at the 3-position with the azido anion, followed by selective hydrolysis of the 5,6-isopropylidene group with acetic acid and benzoylation of the 6-position,

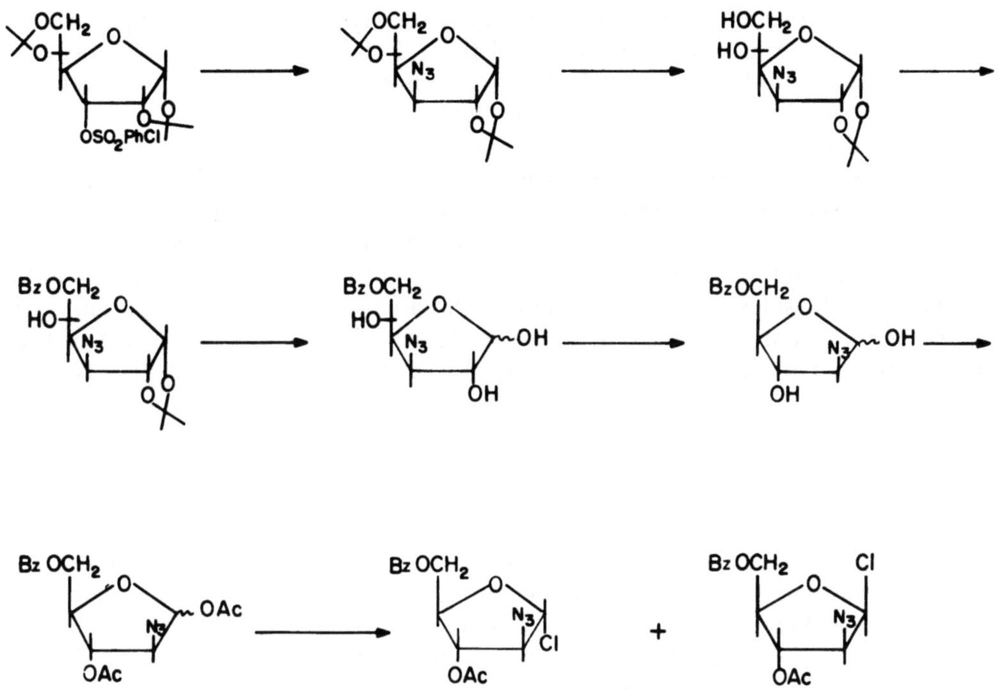

Fig. 1

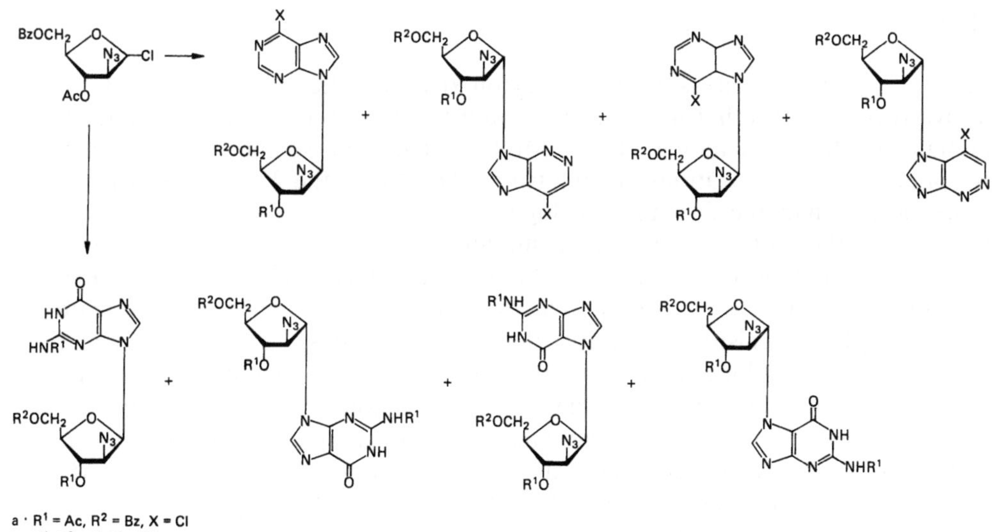

a · R^1 = Ac, R^2 = Bz, X = Cl
b R^1, R^2 = H, X = NH_2

Fig. 2

gave 1,2-isopropylidene-3-azido-6-benzoylglucose. Hydrolysis of the isopropylidene group followed by periodate oxidation of the 1,2-*cis*-diol and acetylation provided 1,3-di-*O*-acetyl-5-*O*-benzoyl-2-azido-2-deoxyarabinofuranose, which was converted to the 1-chloro derivative with titanium tetrachloride.
This sugar derivative was condensed with purine or pyrimidine bases which had been activated by silylation (Fig. 2) or – as in the case of adenine – by chloromercuriation [1, 3]. The isomeric nucleosides were separated by silica-gel chromatography, and were deblocked by treatment with methanolic ammonia or with potassium carbonate in methanol. Catalytic reduction of the 2′-azido group provided the corresponding 2′-amino nucleosides. The hypoxanthine derivatives were prepared by enzymatic deamination of the corresponding ara-A analogues. The synthesis of some of these agents by, in part, different procedures has recently been reported [9–11].

Biologic and Biochemical Procedures

The methods used for assaying the effects of the newly synthesized agents on tumor cell growth in vitro and in vivo and on the in vitro replication of herpes simplex virus have previously been published [2, 6]. The procedures employed for the isolation and assay of dCR kinase have also been described [5]. CdR deaminase was partially purified from KB cells by fractionation with ammonium sulfate to 35%–55% saturation and elution from DEAE cellulose with a 0–1 *M* KCl gradient in 50 m*M* Tris-HCl buffer, pH 8.0, containing 2 m*M* DTT and 10% glycerol. Adenosine deaminase from calf intestinal mucosa was purchased from Sigma Chemical Co., Saint Louis, Missouri.

Results

Table 1 provides a measure of the cytotoxicity of the newly prepared cytosine derivatives. It shows that these agents inhibit the growth of L1210 cells and of three human cell lines, including HeLa, Molt 4 (T-cell leukemia) and B35M (B-cell lymphoma) at concentrations ranging from 0.06–4 μ*M*, the 2′-azido derivative being more potent than the 2′-amino analogue.
Based upon these observations, the compounds were examined for their effect upon leukemia L1210 in vivo, as assayed by the survival of DBA2/Ha mice. The data shown in Table 2, which are representative of multiple experiments, demonstrate that 2′-azidoara-C, administered at various doses and schedules, is capable of giving rise to a high percentage of long-term survivors. Treatment with this compound also provided a significant number of long-term survivors among DBA2/CR mice carrying plasmacytoma P288. The 2′-amino analogue was similarly effective, but only at approximately twice the dose at which the azido derivative was active. At these treatment schedules, the animals suffered no significant weight loss.
The 2′-azido nucleoside was also tested for its ability to interfere with the in vitro replication of herpes simplex virus types I and II and, at 50 μ*M*, was found to reduce plaque formation to 0.2% and 2% of control, respectively.
To gain some information on the metabolic disposition the cytosine derivatives may undergo in the cells, their susceptibility to deamination by an aminohydrolase partially purified from KB cells was examined, and 2′-azidoara-C proved to be resistant to

Table 1. Effect of 2′-azido- and 2′-aminoarabinofuranosyl cytosine on the growth of various cell lines in culture

Cell line	ID_{50} (μM)	
	2′-azidoara-C	2′-aminoara-C
L1210	0.6	4.0
HeLa	0.2	3.0
Molt 4F	0.07	0.4
B35M	0.06	

Table 2. Effect of 2′-azidoara-C on leukemia L1210 in DBA2/HaDD mice[a]

Dose (mg/kg/day IP)	No. of days of treatment	Day of 1st treatment	Average survival time[b]	Surviving mice/ tested mice	Survival (%)[c]
Saline			8.2	0/30	–
20	5	+1	13.5	7/10	70
40	5	+1	–	10/10	100
80	5	+1	16.3	7/10	70
40 + 40	2	+1	23.7	32/35	91

[a] 1×10^6 L1210 cells were inoculated IP per mouse
[b] Excludes survivors
[c] > 30 days

enzyme-catalyzed deamination. Because 2′-aminoara-C undergoes rapid transformation at or above neutral pH to as yet unidentified products, the extent of its susceptibility to ezymatic deamination remains to be established.

Neither the azido nor the amino compound was found to interfere with the growth of L1210 cells resistant to ara-C by virtue of dCR-kinase deletion, suggesting that phosphorylation of the agents may be required for their activation. Phosphorylation was, indeed, demonstrated to occur, as catalyzed by a dCR kinase partially purified from human AML cells. Deoxycytidine was observed to compete with the analogues for phosphorylation, a competition that finds its analogy in intact L1210 cells, which can be protected from the cytotoxic effects of the agents by approximately tenfold higher concentrations of 2′-deoxycytidine.

In parallel with the ara-C derivatives, the 2′-azido and 2′-amino analogues of ara-A were also found capable of inhibiting in vitro cell growth. As shown in Table 3, azidoara-A is 40 times more potent an inhibitor of KB cell growth than is ara-A, whereas the amino analogue is less effective. Similarly, the azido compound is ten times more cytotoxic to L1210 cells than is ara-A. Deoxycoformycin, an inhibitor of adenosine deaminase, increased the potency of all three compounds, suggesting that the newly prepared agents, like ara-A, are substrates for deamination. As determined with adenosine deaminases partially purified from calf intestinal mucosa (Table 4), both compounds served as substrates for this enzyme, the K_m obtained with the 2′-amino analogue being larger and that furnished by the 2′-azido derivative being smaller than the K_m values provided by adenosine or 2′-deoxyadenosine. In contrast,

Table 3. Effect of 2′-azido- and 2′-aminoarabinofuranosyl adenine on the growth of KB and leukemia L1210 cells in vitro

Compound	Concentration for 50% growth inhibition of	
	KB cells	L1210 cells
2′-azidoara-A	2×10^{-6}	4×10^{-6}
2′-aminoara-A	2×10^{-4}	4×10^{-4}
Ara-A	8×10^{-5}	4×10^{-5}

Table 4. Comparative substrate activity of various adenine nucleosides for adenosine deaminase from calf intestinal mucosa

Substrate	K_m (μM)	V_{max} (%)
Adenosine	25	100
2′-Deoxyadenosine	30	100
Ara-A	300	25
2′-Aminoara-A	133	12
2′-Azidoara-A	5	0.18

the V_{max} values for both analogues were smaller than those pertaining to the natural substrates.

The 2′-azido derivatives of arabinofuranosyl uracil, thymine, and hypoxanthine were found inactive in the leukemia L1210 test system.

Discussion

As demonstrated by the results of this investigation, replacement of the 2′-hydroxyl groups of ara-C or ara-A by an azido group decreases the susceptibility of the modified compounds to enzymatic deamination, while preserving their ability to be phosphorylated. Although 2′-azidoara-C is a more effective inhibitor of leukemia L1210 growth in vivo than is ara-C, and 2′-azidoara-A more cytotoxic to two tumor cell lines in vitro than is ara-A, this improved effectiveness cannot be attributed unequivocally to the decreased susceptibility of the compounds to deamination. The rate and extent of their accumulation as the nucleotides, and the effectiveness of their interference with the target enzyme(s) are additional parameters that undoubtedly affect their potency. Nevertheless, the encouraging results assembled so far render these agents worthy of fuller exploration, particularly with respect to their clinical potential.

References

1 Bobek, M (1979) 2′-Azido-2′-deoxy- and 2′-amino-2′-deoxy-β-D-arabinofuranosyl purine nucleosides. Carbohydr Res 70: 263–273

2 Bobek M, Bloch A, Berkowitz P, Bardos TJ (1977) Synthesis and antitumor activity of 1,2-dihydro-1-(2-deoxy-β-D-erythro-pentofuranosyl)-2-oxo-5-methylpyrazine 4-oxide, a structural analogue of thymidine. J Med Chem 20: 458–460
3 Bobek M, Cheng YC, Bloch A (1978) Novel arabinofuranosyl derivatives of cytosine resistant to enzymatic deamination and possessing potent antitumor activity. J Med Chem 21: 597
4 Bobek M, Martin V (1978) The synthesis of anomeric 3-*O*-acetyl-5-*O*-benzoyl-2-azido-2-deoxy-D-arabinofuranosyl chlorides. Versatile sugar intermediates for the synthesis of 2′-azido-2′-deoxy- and 2′-amino-2′-deoxy-β-D-arabinofuranosyl nucleosides. Tetrahedron Lett 22: 1919–1922
5 Cheng YC, Domin B, Lee LS (977) Human deoxycytidine kinase. Purification and characterization of the cytoplasmic and mitochondrial isozymes derived from blast cells of acute leukemia patients. Biochem Biophys Acta 481: 481–492
6 Cheng YC, Domin BA, Sharma RA, Bobek M (1976) Antiviral action and cellular toxicity of four thymidine analogues: 5-ethyl-, 5-vinyl-, 5-propyl-, and 5-allyl-2′-deoxyuridine. Antimicrob Agents Chemother 10: 119–122
7 Ho DHW, Carter CF, Loo TL (1975) Tetrahydrouridine in the uptake and metabolism of arabinosylcytosine by human acute myelocytic leukemia cells. Proc Am Assoc Cancer Res 16: 57
8 LePage GA, Worth LS, Kimball AP (1976) Enhancement of the antitumor activity of arabinofuranosyladenine by 2′-deoxycoformycin. Cancer Res 36: 1481–1485
9 Ranganathan R, Larwood D (1978) Facile conversion of adenosine into new 2′-substituted-2′-deoxy-arabinofuranosyladenine derivatives: Stereospecific synthesis of 2′-azido-2′-deoxy-, 2′-amino-2′-deoxy-, and 2′-mercapto-2′-deoxy-β-D-arabinofuranosyladenines. Tetrahedron Lett 45: 4341–4344
10 Robins MJ, Hawrelak SD (1978) Nucleic acid related compounds. 28. 2′-Amino-araA 9-(2-amino-2-deoxy-β-D-arabinofuranosyl)adenine. Synthesis via nucleoside-aziridine or azido intermediates and biological effects. Tetrahedron Lett 39: 3653–3656
11 Unger FM, Christian R, Waldstatten P (1979) Azido- und Diazido-Derivative von Arabinonukleosiden. Tetrahedron Lett 7: 605–608

Prediction of Clinical Response to 5-Fluorouracil-Containing Chemotherapy: Preliminary Results of in Vitro Assay in Human Breast Cancer

B. Ardalan, J. Macdonald, D. Cooney, M. Lippman, and P. Schein

Summary

An in vitro assay system measuring the production of phosphorylated nucleotide products of 5-FU by human tumor cytosols is described. Samples from 11 patients with breast cancer treated with 5-FU-containing chemotherapy regimens were assayed. Significant differences were seen in quantitative and qualitative patterns of phosphorylation between samples from chemotherapy responding and nonresponding patients. The rate of 5-fluorodeoxyuridylate production and the amount of nucleotide triphosphate produced were significantly $P < 0.05$ increased in chemotherapy-responding patients. This in vitro assay system is a simple, reproducible procedure that requires further evaluation as a potential system for prospectively predicting clinical response to fluorinated pyrimidines.

Introduction

The fluorinated pyrimidine 5-fluorouracil (5-FU), originally synthesized and studied by Heidelberger et al. [6] and Duschinsky and Pleven [3], potently inhibits the growth of a variety of tumor cells [5, 7]. However, in patients with disseminated cancer of the ovary, bowel, and breast, 5-FU is associated with objective partial response in only 20%–30% of cases [8]. Therefore, in vitro predictive assays that would serve to prospectively select patients possessing tumors likely to respond to 5-FU would be very useful. Such assays would result in the sparing of 70%–80% of patients' unnecessary potential toxicity from fluorinated pyrimidines and also in the selection of those patients most likely to benefit from this class of drugs.

Several metabolic steps must occur before fluorinated pyrimidines become active antineoplastic agents [4]. 5-Fluorouracil, for example, must be extensively anabolized first to its nucleoside and then to nucleotide derivatives before demonstrating antimetabolic and antineoplastic activity. The failure to perform these conversions would be expected to be associated with resistance to this drug. Because of the complicated activation of this agent, resistance can emerge in one or several steps in the process of anabolism of the agent to its active nucleotide.

We have recently reported on an assay system that predicted the response of murine tumors to fluorinated pyrimidines [1]. In this assay the ability of cell-free supernatants of tumors to produce phosphorylated products of 5-FU was shown to correlate with in vitro sensitivity of the tumors to 5-FU. In this assay the murine tumors sensitive or resistant to 5-FU in vivo demonstrated distinctly different in vitro 5-FU phosphorylation patterns. For example, when the pattern of phosphorylation in the 5-FU-sensitive tumor P388S was examined, it was seen that nucleotide mono-, di-, and triphosphates were formed. This was in contrast with the resistant tumor P388R, in which only monophosphates were detected. There was no significant difference in the concentration of the monophosphate peak in the sensitive or the resistant lines, whereas differences in the levels of di- and triphosphate peaks were statistically significant. It is of interest that 5-fluorodeoxyuridylate (FdUMP) generation was minimal in the murine tumors tested.

The present communication reports the application of our assay system to human breast cancer specimens. We have correlated the ability of extracts of human tumors to form phosphorylated products of 5-FU with clinical response to chemotherapy.

Materials and Methods

Patients

Eleven patients with metastatic or locally unresectable primary breast cancer were studied. Biopsy specimens were trimmed of excess fat and a portion was submitted for pathologic confirmation. Samples of tumor for 5-FU anabolism assays were frozen in liquid nitrogen. The ability of cell-free tumor extracts to produce phosphorylated products of 5-FU was assayed on prechemotherapy specimens of all patients. The patients were treated with 5-FU-containing combination chemotherapy regimens (cyclophosphamide, methotrexate, and 5-FU; or cyclophosphamide, adriamycin, and 5-FU).

In all patients, response was assessed as follows: complete response required the disappearance of all measurable disease, including healing of all lytic bone lesions, and a return of the patient to a premorbid performance status. Partial response required a shrinkage of 50% of all measurable disease. No new lesions could appear and no growth could be observed in a preexisting lesion for at least 2 months. Any patient not achieving this degree of improvement was described as a nonresponder. All patient records were assessed by investigators unaware of 5-FU in vitro assay results.

Assay System

The basis of our assay system was the incubation of a cytosol fraction of tumor homogenate with ^{14}C-labeled 5-FU. Tumor homogenates were prepared from 50 mg of tumor with a hand homogenizer in 0.01 *M* Tris buffer containing 0.15 m*M* EDTA and 0.5 m*M* dithiothreitol (pH 7.4). The homogenates were centrifuged at 12,000 *g* and the cytosol fraction removed for the assay. The incubation medium consisted of 10 μl of ^{14}C 5-fluorouracil (SA 9.1 mCi/mol), and 10 μl of a buffer mix containing 0.03 *M* of the following sugars: ribose-1-P (R-1-P), 2-deoxyribose-1-P (dR-1-P), and phosphoribosylpyrophosphate (PRPP). The reaction mixture also contained 0.03 *M* phosphoenolpyrophosphate, 10 units of pyruvate kinase and myokinase per 1 ml of buffer mix, and ATP at 10 m*M* (pH 8.0). The reaction was started with the addition of 10 μl of cytosol fraction. To assess differences in the ability of the cytosols to utilize individual sugars as substrates, experiments were performed in which each cytosol was incubated in the above assay system with a single sugar, i.e., R-1-P, dR-1-P, or PRPP.

The reaction mixture was incubated at 37° C for 30 min, since we had demonstrated that production of total phosphorylated products of 5-FU was linear over 30 min. The reaction was stopped by heating to 95° C for 2 min followed by centrifugation at 12,000 *g* for 1 min. The supernatants were then analyzed for phosphorylated products by the methods described below.

Total phosphorylation was assessed utilizing paper chromatography; 5-μl aliquots of the acidified supernatant of the reaction mixture were spotted in duplicate on Whatman 3M paper. Ascending chromatography was performed overnight in a solvent system consisting of isopropanol, toluene, 0.1 *M* EDTA, and concentrated NH_4OH, 320 : 40 : 44 : 4, v/v/v/v. The papers were air dried and the UV-absorbent spots were circled, cut, eluted with 200 μl of 0.1 HCl, and counted at 80% efficiency in a scintillation counter.

The mono-, di-, and triphosphates of 5-fluorouracil were analyzed by high-resolution ion-exchange chromatography. Reaction mixtures were scaled up 20 times, deproteinized, and centrifuged as previously described, and 1-ml aliquots of the clear supernatants were loaded on a 0.8 × 15 cm column of Hamilton HA- × 4 resin, thermoregulated at 37° C. Anions were then eluted at a flow rate of 0.67 ml/min with five stepwise buffers of lithium citrate at pH 2.65–2.72; 0.015 *M* buffer for 90 min, followed by 0.0375 *M*, 0.075 *M*, 0.15 *M*, and 0.225 *M* lithium citrate buffers at the same pH, applied for periods of 60 min each. Under these conditions, 5-FU and 5-fluoro-2-deoxyuridine (5-FUdR) were eluted with the void volumes at 8 min, 5-fluorouridylate (FUMP) and FdUMP at 96 min, the diphosphates FUDP and FdUDP at 245 min, and the triphosphates FUTP and FdUTP at 330 min. Fractions were collected and the peaks of interest were desalted on miniature ammoniac columns of acid-washed charcoal. Nucleotides were eluted from the column using 60% ethanol.

FdUMP generation was determined by using a modification of previously described assays [9] based on the inhibition of thymidylate synthetase by FdUMP. The major modification we made involves the microdistillation of the tritiated water resulting from methylation of 5-^3H-deoxyuridine monophosphate (5-^3H-dUMP). In analyzing the results of these assays, a low rate of anabolism of 5-FU by an individual breast tumor extract was arbitrarily defined as ≥ 1 but < 12 nmol of phosphorylated products of 5-FU/mg protein/h. A high rate of anabolism by a tumor cytosol was defined as ≥ 12 nmol of phosphorylated products of 5-FU/mg protein/h.

Results

Eight of 11 patients were documented to have partial objective responses to 5-FU-containing combination chemotherapy regimens. There were no significant differences in performance status and site of metastases between responding and nonresponding patients. The ability of cytosol fractions from the tumors of these patients to produce phosphorylated products of 5-FU was assayed.

Synthesis of FUdR, FUR, and FUMP

Pyrimidine nucleoside phosphorylases catalyze the reversible phosphorylytic conversion of pyrimidine nucleosides to ribose-1-phosphate (R-1-P) or deoxyribose-1-phosphate (dR-1-P) pyrimidine bases. Moreover, FUMP may be formed directly from 5-FU, via the enzyme phosphoribosyl transferase. To examine the activities of these enzymes in human breast cancer samples under study, [^{14}C] 5-FU was incubated with appropriate cellular extracts in the presence of saturating concentrations of R-1-P, dR-1-P, and PRPP as described previously. There was a significant difference ($P < 0.05$) between the responders and nonresponders in the in vitro conversion rates of 5-FU to FUR, but not to FUdR or FUMP (Table 1).

Table 1. Synthesis of FUdR, FUR, and FUMP from 5-FU and cytosols from human breast cancer in vitro[a]

Precursor	Product	Responders[b]	Nonresponders[b]
dR-1-P	5-FUdR	307.0 ± 121.2	275.2 ± 125.1
R-1-P	5-FUR	272.3 ± 98.2	81.5 ± 29.2
PRPP	5-FUMP	1.43 ± 0.59	1.67 ± 0.72

[a] Cytosol fraction of human breast cancer incubated with [2−^{14}C] 5-FU, and buffer mix containing dR-1-P, R-1-P, or PRPP

[b] Mean ± SD (nmol product formed/mg protein/h)

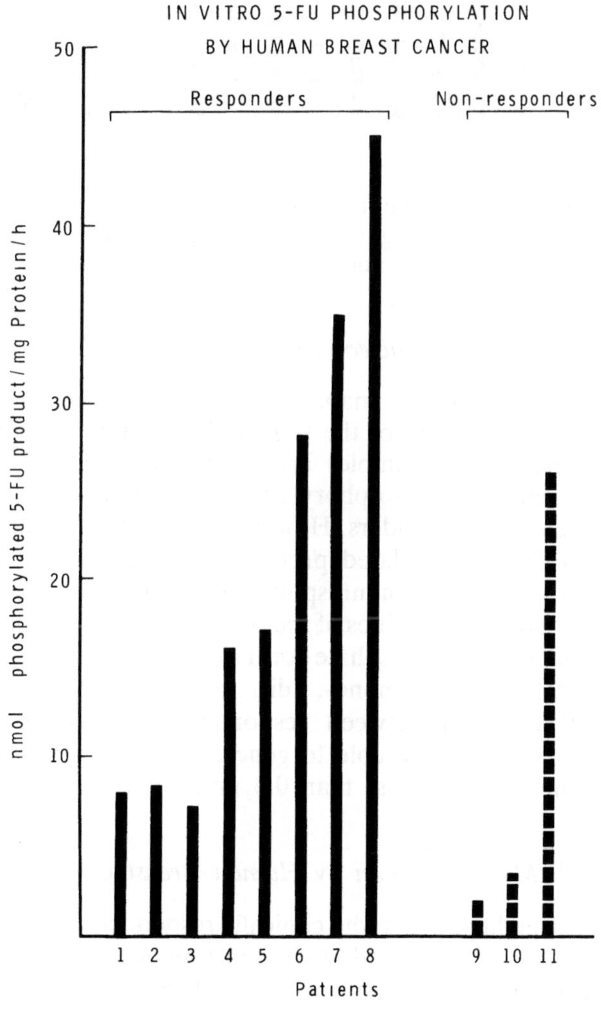

Fig. 1. Total production of phosphorylated nucleotide products of 5-FU by human breast cancer samples

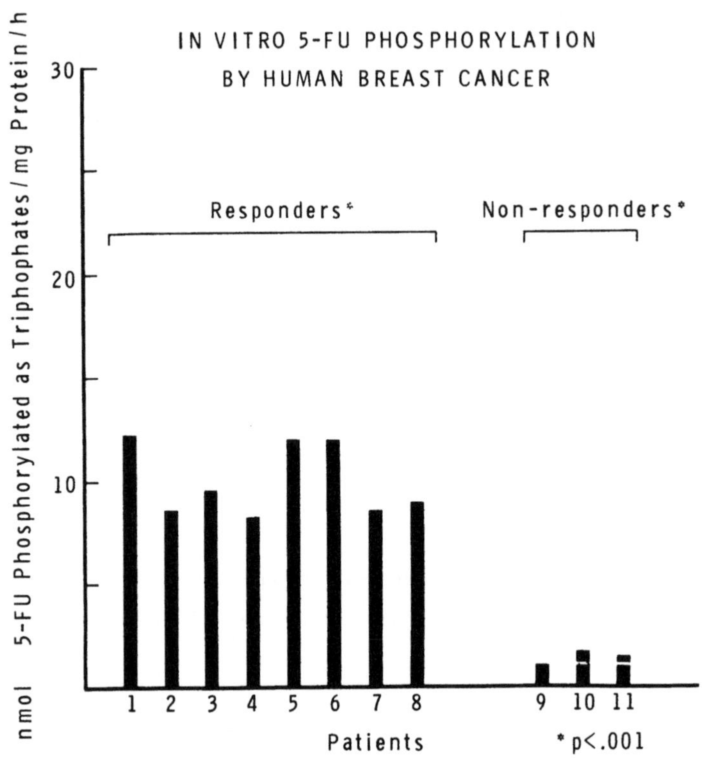

Fig. 2. Production of nucleotide triphosphates by human breast cancer samples. Samples from patients responding to chemotherapy produced significantly higher average amounts of triphosphates than nonresponding patients ($P < 0.001$)

Formation of Nucleotides from [2-^{14}C] 5-FU by Human Breast Cancer Cytosols

The subsequent anabolism of the riboside or deoxyriboside of 5-FU involves phosphorylation of the sugars. The results of total phosphorylation for the assayed breast cancer samples are illustrated in Fig. 1. Generally, in the nonresponding patients, total phosphorylation of 5-FU proceeded at a rate that was slower than that seen with responders. However, one nonresponder, patient 11, generated 25 nmol of 5-FU-phosphorylated products. The differences in total phosphorylation between responding and nonresponding patients were not statistically significant.

To examine activities of the several pyrimidine nucleotide kinases required for di- and trinucleotide phosphate formation, the total phosphorylated products of 5-FU were resolved into mono-, di-, and triphosphates. Highly significant differences ($P < 0.0001$) between responders and nonresponders were seen, since all the responders were able to generate over 8 nmol of FUTP/mg protein/h, and all the nonresponders less than 0.3 nmol of FUTP/mg protein/h (Fig. 2).

FdUMP Generation by Human Breast Cancer Cytosols

The eight patients who clinically responded all generated over 800 pmol of FdUMP/mg protein/h compared with nonresponders, who generated less than 200 pmol of FdUMP/mg protein/h (Fig. 3). This result was significantly different ($P < 0.05$).

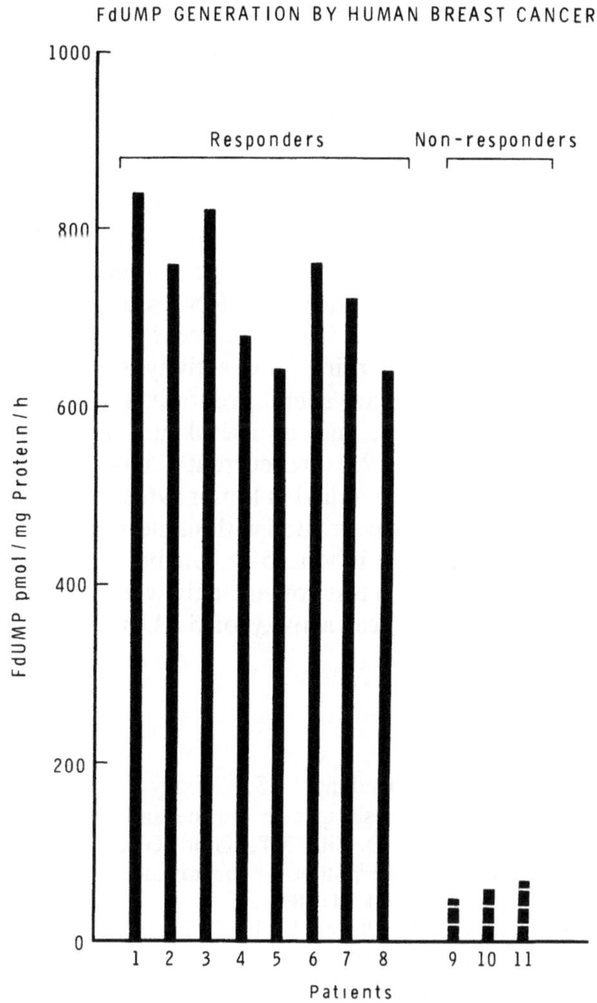

Fig. 3. FdUMP generation by human breast cancer samples. Samples from patients responding to chemotherapy had significantly ($P < 0.05$) increased FdUMP generation in comparison to samples from nonresponding patients

Discussion

It should be stressed that these results are preliminary and have been developed from patients who were treated with combination chemotherapy and not single-agent 5-FU. However, we felt that it was inappropriate to treat advanced breast cancer patients with single-agent 5-FU because of the documented superiority of combination chemotherapy in these patients [2].

These results are of value because they illustrate the applicability of our assay system to human tumor samples and also confirm that the differences in the ability of human tumors to anabolize 5-FU are analogous to those we have seen in the murine system [1]. It should be emphasized that significant differences are seen both in the amount of triphosphate nucleotides of 5-FU formed and in the rate of generation of the potent thymidylate synthetase inhibitor, FdUMP, between responding and nonresponding patients. These data tentatively suggest that resistance to 5-FU in human tumors may result from either the failure of the tumor to produce and sustain adequate amounts of FdUMP to result in inhibition of DNA synthesis or the failure of production of sufficient amounts of FUTP to interfere with RNA synthesis and function. Maximum cytotoxicity in some human tumors might result from a combination of the inhibition of DNA and RNA synthesis and function. This is supported by recently reported animal data suggesting the importance of 5-FU inhibition of RNA as a mechanism of cytotoxicity. SAWYER et al. [10] have shown in the CD8F1 murine mammary tumor model that greater than 90% inhibition of DNA synthesis only occurred at more than 24 h after 5-FU treatment. This finding correlated positively with the amount of fluorinated pyrimidine incorporated into RNA. The mechanism of DNA synthesis inhibition appeared to be secondary to decreased levels of thymidine kinase resulting from 5-FU interference with RNA translation and transcription.

It should be stressed that the current studies reported can only serve as the basis for suppositions concerning 5-FU activity in human tumors. However, the assay systems described, which are simple, reproducible, and can be performed on cryopreserved biopsy specimens, may be useful in helping to develop predictive assays of 5-FU activity in man. We are currently mounting a prospective study in which 5-FU anabolism will be studied in tumor cytosols from colon cancer patients. These patients will subsequently be treated with single-agent 5-FU and response to chemotherapy will be correlated with in vitro 5-FU anabolism studies. Through this type of approach, it will be possible to test convincingly whether our assay system represents a predictive assay of the clinical activity of 5-FU in man.

References

1 Ardalan B, Macdonald JS, Cooney D, Schein PS (1979) Studies on mechanisms of 5-fluorouracil resistance in murine and human tumors. Bull Cancer 66: 55–59

2 Canellos GP, DeVita VT, Gold GL, Chabner BA, Schein PS, Young RC (1976) Combination chemotherapy for advanced breast cancer: Response and effect on survival. Ann Intern Med 84: 389–392

3 Duschnisky R, Pleven E (1957) The synthesis of 5-fluoro-pyrimidines. J Am Chem Soc 79: 4559–4560

4 Friedman MA, Sadee W (1978) The fluoropyrimidines: Biochemical mechanisms and design of clinical trials. Cancer Chemother Pharmacol 1: 77–82

5 Heidelberger C (1965) Fluorinated pyrimidines. Prog Nucleic Acid Res Mol Biol 4: 1–50

6 Heidelberger C, Chaudhuri NK, Pleven E, Scheiner J (1957) Fluorinated pyrimidines, a new class of tumor-inhibiting compounds. Nature 179: 663–666

7 Heidelberger C, Greisbach L, Montag BJ, Mooren D, Cruz O, Schneizer RJ, Grunberg E (1958) Studies on fluorinated pyrimidines. II. Effects on transplanted tumors. Cancer Res 18: 305–317

8 Livingston RB, Carter SK (1970) Single agents in cancer chemotherapy. Plenum, New York

9 Roberts D (1966) An isotopic assay for thymidylate synthetase. Biochemistry 5: 3546–3548

10 Sawyer R, Nayak R, Spiegelman S, Martin D (1979) Mechanism of action of 5-fluorouracil (FU) in the chemotherapy of the murine mammary tumor. Proc Am Assoc Cancer Res and Am Soc Clin Oncol 20: 263

Vindesine: A New Vinca Alkaloid

M. Bayssas, J. Gouveia, F. de Vassal, J.-L. Misset, L. Schwarzenberg, P. Ribaud, M. Musset, C. Jasmin, M. Hayat, and G. Mathé

Summary

Vindesine (VDS) is an analogue of the vinca alkaloids. Its spectrum of antitumoral activity is similar to that of vincristine (VCR), but with milder experimental neurotoxicity, and it inhibits the polymerization of tubulin. Its terminal half-life is 24 h and its plasma clearance is intermediate between those of vinblastine (VLB) and VCR. The maximal tolerated dose is 4–5 mg/m^2/week, the dose-limiting toxicity being myelosuppression (nadir by days 7–8 and recovery by days 11–13). It has already been demonstrated as efficient in childhood acute lymphoid leukemia (ALL), non-Hodgkin's lymphoma, blastic crisis of chronic myeloid leukemia, and esophageal carcinoma. It has also shown activity in Hodgkin's disease, breast and germ cell carcinomas, and melanoma. Intolerance is mainly neurologic, with paresthesias, without motor impairment, or hematologic, with leukopenia, and sometimes alopecia, asthenia, and muscle pains. The results are better if the patients have not been treated previously; continuous infusion could be of interest and there appears to be no cross-resistance with its parent VCR, as documented in ALL.

Vindesine (VDS) or deacetyl vinblastine amide sulfate (DVAS) is an analogue of the vinca alkaloid family. The two other related drugs, vinblastine (VLB) and vincristine (VCR), differ in only one functional group, R_3 [1]. This minor distinction, however, is responsible for profound differences in the oncolytic spectrum, potency, and toxicity of the two compounds. VDS is a semisynthetic derivative of VLB from which it differs by one hydroxyl (R_2) and one carboxyamino group (R_1) on its side chain (Fig. 1).

In the *experimental studies* [1], VDS showed an activity spectrum which was broader than that of VLB in Ridgeway osteosarcoma, Gardner lymphosarcoma, and Ca755 mammary carcinoma, and which was similar to that of VCR. Moreover, the response of P388 leukemia was excellent. Comparative acute toxicity studies of intravenously (IV) administered VLB, VCR, and VDS indicated that VDS was relatively more toxic than VLB and less toxic than VCR. Concerning neurotoxicity with VDS treatment, there was no evidence of functional or structural changes in neural tissue; neurotoxic effects were commonly seen in animals given VCR at lower doses and for shorter test periods. It is concluded that VDS is less toxic in animals, on a mg/kg basis, than is VCR.

An experimental study on P388 leukemia was conducted in collaboration with Dr. Dantchev and M. Paintrand [12]. VDS was given intraperitoneally (IP) at a dosage of 3–5 mg/kg on day 1; mice were killed 10 h after treatment, and their ascites were

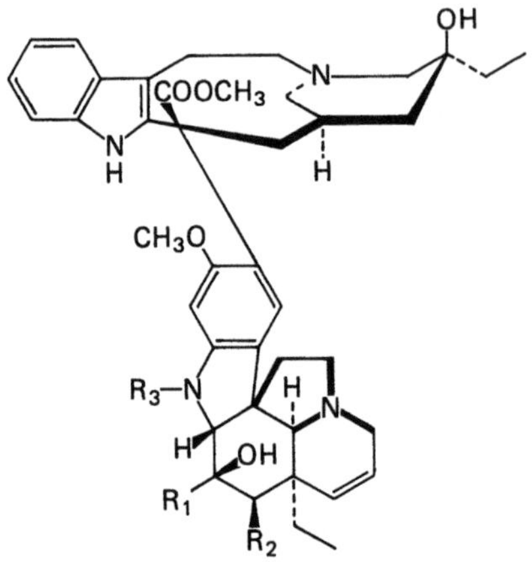

Vindesine (VDS)	*Vinblastine (VLB)*	*Vincristine (VCR)*
$R_1 = CONH_2$	$R_1 = COOCH_3$	$R_1 = COOCH_3$
$R_2 = OH$	$R_2 = OCOCH_3$	$R_2 = OCOCH_3$
$R_3 = CH_3$	$R_3 = CH_3$	$R_3 = CHO$

Fig. 1. General formula of the vinca alkaloids

washed with HBSS, without calcium or magnesium. From 20% to 50% of the P388 cells were blocked from their metaphases and seen in mitosis, compared with only 3% for the saline control: VDS was threefold more potent than VCR and tenfold more potent than VLB. Seen by electron microscopy, an untreated P388 cell contains many microtubules (MT) irradiating from the chromosomes to the centriolar complex; MT disappeared after treatment with VDS and mitosis was completely disorganized. Paracrystals appeared with a honeycomb-like structure and mixed inclusion bodies, consisting of MT strongly associated with ribosomes. The number of these paracrystals increased from VCR to VLB, VDS being intermediate between the two other compounds. In vitro, the three compounds blocked bovine tubulin polymerization and were almost equally effective at 1-μ*M* concentrations [9]. Thus, the differential actions of VLB, VCR, and VDS in vitro seem to be based on some biologic process other than the reaction with tubulin.

In the *pharmacokinetic studies,* a radio-immuno-assay with tritiated VLB was used. VDS was administered by rapid bolus injection, with blood and urine samples collected at specific times. The plasma decay was triphasic [6], which is compatible with a three-compartment open mammillary model (Fig. 2). Vindesine showed very high values for exit rate from the central compartment (11.66 and 9.36 h^{-1}), while the elimination rate constant was principally in the bile and quite low (0.550 h^{-1}), so the tissue distribution was primarily responsible for the rapid clearance from the plasma.

If the three vinca alkaloids are compared, after giving 2 mg of the drug to a 70-kg patient, the terminal or elimination half-lives at approximately 24 h are nearly identical for VDS and VLB and quite different from that of VCR, which lasted more than 6 days: the clearance of VDS is between those of VLB and VCR, the latter having the lowest clearance with the highest serum levels. These data suggest that differences in toxicities of the vinca alkaloids may have a pharmacokinetic basis. The definite differences in the human pharmacokinetics of VDS, VLB, and VCR appear to

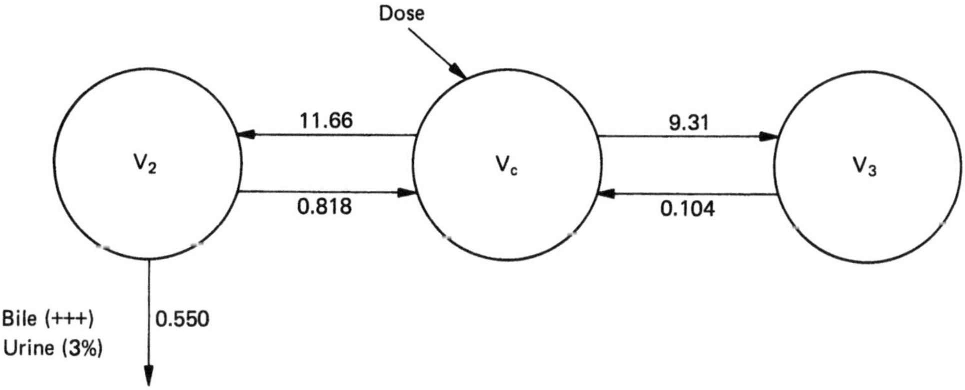

Fig. 2. Vindesine: pharmacokinetics (from [6]); *numbers* indicate constants-units are $hours^{-1}$. V_c = volume of the central compartment; V_2 = volume of the superficial tissue comparment; V_3 = volume of the deep tissue compartment

correlate well both with acute LD_{50} doses and with clinically tolerated doses (Table 1).

VDS was submitted to *clinical studies*. The phase I studies [5] showed that the maximal tolerated dose was 3–4 mg/m²/week for adults and 4–5 mg/m²/week for children. Doses administered on 5 separate days were much more toxic than those given 1 day weekly. The limiting toxicity was myelosuppression with leukoneutropenia; the nadir was reached by days 7–8 and recovery occurred by days 11–13.

Phase II trials were conducted in *leukemia and hematosarcoma;* the dosage used was 4 mg/m²/week. The complete plus partial response rate reported from several investigations [7] was 40% of 95 cases, compared with 53% in our series; in the same series, VDS in Hodgkin's disease showed a 35% response rate [7] in patients who were resistant to MOPP and ABVD, and about 40% in non-Hodgkin's lymphoma. In our studies at Villejuif [2], we used 2 mg/m²/day on 2 consecutive days weekly, by IV push, continuous infusion, or both, successively. The response rate for 19 acute lymphoid leukemias (Table 2) was 63%, which is higher than the range reported in the literature and could be based on pharmacokinetics. There was no response in acute myeloid leukemia; chronic myeloid leukemia blastic crisis was extremely sensitive to VDS and the response rate was 55%. Moreover, the immunoblastic type of leukemia or lymphosarcoma showed a good response. All patients had advanced malignancies and were heavily pretreated.

Continuous infusion for 48 h improved the results after failure of the IV push technique: in our experience [2], 6 of 12 patients entered a complete or partial remission with infusion.

In *solid tumors,* 3 mg/m² VDS used weekly was active against several malignancies (Table 3): (a) Lung carcinoma, in which a 25% response rate (13 patients) was described [8] in non-small cell lung carcinoma (NSCC) [partial responses in adenocarcinoma: 20% (6 patients); epidermoid carcinoma: 21% (3 patients); large cell of undifferentiated carcinoma: (one out of three patients)] and in small cell carcinoma (SCC), the median response duration (MRD) being 5 months. (b) Breast carcinoma: the responses varied from 18% [7] to 29% [15]; in the latter series, 6/11 responder patients (out of 23 in the trial) were not previously treated, and 5 (24 %) were only mild responses; MRD was of 3.5 months. (c) Melanoma: 14% [7] to 17% [13] of the

Table 1. Correlation among pharmacokinetics, experimental data, and clinical dosage[a]

Parameters	VCR	VDS	VLB
Plasma clearance (l/kg/h)	0.053	0.252	0.865
Mean dosage for a 70-kg man (mg)	2.0	7.0	12.0
LD_{50} in mouse (mg/kg)	2.1	6.3	10.0

[a] From Dyke et al. [7]

Table 2. Responses in leukemias and hematosarcomas

Diagnosis	Ref.	Number of patients	CR[b]	CR + PR[c]	Overall[d]
ALL	2	19	7 (37%)	12 (63%)	14 (73%)
CML blastic crisis	2	11	5 (45%)	6 (55%)	
Lymphosarcoma[a]	2	15	0	6 (40%)	8 (53%)
Leukemic		8	0	3 (38%)	3 (38%)
Immunoblastic		3	0	1	2
Prolymphocytic		4	0	2	3
Hodgkin's disease	6	20	1 (5%)	7 (35%)	

[a] According to the WHO classification
[b] CR, complete regression
[c] PR, partial regression or more than 50% decrease in tumor cells
[d] Overall, responses of more than 25% decrease in tumor cells

Table 3. Vindesine: Responses in advanced solid tumors

Diagnosis	Ref.	Number of patients	CR[a]	CR + PR[b]	Overall[c]
Lung	8	53	2 (4%)	13 (25%)	22
SCC		7	2	3	5
NSCC		46	0	10 (22%)	17 (37%)
Breast	7	44	(7%)	(18%)	–
	15	21	2 (10%)	6 (29%)	13 (62%)
Melanoma	7	74	(3%)	(14%)	–
	13	21	1 (5%)	3 (14%)	2 (23%)
	15	12	0	2 (17%)	–
Esophageal	10	22	1 (4%)	3 (13%)	8
	3	9	0	1	3
Germ cell	14	19	0	3 (16%)	–

[a] CR, complete regression of tumor mass
[b] PR, partial regression or more than 50% of the tumor size, without progression elsewhere
[c] Overall, regression of more than 25% of the tumor mass, without progression elsewhere

Table 4. Vindesine: Tolerance

Type	Manifestations	%
Hematologic		
Leukopenia	< $3000/mm^3$	50
	< $2000/mm^3$	20
Thrombocytopenia		5
Neurologic		
Paresthesias		40–60
Hyporeflexia		100
Muscle weakness		24
Constipation		15
Muscle pains		2–14
Loss of taste		2–15
Paralytic ileus		7
Others		
Alopecia		60
Nausea – vomiting		13
Diarrhea		8
Fever		10–60
Fatigue		12
Cutaneous rash		5
Phlebitis		15
Cellulitis		6

evaluable patients responded to treatment with VDS, with an MRD of 4 months. (d) Esophageal squamous carcinoma: there were 3 responses (13%) in one series [10] and one response in 9 patients in another [3], which is interesting for that type of tumor. (e) Germ cell carcinoma: VDS used in 5-day treatment induced a 16% response rate [14]. There was no response in renal carcinoma or in myeloma. VDS could be efficient in teratoma, histiocytosis, and Wilms' tumor.

VDS has been used in *phase III studies* [4], in combination with cisplatin (CDDP), high dose (100 mg/m^2/3 weeks) or low dose (60 mg/m^2/week). In non-small cell lung carcinoma, the responses (45%) between the two regimens were not significantly different, but the MRD was longer with high-dose CDDP; it was 9 months long, compared with 5 months in the low-dose CDDP group.

The response rate was higher when vindesine was used as first-line treatment in poorly responsive malignancies such as non-small cell carcinoma, in which it was 33% in previously untreated patients, compared with 22% overall [8].

Intolerance was mainly hematologic and neurologic (Table 4). The dose-limiting toxicity was leukopenia and, to a lesser degree, general intolerance and fatigue. Hematologic aspects included leukoneutropenia, which was generally mild: 50% under 3,000/mm^3, being less than 2,000/mm^3 in 17%–20%, with the nadir by day 7 and recovery by days 11–12; thrombocytopenia was rare (2%–5%), but thrombocytosis with increase of more than 50,000–100,000/mm^3 occurred in 20%–27% of the patients. Neurotoxic side effects were found in about 40%–60% of the patients, with loss of reflexes occurring at a dosage of 4 mg/m^2; at the median dosage of 19 mg/m^2, generally mild paresthesia occurred, but it was not progressive with treatment and it

Table 5. Vindesine: Apparent absence of cross-resistance with vincristine

Diagnosis	Number of resistant patients	Complete response + Partial response	
ALL	13	4	2
CML blastic crisis	4	1	2
Leukemic lymphosarcoma	5	1	2
Total	22	6	6 = 12/22 (55%)

was rapidly reversible when VDS was stopped. Constipation (15%), jaw pain (2%–7%), muscle pain (2%–14%), and taste loss (2%–5%) were the other signs; paralytic ileus was found in 7% of the cases, retroceding briefly under supportive care. There were no severe motor problems, but motor weakness mostly without impaired function. The electromyographic studies showed no important changes. Alopecia, fever, nausea and vomiting, and superficial phlebitis also occurred. Some diarrhea, cellulitis and cutaneous rash were described.

One of the most important characteristics of VDS is the *apparent absence of cross-resistance with VCR*. Resistance was defined as no improvement in the bone marrow (with the same cellularity) [6] after three cycles of VCR at a dosage of 1.4 mg/m^2, combined with prednisone and asparaginase; we showed [2] that about 50% of the patients entered remission after VCR failure, in acute lymphoid leukemia (which was also found by Dr. Krivit [11]), blastic crisis of chronic myeloid leukemia, and leukemic lymphosarcoma (Table 5).

VDS is a new vinca alkaloid of interest; it was investigated as an analogue, and was introduced into clinical studies after experimental demonstration of its broader spectrum of activity and its milder neurotoxicity. It is active in acute lymphoid leukemia, lymphosarcoma, lung carcinoma, breast carcinoma, melanoma, and esophageal carcinoma and has already been included in phase III trials. The neurologic side effects are tolerable and seem mild, with characteristics which differ from VCR.

New modalities of administration, such as continuous infusion, remain to be studied, and there might be no crossresistance with VCR.

References

1 Barnett CJ, Cullinan GJ, Gerzon K, Hoying, RC, Jones WE, Newlon WM, Poore GA, Robinson RL, Sweeney MJ, Todd GC, Dyke RW, Nelson RL (1978) Structure-activity relationship of dimeric Catharanthus alkaloids. I. Desacetylvinblastine amide (vindesine) sulfate. J Med Chem 21: 88–96

2 Bayssas M, Gouveia J, Ribaud P, Musset M, De Vassal F, Pico JL, De Luca L, Misset JL, Machover D, Belpomme D, Schwarzenberg L, Jasmin C, Hayat M, Mathé G (1979) Phase-II trial with vindesine for regression induction in patients with leukemias and hematosarcomas. Cancer Chemother Pharmacol 2: 247–255

3 Bedikian AY, Valdivieso M, Bodey GP, Freireich EJ (1979) Phase II evaluation of vindesine in the treatment of colorectal and esophageal tumors. Cancer Chemother Pharmacol 2: 263–266

4 Casper ES, Gralla RJ, Golbey RB (1979) Vindesine (DVA) and cis-dichloro diammine platinum II (DDP) combination chemotherapy in non-small cell lung cancer (abstr C-190). Proc Am Soc Clin Oncol 20: 337
5 Currie VE, Wong P, Krakoff IH, Young CW (1978) Phase I trial of vindesine in patients with advanced cancer. Cancer Treat Rep 62: 1333–1336
6 Dyke RW, Nelson RL (1977) Phase I anti-cancer agents. Vindesine (desacetyl vinblastine amide sulfate). Cancer Treat Rev 4: 135–142
7 Dyke RW, Nelson RL, Brade WP (1979) Vindesine. A short review of preclinical and first clinical data. Cancer Chemother Pharmacol 2: 229–232
8 Gralla RJ, Tan CTC, Young CW (1979) Vindesine. A review of phase-II trials. Cancer Chemother Pharmacol 2: 271–274
9 Himes RH, Kersey RN, Heller-Bettinger I, Samson FE (1976) Action of the vinca alkaloids vincristine, vinblastine, and desacetyl vinblastine amide in microtubules in vitro. Cancer Res 36: 3798–3802
10 Kelsen DP, Bains M, Golbey R, Woodcock T (1979) Vindesine in the treatment of esophageal carcinoma (abstr C-193). Proc Am Soc Clin Oncol 20: 338
11 Krivit W, Chilcote R, Pyesmany A, Anderson J, Hammond D (1979) An initial report of a phase-III trial comparing vindesine and vincristine for acute lymphocytic leukemia of childhood. Cancer Chemother Pharmacol 2: 267–270
12 Paintrand MR, Dantchev D, Bayssas M, Bourut C, Reiss F, Hayat M, Mathé G (to be published) Comparative actions of vindesine, vinblastine and vincristine in an electron microscopical study in mice, using P388 leukemic cells. Europ J Cancer
13 Retsas S, Newton KA, Westbury G (1979) Vindesine as a single agent in the treatment of advanced malignant melanoma. Cancer Chemother Pharmacol 2: 257–260
14 Reynolds TF, Cvitkovic E, Golbey RB, Young CW (1979) Trial of vindesine (DVA) in patients with germ cell tumors (abstr C-196). Proc Am Soc Clin Oncol 20: 338
15 Smith IE, Hedley DW, Powles TJ, McElwain TJ (1978) Vindesine: A phase II study in the treatment of breast carcinoma, malignant melanoma, and other tumors. Cancer Treat Rep 62: 1427–1433

The Epipodophyllotoxin Derivatives VM-26 and VP-16-213, 1976–1979, a Review

N. I. Nissen, P. Dombernowsky, H. H. Hansen, and A. G. Pedersen

Summary

The epipodophyllotoxin derivatives VM 26 and VP 16-213 are currently entering phase III studies. The mechanism of their action is incompletely understood, but the greatest lethal effect is experienced in the late S and G_2 phases. In transplanted tumors both drugs have shown marked schedule dependency and human studies also support this.

As a single agent VP 16-213 is among the most active drugs in small-cell carcinoma of the lung. Significant clinical activity (> 20% response frequency) has been observed for both drugs in Hodgkin's disease, non-Hodgkin lymphomas and possibly in other more rare tumors (monocytic leukemia, hepatoma and teratoma).

Although further clinical studies of both drugs would be ideal, it seems possible at present to justify a discontinuation of VM-26 in order to concentrate the efforts on VP 16-213. Further studies are needed to define optimal dose and schedule and place in combination chemotherapy.

Introduction

The antineoplastic epipodophyllotoxin derivatives VM-26 and VP-16-213 have now been in clinical use for 7–8 years and, although many aspects have not yet been sufficiently examined, a picture of their place in cancer chemotherapy is slowly emerging. Rozencweig et al. [35] thoroughly summarized the literature up to 1976. The present review therefore focuses on some of the more recent findings.

Mechanism of Action and Pharmacology

In 1976, a summary of the available information indicated that VM-26 and VP-16-213, in contrast to podophyllotoxin, had no effect on microtubules and, although metaphase arrest occurred, this effect was minor compared with the premitotic block which prevented cells from entering the mitotic phase [35].

The site of the block has now been further defined. In human lymphoma cells in vitro, the two drugs delayed the passage of cells through late S and through the G_2 phase, and it was shown with synchronized cells that this was also the site for the main lethal action of the drugs [15].

The same conclusion was reached with mastocytoma cells in vitro [21], and it was pointed out that this mechanism was unique when compared with other cytostatic agents, but quite similar to the effect of ionizing radiation.
The mechanism of the blocking effect is still obscure. A demonstrated inhibition of nucleoside transport [27] is one possibility.
Cellular uptake of the two drugs occurs in L1210 cells by a membrane-controlled passive diffusion [2, 3]; 20% of the drug is irreversibly retained in the cell. At steady state, the intracellular concentration of VM-26 is ten times higher than that of VP-16-213, a fact which in part explains the difference in equitoxic doses of the two drugs in whole organisms [3].
Another explanation for the difference are the plasma and renal clearances, which, as previously summarized [35], are three and six times greater, respectively, for VP-16-213 than for VM-26. At the same time, VP-16-213 has a much lower affinity to human albumin than VM-26.

Mode of Administration and Schedules

In the first trials, both VM-26 and VP-16-213 were administered only intravenously (IV) by infusion for 30 min. As summarized by Rozencweig et al. [35], lipophilic capsules of VP-16-213 for oral use were abandoned due to erratic absorption and, in addition to the IV preparation, two forms of oral (PO) preparation of VP-16-213 are now available: drink ampules and new gelatin capsules, both of which are well tolerated and absorbed [8, 26, 29].
While several studies have demonstrated the schedule dependency of the antineoplastic activity in transplanted tumors [35], only one study has examined this question prospectively in humans. Cavalli et al. [9] randomized patients with small cell carcinoma of the lung to treatment with VP-16-213 once weekly IV, or on days 1, 3, and 5 every week PO, *or* on days 1–5 every 3 weeks PO. Response frequency was significantly inferior with the weekly IV dose (20%) compared with the other two schedules (65% and 42%, respectively).
Comparison of other published reports with respect to the relation between schedules and obtained results is difficult, as both IV and PO administrations are used, and as both patients with and without prior treatment are included, but there is a trend that weekly or twice weekly treatment is less effective than treatment 3–5 days per week with or without treatment-free weeks between the courses.

Antitumor Effect

Except for the possible fallacies in interpreting reports where methods of selection of patients and response criteria differ, where previous treatment can vary from none to ten drugs, where treatment schedules vary, and where some double reporting of patients has occurred, the antineoplastic effect of the two drugs in the best-investigated and most-sensitive disease categories is shown in Tables 1–3.
In *carcinoma of the lung*, the *small cell type* is very sensitive to VP-16-213 with an overall response frequency of 41%. Table 1 demonstrates the wide variation in results in different studies. The table includes the previously mentioned prospective study [9], and it is seen that also in other studies the weekly or twice weekly schedule produced

Table 1. VP-16-213 and VM-26 in carcinoma of the lung

Study	Administration (IV/PO)	Schedule	Dose (mg/m^2)	Number of patients	Number with PR or CR	% Response
VP-16-213 in small cell carcinoma						
Cohen et al. [13]	IV	once/week	300	16	4	25
Cavalli et al. [9]	IV	once/week	250	20	4	20
Nissen et al. [32]	IV	twice/week	60–135	20	2	10
Jungi and Senn [25]	IV	days 1–5	60	11	5	46
Eagan et al. [16]	IV	days 1, 3, 5	125–140	13	7	54
Tucker et al. [43]	IV	days 1–5	60	47	24	51
Falkson et al. [20]	PO	days 1–5	100–200	10	2	20
Hansen et al. [22]	PO	days 1–4 (5)	200	40	20	50
Cavalli et al. [9]	PO	days 1–5	170	19	8	42
Cavalli et al. [9]	PO	days 1, 3, 5	170	17	11	65
Total				213	87	41
VM-26 in small cell carcinoma						
Samson et al. [36]	IV	days 1–5	20–30	11	0	0
VP-16-213 in other cell types						
Eagan et al. [17]	IV	days 1, 3, 5	140	44	8	18
Nissen et al. [32]	IV	twice/week	60–135	60	2	3
Falkson et al. [20]	PO	days 1–5	100–200	9	1	11
Total				113	11	10
VM-26 in other cell types						
Bhuchar et al. [6]	IV	days 1–5	40	12	0	0
Samson et al. [36]	IV	days 1–5	20–30	44	1	2
Total				56	1	2

results inferior to those obtained in series, in which the treatment was administered 3–5 days per week. The only exception is the study by Falkson et al. [20], in which the poorly absorbable lipophilic capsule [8, 30] was used.

In other *histologic cell types* of *bronchogenic carcinoma*, VM-26 led to remission in only one (2%) of 56 patients and VP-16-213 induced remission in 11 (10%) of 113.

Table 2. VP-16-213 and VM-26 in Hodgkin's disease

Study	Administration (IV/PO)	Schedule	Dose (mg/m^2)	Number of patients	Number with PR or CR	% Response
VP-16-213						
Nissen et al. [31]	IV	days 1–7	22–34	2	1	50
Nissen et al. [31]	IV	twice/week	18–30	3	2	67
EORTC [19]	IV or PO	days 1–5	50	15	2	13
		days 1–5	100			
Falkson et al. [20]	PO	days 1–5	100–200	2	0	0
Cecil et al. [10]	IV	days 1–5	35–45	17	3	18
Nissen et al. [32]	IV	twice/week	60–135	7	2	22
Total				46	10	22
VM-26						
Trempe et al. [42]	IV	days 1–3 (10)	30–60	4	2	50
Dombernowsky et al. [14]	IV	twice/week	30–90	8	3	38
EORTC [18]	IV	days 1–10 (20)	30	22	6	27
Sonntag et al. [40]	IV	twice/week	50	10	3	30
Sonntag et al. [40]	IV	days 1, 3, 5	40	6	4	67
Chiuten et al. [12]	IV	once/week	100	9	2	22
Total				59	20	34

In *Hodgkin's disease* (Table 2), the reported series are very small and many are phase I type studies with examination of several dose levels. When the studies were combined, VM-26 led to complete remission (CR) or partial remission (PR) in 34% of the patients, while VP-16-213 induced remission in 22%. The nature of the many small studies makes it difficult to conclude whether there is a real difference in the activity of

Table 3. VP-16-213 and VM-26 in non-Hodgkin's lymphoma

Study	Administration (IV/PO)	Schedule	Dose (mg/m^2)	Number of patients	Number with PR or CR	% Response
VP-16-213						
Nissen et al. [31]	IV	days 1–7	22–34	11	3	27
EORTC [19]	IV or PO	days 1–5	50 100	29	6	21
Jacobs et al. [24]	IV	days 1–5	60	27	17	63
Falkson et al. [20]	PO	days 1–5	100–200	7	2	29
Cecil et al. [10]	IV	days 1–5	35–45	35	0	0
Bender et al. [5]	IV	days 1–5	60	19	8	42
Jacobs et al. [23]	IV	days 1–5	60	34	27	79
Nissen et al. [32]	IV	twice/week	60–135	24	6	25
Total				186	69	37
VM-26						
Trempe et al. [42]	IV	days 1–3 (10)	30–60	2	0	0
Dombernowsky et al. [14]	IV	twice/week	30–90	2	0	0
EORTC [18]	IV	days 1–10 (20)	30	44	19	43
Sonntag et al. [40]	IV	twice/week	50	7	2	14
Chiuten et al. [12]	IV	once/week	100	25	6	24
Total				80	27	34

the two drugs in this disease. It is also impossible to make conclusions as to optimal schedule.

In *non-Hodgkin's lymphomas* (Table 3), the reported series are somewhat larger, but the disease group is more heterogeneous and many of the older studies did not use the present histologic classifications. The combined results show equal activity of the two drugs, 34% CR + PR for VM-26 and 37% for VP-16-213, but a prospective direct comparison within one study has not been made. When only the larger VP-16-213 series are considered, there is a trend that treatment 5 days per week is superior to twice weekly administrations. VP-16-213 was active both in diffuse histiocytic and diffuse poorly differentiated lymphocytic lymphomas [5, 23, 24], while definite data for VM-26 in this respect are lacking.

An extensive review of all other tumor areas is not possible within the allotted space, but a few conclusions can be drawn when the older literature summarized by Rozencweig et al. [35] is supplemented with review of more recent data.

In previously treated *acute nonlymphocytic leukemia*, both drugs show moderate activity. The response figures in the previous review, one of seven patients for VM-26 and 11 of 30 for VP-16-213, can be supplemented by the totals from three more recent series: one of 14 for VM-26 and 18 of 113 for VP-16-213 [7, 11, 39]. As previously pointed out by Mathé et al. [28], the myelomonocytic type of leukemia seems more responsive to VP-16-213 than the myeloblastic type.

Acute lymphocytic leukemia refractory to standard treatment shows also very moderate sensitivity to the podophyllotoxin derivatives: four of 28 responses with VM-26 and two of 19 with VP-16-213 [7, 11, 34].

Among the childhood tumors, responses have been seen in recent studies of *neuroblastoma*: 13 of 44 with VM-26, three of 11 with VP-16-213 [7, 32 33]; *Wilms' tumor*: one of six with VM-26, two of six with VP-16-213 [7]; *rhabdomyosarcoma*: none of six with VM-26, three of 11 with VP-16-213 [7, 32].

In *colorectal cancer*, VM-26 led to response in two of 14 [37], and VP-16-213 induced remissions in five of 81 patients [32].

In *brain tumors*, the early promising results [35] have not been confirmed: none of 20 patients responded to treatment with VM-26 [7, 41], and VP-16-213 has not been sufficiently studied.

Previously reported [35] negative results have also been obtained in recent studies of *breast cancer*: one of 17 with VM-26 [37] and one of 24 with VP-16-213 [32]; *melanoma*: none of 21 with VM-26 [4], none of 48 with VP-16-213 [1, 10]; *ovarian carcinoma*: one of 19 with VM-26 [36, 37], three of 42 with VP-16-213 [32, 38]; and *bladder carcinoma*: none of 13 with VP-16-213 [32].

Discussion

The antineoplastic spectra of VM-26 and VP-16-213 are almost identical. In a comparative study of the drugs in 260 children with neoplasms refractory to standard treatment, the CR + PR frequency was 18% for both drugs. VM-26 appeared more active than VP-16-213 in ALL (four of 15 versus one of 11) and neuroblastoma (ten of 31 versus one of five), while the opposite was true for ANLL (one of 14 versus nine of 50) [7]. However, the small numbers hardly justify a definite conclusion.

When Tables 1–3 are considered, the only difference in antineoplastic activity of the two drugs appears to be in small cell carcinoma of the lung, where VP-16-213 is highly active, while the study with VM-26 was negative. The difference in response rate in Hodgkin's disease is based upon addition of several small series, and it can hardly be taken as an expression of a difference in antitumor activity.

Although further comparative studies of the two drugs would be ideal, it seems almost possible at present to justify a discontinuation of VM-26 in order to concentrate efforts

on further studies of VP-16-213. Especially, the place of the drug in clinical combination chemotherapy needs to be further defined.
The question of which schedule to recommend has been partly answered for small cell carcinomas and lymphomas, but very limited information is available for other tumors.

Conclusion

The epipodophyllotoxins have significant clinical activity (> 20% response frequency) in small cell carcinoma of the lung (only VP-16-213), Hodgkin's disease, non-Hodgkin's lymphomas, childhood tumors, and possibly in other more rare tumors (monocytic leukemia, hepatoma, teratoma), and further studies are needed to define optimal dose and schedule, and optimal place in combination chemotherapy.
In other disease areas, the remission frequency is at the 10% level or below, and unless more positive results appear from current studies, continued research is hardly justified.

References

1 Ahmann DL, Bisel HF, Edmonson JH, Hahn RG, O'Connell MJ, Frytak S (1976) Phase II study of VP 16-213 versus dihydrogalactitol in patients with metastatic malignant melanoma. Cancer Treat Rep 60: 1681–1682
2 Allen LM, Shirley M (1977) Mechanism of cellular transport of two epipodophyllotoxin glucopyranoside derivatives, VM 26 and VP 16. Proc Am Assoc Cancer Res 18: 22
3 Allen, LM (1978) Cellular pharmacokinetics of two epipodophyllotoxin glucopyranoside derivatives, VM 26 and VP 16: Uptake in the presence and absence of human serum albumin. Proc Am Assoc Cancer Res 19: 125
4 Bellet RE, Catalano RB, Mastrangelo MJ, Berd D, Koons LS (1978) Phase II trial of VM 26 in patients with metastatic malignant melanoma. Cancer Treat Rep 62: 445–447
5 Bender RA, Anderson T, Fisher RI, Yong RC (1978) Activity of the epipodophyllotoxin VP-16 in the treatment of combination chemotherapy-resistant non-Hodgkin lymphoma. Am J Hematol 5: 203–209
6 Bhuchar VK, Boyle LE, Lanzotti VJ (1978) VM 26 in non-oat cell bronchogenic carcinoma. Proc Am Soc Clin Oncol 19: 407
7 Bleyer WA, Chard RL, Kriwit W, Hammond D (1978) Epipodophyllotoksin therapy of childhood neoplasia: A comparative phase 2 analysis of VM 26 and VP 16-213. Proc Am Soc Clin Oncol 19: 373
8 Brunner KW, Sonntag RW, Ryssel HJ, Cavalli F (1976) Comparison of the biologic activity of VP 16-213 given iv and orally in capsules or drink ampules. Cancer Treat Rep 60: 1377–1379
9 Cavalli F, Sonntag RW, Jungi F, Senn HJ, Brunner KW (1978) VP 16-213 monotherapy for remission induction of small cell lung cancer: A randomized trial using three dosage schedules. Cancer Treat Rep 62: 473–475
10 Cecil JW, Quagliana JM, Coltman CA, Al-Sarraf M, Thigpen T, Groppe CW (1978) Evaluation of VP 16-213 in malignant lymphoma and melanoma. Cancer Treat Rep 62: 801–803
11 Chard RL, Hammond D (1977) 4′-Demethylepipodophyllotoxin-β-D-ethylidene glucoside (VP 16–213) phase II study for refractory acute leukemias of childhood. Proc Am Soc Clin Oncol 18: 354

12 Chiuten DF, Bennett JM, Creech RH, Glick J, Falkson G, Brodovsky HS, Begg CB, Muggia FM, Carbone PP (1979) VM 26, a new anticancer drug with effectiveness in malignant lymphoma: An Eastern Cooperative Oncology Group study. Cancer Treat Rep 63:7–11

13 Cohen MH, Broder LE, Fossieck BE, Ihde DC, Minna JD (1977) Phase II clinical trial of weekly administration of VP 16-213 in small cell bronchogenic carcinoma. Cancer Treat Rep 61:489–490

14 Dombernowsky P, Nissen NI, Larsen V (1972) Clinical investigation of a new podophyllin derivative, VM 26, in patients with malignant lymphomas and solid tumors. Cancer Chemother Rep 56:71–82

15 Drewinko B, Barlogie B (1976) Survival and cycle-progression delay of human lymphoma cells in vitro exposed to VP 16-213. Cancer Treat Rep 60:1295–1306

16 Eagan RT, Carr DT, Frytak S, Rubin J, Lee RE (1976) VP 16-213 versus polychemotherapy in patients with advanced small cell lung cancer. Cancer Treat Rep 60:949–951

17 Eagan RT, Ingle JN, Creagan ET, Frytak S, Kvols LK, Rubin J, McMahon RT (1978) VP 16-213 chemotherapy for advanced squamous cell carcinoma and adenocarcinoma of the lung. Cancer Treat Rep 62:843–844

18 European Organization for Research on the Treatment of Cancer, Cooperative Group for Leukaemias and Haematosarcomas (1972) Clinical screening of epipodophyllotoxin VM 26 in malignant lymphomas and solid tumors. Br Med J 2:744–748

19 European Organization for Research on the Treatment of Cancer, Clinical Screening Group (1973) Epipodophyllotoxin VP 16-213 in treatment of acute leukaemias, haematosarcomas and solid tumors. Br Med J 3:199–202

20 Falkson G, Dyk JJ van, Eden EB van, Merwe AM van de, Berg JA van den, Falkson HC (1975) A clinical trial of the oral form of 4′demethyl-epipodophyllotoxin-β-D-ethylidene glucoside, VP 16-213. Cancer 35:1141–1144

21 Grieder A, Maurer R, Stähelin H (1977) Comparative study of early effects of epipodophyllotoxin derivatives and other cytostatic agents on mastocytoma cultures. Cancer Res 37:2998–3005

22 Hansen M, Hirsch F, Dombernowsky P, Hansen HH (1977) Treatment of small cell anaplastic carcinoma of the lung with the oral solution of VP 16-213 (NSC 141540, 4′-demethylepipodophyllotoxin 9-(4,6-0-ethylidene-β-D-glucopyranoside). Cancer 40:633–637

23 Jacobs P, King H, Cassidy F, Dent D (1979) The treatment of diffuse lymphocytic lymphoma (large cell) with VP 16-213. Proc Am Assoc Cancer Res 20:289

24 Jacobs P, King HS, Sealy GRH (1975) Epipodophyllotoxin (VP 16-213) in the treatment of diffuse histiocytic lymphoma. S Afr Med J 49:483–485

25 Jungi WF, Senn HJ (1975) Clinical study of the new podophyllotoxin derivative, 4′-demethylepipodophyllotoxin 9-(4,6-0-ethylidene-β-D-glucopyranoside) (NSC-141540; VP 16-213), in solid tumors in man. Cancer Chemother Rep 59:737–742

26 Lau ME, Hansen HH, Nissen NI, Pedersen H (1979) Phase I trial of a new form of an oral administration of VP 16-213. Cancer Treat Rep 63:485–487

27 Loike JD, Horwitz SB (1976) Effects of podophyllotoxin and VP 16-213 on microtubule assembly in vitro and nucleoside transport in HeLa cells. Biochemistry 15:5435–5443

28 Mathé G, Schwarzenberg L, Pouillart P, Oldham R, Weiner R, Jasmin C, Rosenfeld C, Hayat M, Misset JL, Musset M, Schneider M, Amiel JL, De Vassal F (1974) Two epipodophyllotoxin derivatives, VM 26 and VP 16-213, in the treatment of leukemias, hematosarcomas, and lymphomas. Cancer 34:985–992

29 Nissen NI, Dombernowsky P, Hansen HH, Larsen V (1976) Phase I clinical trial of an oral solution of VP 16-213. Cancer Treat Rep 60:943–945

30 Nissen NI, Hansen HH, Pedersen H, Strøyer I, Dombernowsky P, Hessellund M (1975) Clinical trial of the oral form of a new podophyllotoxin derivative, VP 16-213 (NSC-141540), in patients with advanced neoplastic disease. Cancer Chemother Rep 59:1027–1029

31 Nissen NI, Larsen V, Pedersen H, Thomsen K (1972) Phase I clinical trial of a new antitumor agent, 4'demethylepipodophyllotoxin 9-(4,6-0-ethylidene-β-D-glucopyranoside) (NSC-141540; VP 16-213). Cancer Chemother Rep 56: 769–777
32 Nissen NI, Pajak TF, Leone LA, Bloomfield C, Kennedy BJ, Ellison RR, Silver RT, Jones B, Holland JF, Falkson FK, Lee S (1980) Clinical trial of VP 16-213 (NSC 141540) iv twice weekly in advanced neoplastic disease. A study by the Cancer and Leukemia Group B. Cancer 45: 232–235
33 Rivera G, Green A, Hayes A, Avery T, Pratt C (1977) Epipodophyllotoxin VM-26 in the treatment of childhood neuroblastoma. Cancer Treat Rep 61: 1243–1248
34 Rosenstock JG, Donaldson MH (1976) Phase I–II trial of VM-26 (NSC-122819) in the treatment of children with late-stage leukemia. Cancer Treat Rep 60: 265–267
35 Rozencweig M, Von Hoff DD, Henney JE, Muggia FM (1977) VM 26 and VP 16-213: A comparative analysis. Cancer 40: 334–342
36 Samson MK, Baker LH, Talley RW, Fraile RJ (1978) VM 26 (NSC-122819): A clinical study in advanced cancer of the lung and ovary. Eur J Cancer 15: 1395–1399
37 Schulz JJ, Spremulli EN, Wampler GL (1978) Phase II trial of 4'-demethylepipodophyllotoxin-9-(4,6-0-2-thenylidene-β-D-glucopyranoside) (VM-26). Proc Am Soc Clin Oncol 19: 346
38 Slayton R, Petty W, Blessing J (1979) Phase II trial of VP-16 in treatment of advanced ovarian adenocarcinoma. Proc Am Assoc Cancer Res 20: 190
39 Smith IE, Gerken ME, Clink HM, McElwain TJ (1976) VP 16-213 in acute myelogenous leukaemia. Postgrad Med J 52: 66–70
40 Sonntag RW, Senn HJ, Nagel G, Giger K, Alberto P (1974) Experience with 4'-demethylepipodophyllotoxin 9-(4,6-0-2-thenylidene-beta-D-glucopyranoside); VM 26; NSC-122819 in the treatment of malignant lymphosis. Eur J Cancer 10: 93–98
41 Sullivan MP, Eys J van, Herson J, Starling KA, Ragab A, Sexhauer C (1978) Nonresponsiveness of brain tumors to VM-26 therapy in children. Cancer Treat Rep 63: 155–156
42 Trempe G, Sykes M, Young C, Krakoff I (1970) Phase I trial of the podophyllotoxin derivative VM 26. Proc Am Assoc Cancer Res 11: 79
43 Tucker RD, Ferguson A, Wyk C van, Sealy R, Hewitson R, Levin W (1978) Chemotherapy of small cell carcinoma of the lung with VP 16-213. Cancer 41: 1710–1714

Antitumor Activity, Pharmacology, and Toxicity of Ellipticines, Ellipticinium, and 9-Hydroxy Derivatives: Preliminary Clinical Trials of 2-Methyl-9-Hydroxy Ellipticinium (NSC 264-137)

C. Paoletti, J.-B. Le Pecq, N. Dat-Xuong, P. Juret, H. Garnier, J.-L. Amiel, and J. Rouesse

Summary

Ellipticine and some derivatives are highly cytotoxic substances which kill L1210 cells at concentrations ranging form 10^{-8} to $10^{-6}M$. Some compounds in this series bind with high affinity to DNA (affinity constant between 10^7 M^{-1} and 10^5 M^{-1}) by intercalation between base pairs. The antitumoral properties of these derivatives are thought to be related to their DNA-binding ability. Both 9-hydroxylation of ellipticine and quaternarization of 2-pyridinic nitrogen tend to increase DNA binding and antitumor activity.

2-Methyl-9-hydroxyellipticine (NSC 264-137) was selected for a phase I and later for a phase II trial in human cancer. This drug does not affect blood cell counts in animals or in man. It is not mutagenic in the Ames' test nor teratogenic in mice, but is endowed with anti-inflammatory properties and induces a marked decrease of motoricity in mice. Transient bradycardia and decrease of blood pressure are the most noticeable cardiovascular effects in dogs.

This compound administered at 80–100 mg/m²/week in 1-h intravenous (IV) infusion induces objective remissions in about 25% of patients suffering from advanced breast cancer refractory to all other treatment. These remissions, which occurred after 3–4 weeks, lasted for 1–18 months. This drug seems particularly to improve the condition of patients suffering from oesteolytic breast cancer metastasis. Activity against anaplastic thyroid carcinoma and ovarian carcinoma has also been observed in some cases.

Toxic side effects are nausea and vomiting (one-third of the patients), hypertension (less than 10% of the patients), muscular cramp (one-third of the patients), fatigue which can be very pronounced (in most patients after 3 months of treatment), mouth dryness, and mycosis of the tongue and esophagus (less than 20% of the patients).

Introduction

Ellipticine and 9-methoxyellipticine (Fig. 1) are alkaloids existing in plants of the Apocynacae family which are to be found in several countries located near the Indian Ocean. The relatively simple structure of these substances prompted chemists to devise several procedures to gain access to these molecules which derive from the pyridocarbazole nucleus [44]. The antitumoral properties of ellipticine were discovered in 1967 by Dalton et al. [9]. This finding was confirmed by researchers in

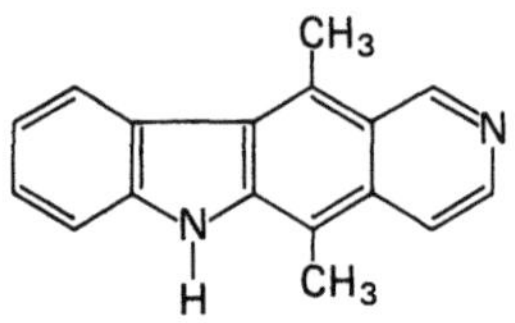

Ellipticine (NSC 71795)

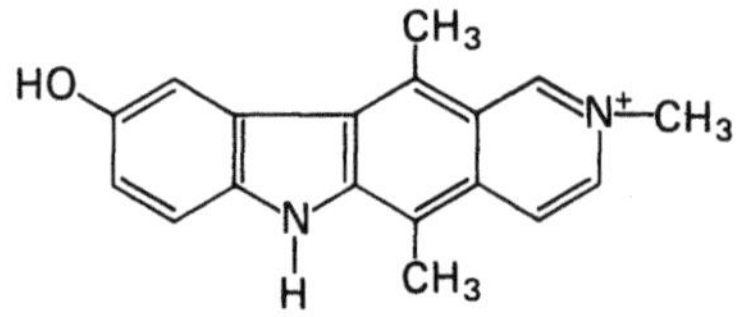

2–Methyl–9–hydroxyellipticinium (NSC 264137)

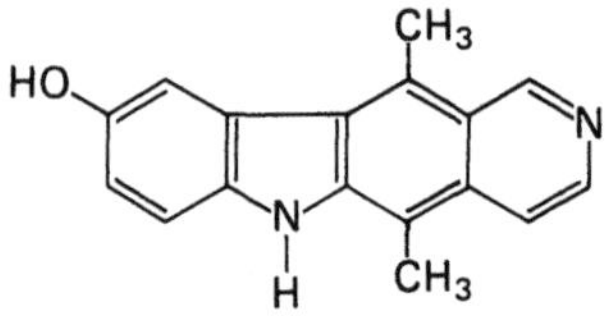

9–Hydroxyellipticine (NSC 210717)

Fig. 1. Structure of ellipticine, 9-hydroxyellipticine and 2-methyl-9-hydroxyellipticinium

the United States [44] and was complemented by toxicologic evaluations in animals, which revealed secondary toxic effects such as cardiovascular problems, hemolysis [18, 42] and nervous toxicity, especially in the cerebellum. Meanwhile, in 1970, MATHÉ et al. first reported the antitumor activity of 9-methoxyellipticine, a natural derivative of ellipticine, in acute myeloblastic leukemia in man [1, 25, 34]. Then, a study of the mechanism of the antitumoral action of these substances in relation to their structure was undertaken at the Institut Gustave-Roussy in Villejuif (France). The DNA-intercalating property of 9-methoxyellipticine was demonstrated [11], thus advancing the hypothesis that DNA might constitute the target of the substances. The search for new derivatives therefore with stronger affinity for DNA led to the synthesis of new ellipticine derivatives, such as 9-hydroxyellipticine [17, 26, 27] and 2-methyl-9-hydroxyellipticinium [28, 37] (Fig. 1). These products showed a broad range of antitumoral activity against experimental tumors when tested by several laboratories and the Pharmacological Screening Group of the European Organization for Research and Treatment of Cancer (EORTC).

Clinical tests were initiated in Caen (France) in 1977 by JURET et al. [21] using 2-methyl-9-hydroxyellipticinium (NMHE). After completion of a phase I study, the phase II trial was started by the early clinical trial group of EORTC, Caen's and Villejuif's group. Some of the preliminary clinical results have been published [6, 21, 22]. In this paper, we present a general overview of the main properties of ellipticine derivatives with special reference to 2-methyl-9-hydroxyellipticinium (NMHE, NSC 264137) which has shown preliminary favorable results in an ongoing phase II clinical trial.

Cytotoxicity and Antitumoral Properties

Ellipticine and several of its derivatives act on a broad range of experimental tumors. Table 1 summarizes the activity of 9-hydroxyellipticine and NMHE on several mice and rat tumors. In vitro studies on L1210 cells show that the toxic effect of these compounds is rapid and induces a marked rearrangement of the cellular architecture, with the appearance of giant cells (Fig. 2) [36]. DNA synthesis is preferentially

Table 1. Effect of 9-hydroxyellipticine (9 OHELL) and 2-methyl-9-hydroxyellipticinium (2 $N^{+}CH_3$–9 NMHE) on experimental tumors

	9 OH-ELL	2 $N^{+}CH3$– 9 OH-ELL	
Mice			
Leukemia L1210	+	++	Villejuif[a] (Institut Gustave-Roussy)
Leukemia P388	+	++	Toulouse[a] (Lab. Pharmacol. CNRS)
Lewis lung carcinoma	±	±	Villejuif[a] (Institut Gustave-Roussy)
Myeloma (ADJ-PCGA)	+		London[a] (Chester Beatty)
Osteosarcoma		–	Rijswick[a] (Radiob. Inst.)
Ependymoblastoma		++	Brussels[a] (Inst. J. Bordet)
Melanoma B16	+	+	New York (Lederle)
Rat			
Yoshida lymphosarcoma (in vitro)		++	Manchester[a] (Dr. Fox)
Gardner lymphosarcoma OG		++	Houston (Wadley Inst.)
Squamous cell carcinoma		+	Rijswick[a] (Radiob. Inst.)
EHTH myeloid leukemia		–	Budapest[a] (Oncol. Inst.)

[a] EORTC screening and pharmacology group

inhibited while protein synthesis remains unaffected [12]. Figure 3 shows that the first toxic effect observed on the cells in vitro is a decrease of the rate of cell multiplication without appearance of cell lysis or immediate death. These cells, however, lose their ability to clone in vitro on agar medium and to promote tumor when grafted to mice (Table 2). Thus the antitumoral efficacy of ellipticine derivatives resides in a direct and preferential cytotoxic action upon malignant cells rather than in an indirect effect. The relation between the concentration of 2-methyl-9-hydroxyellipticinium and the amplitude of the effect upon the rate of cell division of L1210 cells is provided in Fig. 3. Table 3 presents the ID_{50}, the inhibiting concentration of various ellipticine derivatives which reduced the rate of L1210 cell multiplication by 50%. The most active derivatives in the series are capable of significantly decreasing the rate of multiplication of L1210 cells at ng/ml concentrations ($10^{-8}M$). This activity is close to that of the most cytotoxic antitumoral drugs (e.g., actinomycin, Table 3).

Mechanism of Action and Metabolism

The nature of the ultimate intracellular target of ellipticine and its derivatives is uncertain and might therefore vary from one derivative to another. Still, it appears that ellipticine and all of its active derivatives show a relatively high affinity for deoxyribonucleic acid. In this series, this affinity lies in a range of two orders of

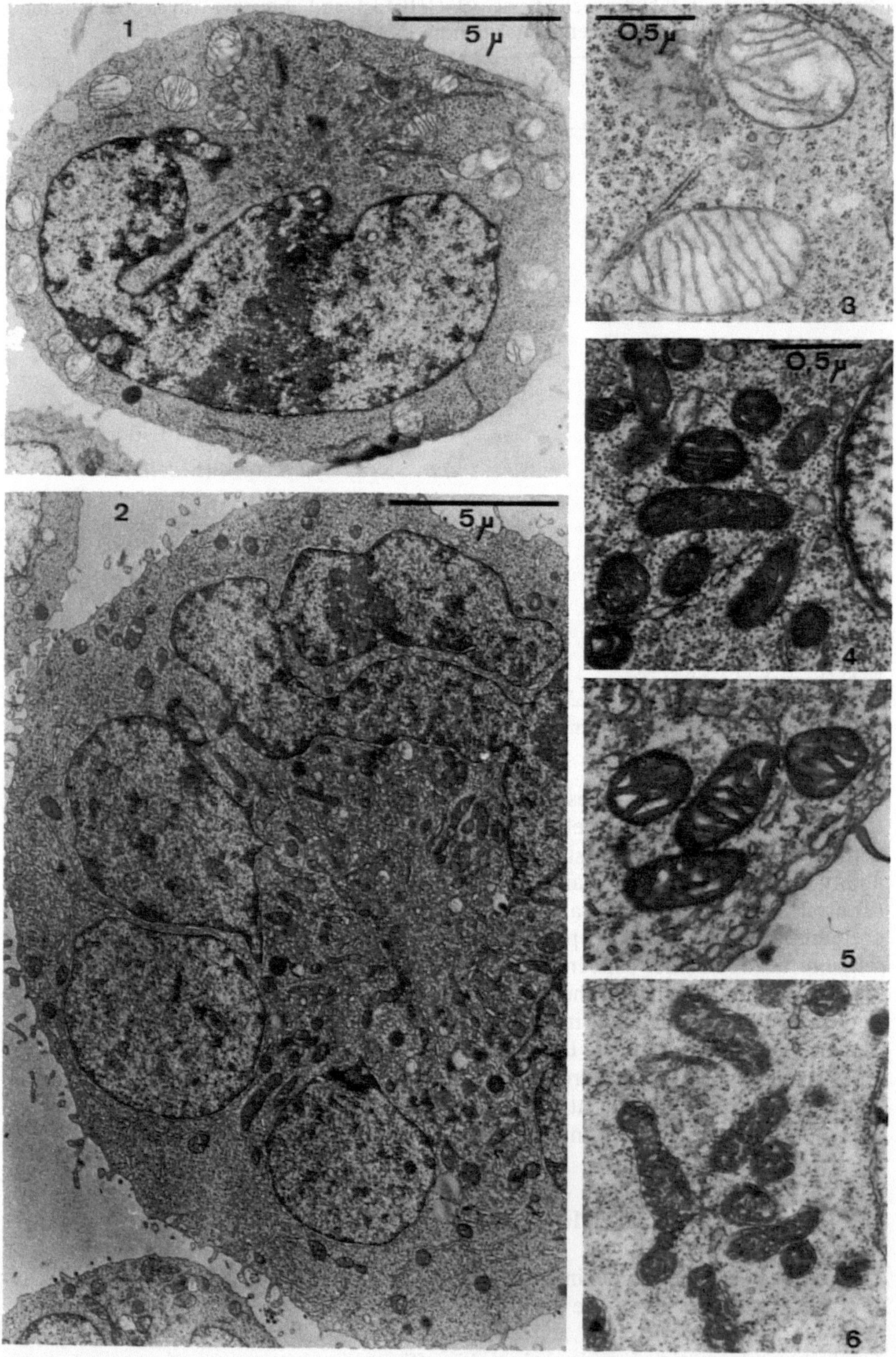
1
5 µ
O,5 µ
3
O,5 µ
4
5
2
5 µ
6

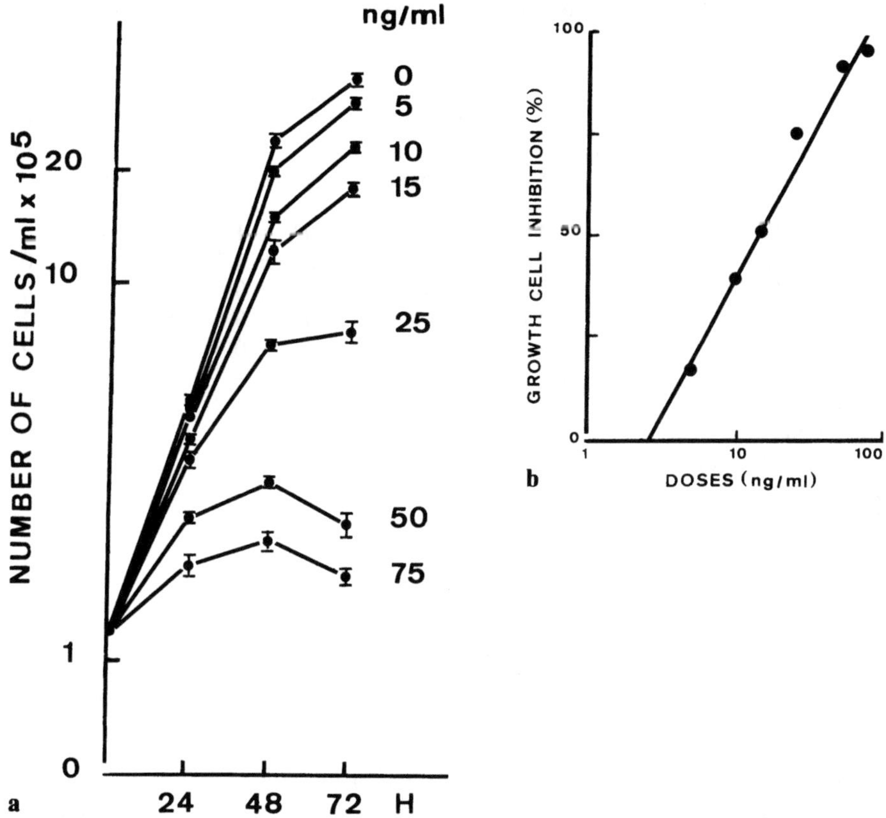

Fig. 3a, b. Effects of 2-methyl-9-hydroxyellipticinium on L1210 cell growth in culture. **a** growth versus time: each *point* represents the average of four replicata samples; *bars* indicate SEM; **b** dose-effect relationship: the *regression line* is drawn as the percentage inhibition of the growth as a function of the logarithm of the dose, after 48 h culture

magnitude (Table 3). Moreover, as previously stated, they inhibit the synthesis of DNA of malignant cells in culture at concentrations which do not modify RNA or protein synthesis [12]. Ellipticine and several derivatives induce changes of the DNA structural integrity in cells; these changes are indicated by the reduction of the rate of migration of DNA fragments when centrifuged in alkaline sucrose gradients after lysis of cells previously exposed to these cytotoxic agents [38]. This phenomenon can be explained either by an induction of breaks in DNA or by the formation of alkaline-sensitive zones in DNA. Finally, some ellipticine derivatives are mutagens in prokaryotes (*Salmonella*) [23] as well as in eukaryotes (*Saccharomyces*) (Pinto, Guerineau and Paoletti, unpublished results).

◀ **Fig. 2.** Cellular damages induced in vitro by 2-methyl-9-hydroxyellipticinium (NMHE) on L1210 cells. Cells were exposed to $7 \times 10^{-8} M$ of NMHE for 48 h. Growth inhibition was about 80%. Note enlarged nucleus and "condensed" configuration of mitochondria at different stage of damage: **1,** control cell; **2,** treated cell; **3,** mitochondria of control cell; **4, 5, 6,** mitochondria of treated cell at different stage of damage (After Paoletti et al. [36])

Table 2. Mice bioassay of L1210 cells grown in vitro in presence of 2-methyl-9-hydroxyellipticinium (after Paoletti et al. [36])

Drug concentration		Growth inhibition after 48 h culture	No. of inoculated mice[a]		Median survival time		No. of cured mice[d]	% L1210 cells killed
ng/ml	M		Control	Treated	Control	Treated		
0.5	1.8×10^{-9}	0	12	12	$10.8^{b} \pm 1.2$	9.8 ± 0.6	0	0
2.0	7.2×10^{-9}	14.4	12	12	10.8 ± 1.2	9.6 ± 0.6	0	0
5.0	1.8×10^{-8}	21.7	42	34	10.4 ± 0.5	11.4 ± 0.5	0	84
15.5	5.6×10^{-8}	73.0	40	31	9.8 ± 0.5	$15.1^{c} \pm 1.0$	2	99.997
25.0	9.0×10^{-8}	87.7	30	24	10.2 ± 0.6	$20.9^{c} \pm 2.1$	9	99.999

[a] 10^5 cells/mouse by IP route
[b] Mean ± SE
[c] Cured mice excluded
[d] Survival longer than 45 days

Table 3. Effects on L1210 cells in vitro and in vivo and DNA binding of ellipticine and derivatives (after Le Pecq et al. [26] and Paoletti et al. [36])

Compounds	ID_{50}[a]		ILS (%) in term of LD_0[b]			LD_0[c] (mg/kg)	DNA affinity[d]
	ng/ml	μM	1	1/2	1/5		
9-OHE	3.9	0.015	53	58	28	50	2.0×10^6
$6\text{-}CH_3\text{-}9\text{-}OHE$	6.0	0.022	–	–	–	–	1.2×10^7
$2\text{-}C_5H_9\text{-}9\text{-}OHE$[e]	9.6	0.033	57 47%[f]	88 32%[f]	119 15%[f]	50	1.0×10^6
$2\text{-}6\text{-}diCH_3\text{-}9\text{-}OHE$[e]	11.9	0.041	78	75	55	15	4.0×10^6
$2\text{-}CH_3\text{-}9\text{-}OHE$[e]	13.8	0.05	62	53	28	5	1.3×10^6
$9\text{-}NH_2E$	138	0.53	18	0	–	150	1.2×10^6
$9\text{-}OCH_3E$	164	0.60	70[g]	–	–	70	1.0×10^5
E	242	0.99	68	40	12	50	1.5×10^5
$2\text{-}CH_3E$	437	1.68	18	22	17	13	2.3×10^5
9-FE	1035	3.94	h	–	–	> 250	6.4×10^5
7-OHE	1421	5.44	h	–	–	h	1.0×10^5
9-BrE	4115	12.7	Inactive			> 500	4.0×10^5
Actinomycin D	1.24	0.001	45[i]	–	36	0.87[i]	2.3×10^6[j]

[a] Dose which reduces the cell growth by 50% after 48 h as compared with controls
[b] Increase in lifespan (ILS) over controls (10^5 cells/mouse IP; single injection 24 h after cell grafting
[c] Highest nonlethal dose (IP treatment)
[d] Measurement carried out at 25° C in 0.1 M NaCl-0.1 M Tris-HCl (pH 7.4)
[f] Percentage of cured mice: survival longer than 45 days
[g] Results from Ref. 16
[h] Insufficient supply of drugs for testing
[i,j] Results from Refs. 13 and 35

If a high affinity for DNA seems to be required for expression of an antitumoral effect, however, this feature does not constitute enough of a condition. For example, 9-aminoellipticine and 9-fluoroellipticine have affinities practically identical to those of 9-hydroxyellipticine and 2-methyl-9-hydroxyellipticinium, yet the former does not display antitumoral properties comparable to those of the latter two compounds. It likewise appears that one or several other characteristics of these molecules must intervene to reinforce their pharmacologic action. In this respect it can be remarked that hydroxylation of ellipticine in position 9 leads to a compound about 40-fold more cytotoxic upon leukemia L1210 grown in vitro and more antitumoral in weak doses than ellipticine itself (Table 3). Two hypothesis actually take into account this observation. The first is based on the increase in affinity for DNA following hydroxylation in position 9.

The second hypothesis is founded on the oxidoreduction properties of 9-hydroxyellipticine derivatives. These compounds can be oxidized to para-imine quinone derivatives with the departure of two hydrogen atoms. An intermediate step in this process can occur with the departure of a single hydrogen atom and can lead to a phenoxylike radical. If such reactions can occur in vivo, formation of toxic radicals will be promoted. Such radicals could cause irreversible damage eventually to DNA and would account for the occurrence of breaks in the polynucleotide chain, as previously mentioned [38].

Two experimental observations favor this hypothesis. On the one hand, 9-hydroxyellipticine derivatives are excellent substrates for peroxydases which transform them into corresponding imine quinone derivatives [2]. These enzymes are known to generate obligatorily intermediate short-lived radicals. On the other hand, these radicals have been directly detected by using EPR spectroscopy.

In this tentative model, the effectiveness of 9-hydroxyellipticine derivatives would lie in the conjunction of two remarkable properties of these molecules: the one, their high affinity for DNA – and probably for other biologic macromolecules – which assigns them the role of vectors; the other, their aptitude to generate transitory radical forms which could constitute true cytotoxic reactants. Both properties would be necessary for these substances to act, yet neither alone would be enough. Bachur et al. [4] have proposed a similar model for several quinone antibiotics.

This reactional scheme of the interaction of active ellipticine derivatives on supposed ultimate target, DNA, opens up many interesting prospects, since it is based on a cytotoxic action mechanism which might be shared with several other antitumoral substances which possess a para-quinone or a para-quinonelike structure: mitomycin C, anthracyclines, lapachol, and streptonigrin. The bioreduction of these substances leads to unstable intermediary metabolic forms which could be responsible for their cytotoxic activity. The derivatives of ellipticine, hydroxylated in position 9, are equivalent to these reduced forms. Their advantage is that they are stable enough to be prepared. This hypothetical model was upheld by experimental arguments in the case of mitomycin C [4, 45], the anthracyclines [3, 4, 14], and streptonigrin [4, 47]. After IV injection, ellipticine is quickly oxidized in the liver by cytochrome P450 mixed oxygenases which already intervene in the metabolism of various anticancerous drugs [5, 43]. The oxidation of ellipticine occurs after binding of the drug to the active oxygenase sites. The interaction of ellipticine derivatives with microsomes and cytochrome P450 has been studied in vitro [31]. It was shown that the pyridinic nitrogen of ellipticine interacts with the iron atom of cytochrome P450. Quaternary ammonium derivatives of ellipticine are, as expected, unable to bind to microsomes.

On the other hand, microsomal preparations are also able to hydroxylate ellipticine in vitro with a yield of about 10%–15% [30]. 9-Hydroxyellipticine is mainly formed, and 7-hydroxyellipticine is also obtained, but in a small proportion [30]. In vivo, ellipticine is also metabolized. The two main metabolites in mice are the glucuroconjugate and the sulfoconjugate of 9-hydroxyellipticine. Conjugates of 7-hydroxyellipticine appear, as well as minor constituents [15, 30]. 9-Hydroxyellipticine, when injected IV in mice, is excreted by the bile mainly as glucuroconjugate, which accounts for a least 90% of all metabolites [47].

2-Methyl-9-hydroxyellipticinium is not metabolized in mice or in man, and is excreted as such through bile (75%) and urine (25%) [47]. This observation agrees with the fact that this compound cannot bind to microsomes and is not metabolized in vitro. A comparative pharmacokinetics and metabolic study of various ellipticine derivatives will be reported elsewhere [47]. The metabolic fate of the various ellipticine derivatives can therefore be quite variable, which could be important in determining the pharmacologic activity of these compounds. Also, ellipticine itself leads in vivo to two metabolites which have very different properties. The in vitro cytotoxicity of 9-hydroxyellipticine on L1210 cells is 40-fold greater than that of ellipticine, as the cytotoxicity of 7-hydroxyellipticine on L1210 cell is sixfold weaker than that of ellipticine. The cytotoxicity of ellipticine could therefore be affected strongly by metabolization. On the other hand, ellipticine is a strong inducer of liver microsomal P448 mixed oxygenases [29], some derivatives are potent inhibitors of cytochrome mixed oxygenases and, consequently, of drug metabolism [32, 33].

Toxicity and Pharmacologic Properties

The toxicity of ellipticine derivatives varies depending upon the nature of the derivative. Of nine compounds in this series tested on mice, the LD_0 after intraperitoneal (IP) injection fluctuated from 5 mg/kg to more than 500 mg/kg in a range of values greater than 100 (Table 3). In most cases, delayed animal death occurred between 5 and 10 days after injection of the product.

The main results of the acute toxicologic study of 2-methyl-9-hydroxyellipticinium presently being tested in man are reported in Table 4. The maximum dose tolerated by mice after IV injection is 26 mg/m^2. Note that the toxic effect of the first IP injection did not disappear until 5 days later. It was necessary therefore to wait until after this delay in order to find a LD_0 equal to 5 mg/kg, when using mice which had already received one 5-mg/kg injection (LD_0 for nontreated animals). The compound was relatively well supported after chronic administration. No mice died after 0.7 mg/kg (LD_0/8) injected every 5 days over a 120-day period.

2-Methyl-9-hydroxyellipticinium is neither embryotoxic nor teratogenic in mice (unpublished results of our laboratory). One important observation is the absence of marked effects of this ellipticinium derivative on hemopoïetic cells (Table 5). An increase in the relative number of polynuclear granulocytic leukocytes and a mild decrease in the relative number of platelets are the only significant features. In rats, 2-methyl-9-hydroxyellipticinium also induced an increase in the proportion of polynuclear leukocytes as well as a relative and moderate increase in the number of lymphocytes.

This lack of hematologic toxicity contrasts strikingly with the severe side effects on hemopoïesis induced by most anticancer agents. Ellipticine is able to hemolyze, in

Table 4. Toxic doses of 2-methyl-9-hydroxyellipticinium (NMHE, NSC 264137) on mice

Route of administration of unique dose	Dose (mg/kg)		
	LD_0	LD_{50}[a]	LD_{100}[a]
IV	8.6	15.2	20.6
IP	5.1	10.2	19.2
per OS	> 250	–	–

[a] Death at 8–9 days after injection. No obvious histologic damages at any level. Each experiment on 125 mice

Table 5. Effect of 2-methyl-9-hydroxyellipticinium (NMHE, NSC 264137) on mice blood cell counts

Unique IP injection	At LD_0 (5.1 mg/kg)
Red cells =	24% Max. decrease at day 9
White cells =	
Total	14% Max. increase at days 13–15
Neutro	84% Max. increase at day 5 (Increase over about 10 days)
Lympho	No significant change
Platelets	32% Max. decrease at day 7
IP injections every 5 days	At ~ $LD_0/8$ (0.7 mg/kg) for 15, 30, and 45 days
Red cells = / White cells = / Platelets =	No significant change

Control values per mm^3 (DBA/2 female mice):

	Red cells	= 12,500,000 ± 980,000
	Leuko	= 14,000 ± 3,400
	Platelets	= 1,400,000 ± 160,000
In %	Neutro	= 20 ± 7.3
	Lympho	= 78 ± 7.7

vitro and in vivo, the blood of dogs and rhesus monkeys [18, 19, 24]. This hemolysis is blocked by the simultaneous administration of citric acid [33]. 9-Methoxyellipticine, which was the first compound tried on man, does not induce hemolysis [18]. Ellipticine and some derivatives are mutagenic upon prokaryote [23] and eukaryote organisms [41], but NMHE is not [23].

The main pharmacologic properties of 2-methyl-9-hydroxyellipticinium are summarized in Table 6. The anti-inflammatory properties of 9-hydroxyellipticine on skin erythema of the guinea pig, on rat edema induced by carragenin, and on the rat polyarthritis induced by the Freund adjuvant have been described. This drug slows the inflammatory process of immunologic as well as on nonimmunologic origin [8]. These properties have also been found with 2-methyl-9-hydroxyellipticinium (NMHE) (LABAZ Laboratories, personal communication). 9-Methoxyellipticine exerts sig-

Table 6. Some pharmacologic effects of 2-methyl-9-hydroxyellipticinium (NMHE) (data obtained by CROS et al. [8] and Labaz Laboratories in Brussels)

Effect	Animal species	Threshold	Dose
Depression of motoricity[a]	Mice	$LD_0/10$	IP
Potentialization of barbiturate sleep	Mice	$0.4\ LD_0$	IP
Analgesia	Mice	$2\ LD_0$	IV
Anti-inflammatory	Rats	2 mg/kg	IM
Liberation of histamine	Dogs		IV
Liberation of serotonin	Dogs		IV
Potentialization of histamine and serotonin effects	Dogs		IV
Decrease of blood pressure[a]	Dogs	2 mg/kg	IV
Increase of respiratory frequency	Dogs	2 mg/kg	IV

[a] Also observed in patients

Table 7. Antagonists of side effects of 2-methyl-9-hydroxyellipticinium (NMHE) in dogs (data obtained by Labaz Laboratories in Brussels)

Antagonized effect	Drug	Dose	Assumed mechanism
Decrease of blood pressure	Phenergan	2.5 mg/kg IV	Blockade of histamine receptors
	Sandomigran	5 mg/kg IV	Blockade of serotonin receptors
Increase of respiratory frequency	Indomethacin	1 mg/kg IV	Inhibition of prostaglandin synthesis

nificant thymolytic action [10], which may approximate the immunosuppressive effect of this compound and of some other ellipticine derivatives (F. SPREAFICO, personal communication).

Actometric measurement revealed a 50% decrease in motoricity in mice 40–45 min after IV injection of 0.45 mg/kg of NMHE, i.e., at $LD_0/20$.

The cardiovascular action of ellipticine [18, 20] and 9-hydroxyellipticine [39, 40, and unpublished data from our group] was studied in dogs and monkeys. The following effects were noted: a decrease in blood pressure, bradycardia, and an increase in carotid artery flow for low or moderate levels of the drugs. All these effects were reversible. The manner in which the drugs are injected influences the amplitude of the variation of blood pressure (Fig. 4). Some respiratory depression was also reported [20, and unpublished data from our group]. Furthermore, in the case of NMHE, some of the adverse side effects could be antagonized in dogs (Table 7) (unpublished data obtained by DE CLAVIERE et al., Labaz Laboratories, Brussels).

Clinical Trials

The first clinical trial of an ellipticine derivative was undertaken by MATHÉ et al. [34]. Several remissions of acute myeloblastic leukemia occurred after treatment with

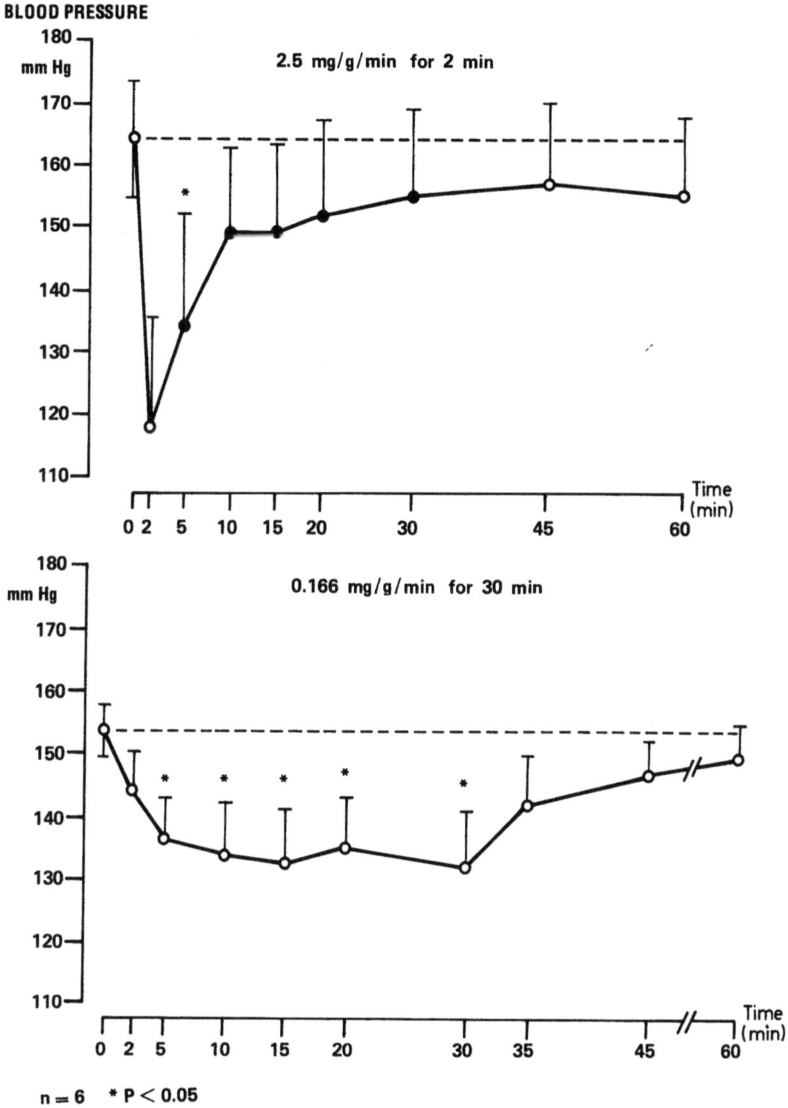

Fig. 4. Variation of blood pressure of dogs after one injection of 2-methyl-9-hydroxyellipticinium (5 mg/kg or 95 mg/m^2). Data from Laboratoires LABAZ (France) in Brussels (De Claviere et al.)

9-methoxyellipticine [1, 34]. Subsequently, a clinical trial of 9-hydroxyellipticine was undertaken at the Institut François Baclesse in Caen and at the Institut Gustave-Roussy in Villejuif. No therapeutic effectiveness was recorded, probably because the amount of drug which could be injected IV into patients was not sufficient, due to its relatively limited solubility. NMHE does not present this inconvenience. In addition, the chemotherapeutic index of this drug tested in the leukemia L1210 system was improved when compared with that of 9-hydroxyellipticine. Phase I clinical testing of NMHE has been carried out by Juret et al. [21, 22] at the Institut François Baclesse in Caen. It has been established that the drug can be administered in doses of up to

Table 8. Toxicity symptoms in 170 patients treated with 2-methyl-9-hydroxyellipticinium (NMHE) (80–100 mg/m^2/weekly, except for the first 15 patients: 2–60 mg/m^2 weekly)

	Total no. of patients	Hemato-toxicity	Hepatic-toxicity	Renal toxicity	Others	
t_0 No toxic reaction	98	0	0	0	0	
t_1 Slight toxic reaction not requiring modification of treatment	49	0	0	0	0	Minor side effects detailed in another table
t_2 Toxic reaction requiring modification of treatment	12	0	0	0	0	
t_3 Toxic reaction requiring cessation of treatment	8	0	0	0	0	
t_4 Lethal toxic reaction	3[a]	0	0	2	1	Sudden death at the start of the 6th injection

[a] Relation with the treatment was suspected but could not be demonstrated

Table 9. Main side effects in 170 patients treated with 2-methyl-9-hydroxyellipticinium (NMHE)

Nausea, vomiting	$^{1}/_{3}$ patients
Fever	10 patients – usually < 38° 1 case 39° after each injection
Hypotension	13 patients – usually < 3 cm and lasting 1–2 h
Vein phlebitis	20 patients
Cramps	$^{1}/_{3}$ patients when treated for 2 months or longer – disappeared usually when patients were given Hexaquine
Fatigue	Usual in patients treated longer than 3 months
Asialia, mouth dryness	$^{1}/_{4}$ of patients
Mycosis of the tongue of the esophagus	20 cases due to *candida albicans* 1 case or *candida tropicalis*

120 mg/m^2/week. This drug seems to be much less toxic in man than in mice. The equivalent dose in mice will be lethal (LD_{100} in mice, 60 mg/m^2 for a single injection). The same phenomenon was observed with 9-hydroxyellipticine. At least a 1-h IV perfusion is preferable to a bolus administration, which sometimes induces local venous toxicity and a more sudden and pronounced decrease in blood pressure as shown in the dog (Fig. 4).

Some patients were treated for longer than 16 months without any major or irreversible problems, except for three deaths which occurred after more than 1 year of treatment. However, a causal relation between these deaths and the prolonged administration of the drug was not established.

After weekly therapeutic doses of 80 mg/m^2, symptoms of toxicity occurred. These are indicated in Tables 8 and 9, and discussed in three communications [6, 21, 22]. A very useful feature of this drug already found in animals is that it does not affect red or white blood cell counts or platelets in man. The EORTC early clinical group preliminary observations dwell on the mouth dryness as sometimes being quite severe, and on pronounced asthenia. This group likewise describes a few cases of hemolysis and alopecia, which we have not found in our group [6].

A phase II evaluation of the therapeutic action of 2-methyl-9-hydroxyellipticinium has been undertaken by the EORTC early clinical group. Table 10 summarizes the data obtained according to the usual measurable criteria. This drug was shown to be a new effective antitumoral agent in about 20% of patients suffering from advanced breast cancer which was refractory to all other treatment [6, 21, 22]. 2-Methyl-9-hydroxy-ellipticinium also displayed some activity against anaplastic thyroid carcinoma (three of seven patients), soft-tissue sarcoma, and ovarian carcinoma. Although the number of cases is still too small to reach definitive conclusions, preliminary observations indicate that this drug might also affect the evolution of kidney carcinoma, Ewing sarcoma, neuroblastoma, and placental choriocarcinoma. No favorable reactions were recorded in 13 patients suffering from gastrointestinal cancer.

The preliminary observation of therapeutic effects on advanced human tumors of 2-methyl-9-hydroxyellipticinium combined with the absence of severe toxicity at therapeutic doses and, mainly, the absence of hematologic toxicity indicate that the

Table 10. Preliminary results of phase II clinical studies of 2-methyl-9-hydroxyellipticinium (NMHE) obtained by various institutions (patients refractory to any other treatment)

Institution	Number of evaluable patients[b,c]	Localization		Stabilization[a]		Remission[a]			
					(%)	Partial		Complete	(%)
						< 50%	> 50%		
F. Baclesse (Caen, Dr. P. Juret)	78	Breast	48	7	(15)	3	5	1	(19)
		Thyroid (anaplastic)	7	1	(23)	1	1	0	(10)
		Others	23	6		0	1	0	
EORTC General Hospital Oviedo, Dr. A. Brugarolas St. Jahn Hospital Bruges, Dr. A. Clarysse Jules Bordet Institute Bruxelles, R. de Jager	18	Breast	18	6	(33)	1	1	1	(17)
Gustave-Roussy Institute Villejuif, Professor J. L. Amiel, Dr. J. Rouesse	48	Breast	17	2	(12)	4	0	0	(24)
		Others	31	3	(10)	4	4	0	(25)

[a] Lasting for one to 18 months
The drug was prepared and delivered by Labaz Laboratories (SANOFI), France
[b] May 1979
[c] Total number of patients: Caen, 100: Villejuif, 82

properties of this compound deserve a more complete evaluation. The new analogues in this series also deserve further study.

Acknowledgements. This work done under the auspice of EORTC (screening and pharmacology group) has been financed and supported by the Association pour le Développement de la Recherche sur le Cancer (Chairman: Mr. J. CROZEMARIE, Villejuif) and by the Institut Gustave-Roussy (Director: Professor P. DENOIX). CNRS, INSERM, University Paris VI and Paris XI, and DGRST also contributed notably to the research, as did the Fondation pour l'Aide à la Recherche Médicale, le Commissariat à l'Energie Atomique, and the Sécurité Sociale. The Labaz Laboratory (SANOFI Group) (A. CIER and P. JOLY) produced, quality-checked, and delivered the 2-methyl-9-hydroxyellipticinium (NMHE) used in the clinical trials. The results briefly presented and outlined in this work were the fruit of a collective effort involving many scientists, technicians, and clinicians in various laboratories of the CNRS (LA 147), of INSERM (U-140) in Villejuif, and in the Laboratoire de Pharmacologie et de Toxicologie Fondamentales of the CNRS in Toulouse. To all, we express our thanks.

References

1 Ansari BM, Thompson EN (1975) Methoxy 9 ellipticine lactate in refractory acute myeloid leukemia. Postgrad Med J 51: 103–105
2 Auclair C, Gouyette A, Paoletti C (1978) Peroxydases catalyzed oxidation of the antitumor drug 9-hydroxy ellipticine. Abstract Coordination Chem and Cancer Chemother Meeting, Toulouse, July 24–26, 1978. Biochimie 60: 1073
3 Bachur NR, Gordon SL, Gee MV (1978) A general mechanism for microsomal activation of quinone anticancer agents to free radicals. Cancer Res 38: 1745–1750
4 Bachur NR, Gordon SL, Gee MV, Kon H (1979) NADPH cytochrome P450 reductase activation of quinone anticancer agents to free radicals. Proc Natl Acad Sci USA 76: 954–957
5 Branfman AR, Bruni RJ, Reinhold VN, Silveira DM, Chadwick M, Yesair DW (1978) Characterization of the metabolites of ellipticine in rat bile. Drug Metab Dispos 6: 542–548
6 Brugarolas A, Gracia M, De Jager R, Mallarmen M, Clarysse A (1979) Hydroxy methyl ellipticinium (9 HME, NSC 264137). Phase I clinical study. Proc 17th Annu Meet Am Assoc Cancer Res 20: C77
7 Chadwick M, Silveira DM, Platz BB, Hayes D (1978) Comparative physiological disposition of ellipticine in several animal species after intravenous administration. Drug Metab Dipos 6: 528–541
8 Cros J, Thibault A, Dat-Xuong N (1975) Action anti-inflammatoire de l'hydroxy 9 ellipticine. CR Acad Sci [D] Paris 281: 1139–1142
9 Dalton LK, Demerac S, Elmes BC, Loder JW, Swan JM, Teitei T (1967) Synthesis of the tumour-inhibitory alkaloids ellipticine 9-methoxy ellipticine and related pyrido (4,3-*b*) carbazoles. Aust J Chem 20: 2715–2727
10 Dufer J, Desplaces A, Aurousseau M (1973) Etude cytochimique des leucocytes de rats traités par la methoxy 9 ellipticine. Ann Pharm Fr 31: 441–450
11 Festy B, Poisson J, Paoletti C (1971) A new intercalating drug: Methoxy 9 ellipticine. FEBS Lett 17: 321–323
12 Garcia-Giralt E, Macieira-Coelho A (1970) Methoxy 9 ellipticine. II. Analysis in vitro of the mechanism of action. Eur J Clin Biol Res 15: 539–544
13 Goldin A, Johnson RK (1974) Evaluation of actinomycin in experimental systems. Cancer Chemother Rep 58: 63–77

14 Handa K, Sato S (1976) Stimulation of microsomal NADPH oxidation by quinone group containing anticancer chemicals. Gann 67: 523–528
15 Hardesty CT, Chaney NA, Mead JAR (1972) The effect of route of administration of the distribution of ellipticine in mice. Cancer Res 32: 1884–1889
16 Hartwell JL, Abbotth BJ (1969) Antineoplastic principles in plants: Recent development in the field. In: Garrattini S, Goldin A, Hawking F, Kopin IJ (eds) Advances in pharmacology and chemotherapy, vol 7. Academic, New York, pp 117–209
17 Hayat M, Mathé G, Janot MM, Potier P, Dat-Xuong N, Cave A, Sevenet T, Kan-Fan C, Poisson J, Miet J, Le Men J, Le Goffic F, Gouyette A, Ahond A, Dalton LK, Connors TA (1974) Experimental screening of 3 forms and 19 derivatives of analogs of ellipticine: Oncostatic effect on L1210 leukemia and immunosuppressive effect of 4 of them. Biomedicine 21: 101–106
18 Herman EH, Chadwick DP, Mhatre RM (1974) Comparison of the acute hemolytic and cardiovascular actions of ellipticine (NSC 71795) and some ellipticine analogs. Cancer Chemother 58: 637–643
19 Herman EH, Lee IP, Mhatre RM, Chadwick DP (1974) Prevention of hemolysis induced by ellipticine (NSC 71795) in rhesus monkeys. Cancer Chemother Rep 58: 171–179
20 Herman E, Vick J, Burka B (1971) The cardiovascular actions of ellipticine. Toxicol Appl Pharmacol 18: 743–751
21 Juret P, Tanguy A, Le Talaer JY, Abbatucci JS, Dat-Xuong N, Le Pecq J-B, Paoletti C (1978) Preliminary trial of 9-hydroxy 2-methyl ellipticinium (NSC 264137) in advanced human cancers. Eur J Cancer 14: 205–206
22 Juret P, Tanguy A, Le Talaer JY, Abbatucci JS, Dat-Xuong N, Le Pecq J-B, Paoletti C (1979) L'acétate d'hydroxy 9-methyl 2-ellipticinium (NSC 264137). Etude toxicologique et thérapeutique chez 100 cancéreux. Nouv Presse Med 8: 1495–1498
23 Lecointe P, Lesca P, Cros S, Paoletti C (1978) Some antitumor derivatives of ellipticine deprived of mutagenic properties. Chem Biol Interact 20: 113–121
24 Lee IP (1976) A possible mechanism of ellipticine induced hemolysis. J Pharmacol Exp Ther 196: 525–535
25 Le Men J, Hayat M, Mathé G, Guillon JC, Chenu E, Humbolt M, Masson Y (1970) Methoxy-9-ellipticine lactate. Experimental study (oncostatic and immunosuppressive actions: preclinical pharmacology). Rev Eur Etud Clin Biol 15: 534–538
26 Le Pecq J-B, Dat-Xuong N, Gosse C, Paoletti C (1974) A new antitumoral agent: 9-Hydroxy ellipticine. Possibility of a rational design of anticancerous drugs in the series of DNA intercalating drugs. Proc Natl Acad Sci USA 71: 5078–5082
27 Le Pecq J-B, Gosse C, Dat-Xuong N, Cros S, Paoletti C (1976) Antitumoral activity of 9 hydroxy ellipticine (NSC 210717) on L1210 mice leukemia. Effect of the route of injection. Cancer Res 36: 3067–3076
28 Le Pecq J-B, Gosse C, Dat-Xuong N, Paoletti C (1975) Deux nouveaux dérivés antitumoraux: l'hydroxy-9 methyl-2 ellipticinium et l'hydroxy 9 dimethyl 2,6-ellipticinium. Action sur la leucémie L1210 de la souris. CR Acad Sci [D] Paris 281: 1365–1367
29 Lesca P, Lecointe P, Paoletti C, Mansuy D (1976) Induction des monooxygenases hépatiques par l'ellipticine chez le rat: formation de cytochrome P448. Activité hydroxylante. CR Acad Sci [D] Paris 282: 1457–1460
30 Lesca P, Lecointe P, Paoletti C, Mansuy D (1977) The hydroxylation of the antitumor agent ellipticine by liver microsomes from differently pretreated rats. Biochem Pharmacol 26: 2169–2173
31 Lesca P, Lecointe P, Paoletti C, Mansuy D (1978) Ellipticine as potent inhibitors of aryl hydrocarbon hydroxylase: Their binding to microsomal cytochrome P450 and protective effect against benzo(a)pyrene mutagenicity. Biochem Pharmacol 27: 1203–1209
32 Lesca P, Lecointe P, Paoletti C, Mansuy D (1978) Ellipticines as potent inhibitors of drug metabolism. Protective effect against chemical mutagenesis and carcinogenesis. Biochimie 60: 1011–1018

33 Lesca P, Rafidinarivo E, Lecointe P, Mansuy D (1978) A class of strong inhibitors of microsomal monooxygenases: The ellipticines. Chem Biol Interact 24: 189–198
34 Mathé G, Hayat M, De Vassal F, Schwarzenberg L, Schneider M, Schlumberger JR, Jasmin C, Rosenfeld C (1970) Methoxy 9 ellipticine lactate. III. Clinical screening: Its action in acute myeloblastic leukemia. Rev Eur Etud Clin Biol 15: 541–545
35 Muller W, Crothers DM (1968) Studies of the binding of actinomycin and related compounds to DNA. J Mol Biol 35: 251–290
36 Paoletti C, Cros S, Dat-Xuong N, Lecointe P, Moisand A (1979) Comparative cytotoxic and antitumoral effects of ellipticine derivatives on mouse L1210 leukemia. Chem Biol Interact 25: 45–58
37 Paoletti C, Le Pecq J-B, Dat-Xuong N, Lesca P, Lecointe P (1978) New anticancer derivatives in the ellipticine series. Curr Chemother 1195–1197
38 Paoletti C, Lesca C, Cros S, Malvy C, Auclair C (1978) Ellipticine and derivatives induce breakage of L1210 cells DNA in vitro. Biochem Pharmacol 28: 345–350
39 Pham-Huu-Chanh, Dat-Xuong N, Le Pecq J-B, Paoletti C (1976) Cardiovascular activity of 9 hydroxy ellipticine. Pharmacology 14: 490–498
40 Pham-Huu-Chanh, Sorbara R, Dat-Xuong N, Paoletti C, Le Pecq J-B (1974) Actions cardiovasculaires et toxicités de l'hydroxy 9 ellipticine chez le chien. CR Acad Sci [D] Paris 279: 1039–1042
41 Rakieten N, Cooney D, Davis R (1970) Acute toxicity of ellipticine (NSC 71795) following i.v. and p.o. administration to beagle dogs with special emphasis on its hypotensive action. US Dep Commer Natl Tech Inf Serv, PB 174–743
42 Reinhold VN, Bruni RJ (1976) Aromatic hydroxylation of ellipticine in rats: Lack of an NIH shift. Biomed Mass Spectrom 3: 335–339
43 Sainsbury M (1977) The synthesis of 6H-pyrido (4,3-*b*) carbazoles. Synthesis 7: 437–448
44 Svoboda GH, Poore GA, Montfort M (1968) Alkaloids of ochrosia maculate (*Ochrosia borbonica* G mel). Isolation of the alkaloids and study of the antitumor properties of 9-methoxy ellipticine. J Pharm Sci 57: 1720–1725
45 Tomasz M, Mercado C, Olson J, Catterjie N (1974) The mode of interaction of mitomycin C with deoxyribonucleic acid and other polynucleotides in vitro. Biochemistry 13: 4878–4887
46 Van-Bac N, Moisand C, Gouyette A, Muzard G, Dat-Xuong N, Le Pecq J-B, Paoletti C (to be published) Metabolic and diposition studies of 9-hydroxy ellipticine and 2-methyl 9-hydroxy ellipticinium acetate in animals
47 White HL, White JR (1968) Lethal action and metabolic effects of streptonigrin on *Escherichia coli*. Mol Pharmacol 4: 549–565

*Comparative Pharmacokinetics of Chlorambucil and Melphalan in Man**

D. S. Alberts, S. Y. Chang, H.-S. G. Chen, B. J. Larcom, and T. L. Evans

Summary

We have studied the pharmacokinetics of orally administered chlorambucil and melphalan in patients with hematologic malignancies and solid tumors. With a standard oral dose of 0.6 mg/kg, chlorambucil showed much more rapid systemic appearance than did melphalan and had a mean peak plasma concentration and area under the plasma disappearance curve which was 3–4 times greater than that observed in patients receiving melphalan. Melphalan had extremely variable systemic availability which was not observed with chlorambucil, and was not related to problems in tablet formulation. Chlorambucil undergoes extensive active metabolism to phenylacetic acid mustard, whereas melphalan undergoes rapid chemical degradation and has little, if any, active metabolism. On a pharmacokinetic basis, chlorambucil's greater in vitro stability, its more rapid and predictable systemic availability after oral dosing, and its extremely low urinary excretion make it a more predictible alkylating agent for clinical use than melphalan, especially for patients with reduced renal function.

Introduction

Melphalan and chlorambucil are standard bifunctional alkylating agents for treatment of several hematologic and solid malignancies [8, 9 11]. Although both have ben available for use in man since the early 1960s, their distribution, metabolism, and elimination in cancer patients have been incompletely described. We have developed sensitive and specific assays for both of these drugs in biologic fluids in order to carry out detailed disposition studies [4, 7]. This report describes the preliminary comparisons of melphalan and chlorambucil disposition studies in patients with hematologic and solid malignancies.

---

* Presented in part at the American Society of Clinical Oncology, Washington, D.C., March, 1978. Supported by research grant CA-17094 and T32-GM07533 from the National Institutes of Health, U.S. Public Health Service, Department of Health, Education, and Welfare, and donations by Burroughs Wellcome Company, Research Triangle Park, North Carolina and the Phi Beta Sci National Sororoity, Lima, Ohio

Materials and Methods

Drug Assays. Melphalan was assayed using high-pressure liquid chromatography (HPLC) as previously described by CHANG et al. [4]. This isocratic HPLC procedure is sensitive to a minimum detectable level of 50 ng/ml plasma. The monohydroxy- and dihydroxymelphalan derivatives were separated and quantitated using a 45 : 55 methanol – water (2% acetic acid) solvent system for HPLC. Melphalan, monohydroxy-, and dihydroxymelphalan were quantitated in plasma and urine samples by counting the ^{14}C contents of their respective HPLC eluates. The protein-bound ^{14}C-melphalan in plasma was determined by comparing ^{14}C counts of methanol-soluble ^{14}C and total ^{14}C.

Chlorambucil was assayed using a GC-MS assay developed by CHANG et al. [7]. Deuterated chlorambucil-d8 was used as an internal standard. Chlorambucil was extracted with ethylacetate-hexane (1 : 1, v/v) after the addition of 4% perchloric acid and chlorambucil-d8 as an internal standard. The dried samples were then converted to trimethylsilyl (TMS) derivatives by the addition of 100 μl of bistrimethylsilyl trifluoroacetamide : CH_3CN : CH_2C1_2 (20 : 10 : 1, v/v/v). This mixture was reacted for 10 min at 100° C and the derivative was analyzed by a GC-MS procedure [7]. The assay has a sensitivity limit of 50 ng/ml plasma. At chlorambucil plasma concentrations of 50 and 1,000 ng/ml, the recovery (± SD) was $91.3 \pm 12.8\%$ and $90.5 \pm 3.0\%$, respectively.

In Vitro Melphalan and Chlorambucil Degradation in Hman Plasma. The spontaneous in vitro degradation rates of melphalan and chlorambucil were determined in distilled water and human plasma. Varying amounts of melphalan and chlorambucil were added to 1 ml water or human plasma at 37° C, and aliquots were removed at intervals of up to 12 h and assayed for the parent compounds.

Patients. Nine patients were studied after intravenous (IV) bolus melphalan administration [3] and 14 after oral (PO) dosing [1, 2] with 0.6 mg/kg. Oral chlorambucil pharmacokinetic studies have been completed in five patients. All patients had adequate renal function (i.e., Ccr > 60 ml/min) and had not received another anticancer drug within 4 weeks of these studies. Two of the oral-melphalan-treated patients and none of the chlorambucil patients had received narcoticies before or during these studies. All patients were fasted after midnight prior to the oral drug studies.

Drug Formulation, Dosage, and Administration. Melphalan and chlorambucil tablets and melphalan powder (Burroughs-Wellcome Co., Research Triangle Park, North Carolina) were used in these studies. ^{14}C-melphalan labeled in the ethyl moiety was provided by Dr. ROBERT ENGLE, Developmental Therapeutics Program, DCT, NCI, NIH, Bethesda, Maryland, and synthesized by the Stanford Research Institute, Palo Alto, California. Purity averaged 95% for melphalan. Specific activity was 33 μCi/mg (10.4 mCi/m*M*). For the melphalan studies 0.6 mg/kg body weight, and ^{14}C-melphalan, approximately 100 μCi, were administered together as a PO or IV dose. For chlorambucil studies 0.6–1.2 mg/kg was administered as a single bolus oral dose.

Blood and Urine Sampling. Blood (10 ml) was obtained from a heparin lock and collected in tubes containing 100 IU of heparin. Samples were taken just prior to the start of therapy at 5, 10, 15, 30, 45, and 60 min, and 2, 3, 4, 6, 8, and 24 h following drug administration.

The samples were placed on ice for a short period prior to centrifugation for 10 min at 3,000 rpm and 4° C. The separated plasma samples were stored at −70° C until they were assayed. Fractional urine collections were taken for the first 8 h and then at longer intervals for up to 24 h. Urine was stored at −70° C in sterile container, acidified with concentrated HCl.

Data Analysis. Melphalan and chlorambucil plasma concentration versus time data obtained from each patient and the combined data obtained from all patients were fitted to a multiexponential equation using a nonlinear regression computer program [10]. Preliminary parameter estimates were obtained using a recently published computer method [13]. The methods for the calculation of anticancer drug absorption lag time, plasma half-lives, and area under the plasma disappearance curves (CXT) have been described previously [1, 3]. By assuming complete absorption and elimination through liver and kidney only, the hepatic extraction ratios were calculated using the following equation:

$$\text{hepatic extraction ratio} = \frac{Q_b - Q_r}{1{,}500} \qquad (1)$$

where Q_b and Q_r are the total body clearance and renal clearance in ml/min.

Results

The in vitro degradation rate constants for melphalan and chlorambucil at 37° C in water and human plasma are presented in Table 1. Note that melphalan degrades at twice the chlorambucil degradation rate in water and almost three times the chlorambucil degradation rate in plasma. The degradation products of these two

Table 1. In vitro degradation rates of melphalan and chlorambucil in water and plasma at 37° C

Drug	Degradation rate constants[a] (H^{-1})	
	Water	Plasma
Melphalan	0.83	0.33
Chlorambucil	0.43	0.12

[a] $K = \frac{2.3 \log I_0/I_t}{T}$

where I_0 and I_t are the drug concentrations at time zero and time T, respectively compounds are comprised almost completely of their monohydroxy and dihydroxy derivatives [1, 3].

Representative plasma concentration · time curves for three patients given an oral dose of melphalan are shown in Fig. 1. The lag times for melphalan appearance in the systemic circulation (obtained from curve fitting of plasma disappearance data) were 60, 255, and 336 min for the three patients. In one patient who took melphalan under direct observation, there was no evidence of the drug in plasma or urine for up to 24 h of plasma sampling. This patient showed no evidence of drug-induced myelosuppression or antitumor effect. In contrast there was evidence of relatively rapid systemic appearance of chlorambucil after a bolus oral dose in all five of our study patients. Figure 2 shows representative plasma disappearance curves for chlorambucil and its major metabolite, phenylacetic acid mustard, in a patient who received 0.6 mg/kg of the parent compound. Note the rapid achievement of chlorambucil peak plasma levels and the early evidence of metabolism to phenylacetic acid mustard.

Comparative, mean, pharmacokinetic parameters for 14 melphalan patients and five chlorambucil patients administered drugs by oral bolus are presented in Tables 2 and 3. All plasma data have been adjusted to a standard dose of 0.6 mg/kg. As seen in Table 2, melphalan had an average absorption lag time of 59 min in 14 patients, whereas it took only an average of 12 min for chlorambucil to appear systemically. The chlorambucil mean peak plasma concentration and area under the plasma concen-

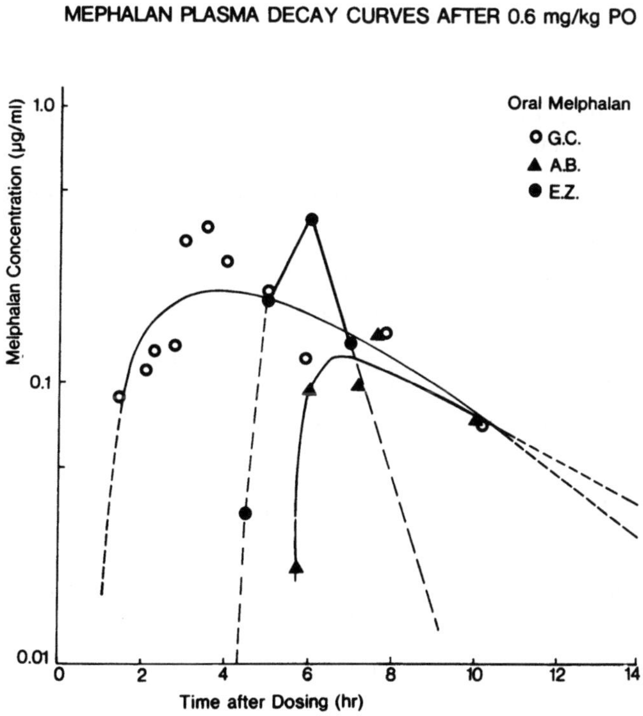

Fig. 1. Plasma disappearance curves for three patients who received an oral bolus dose of melphalan, 0.6 mg/kg

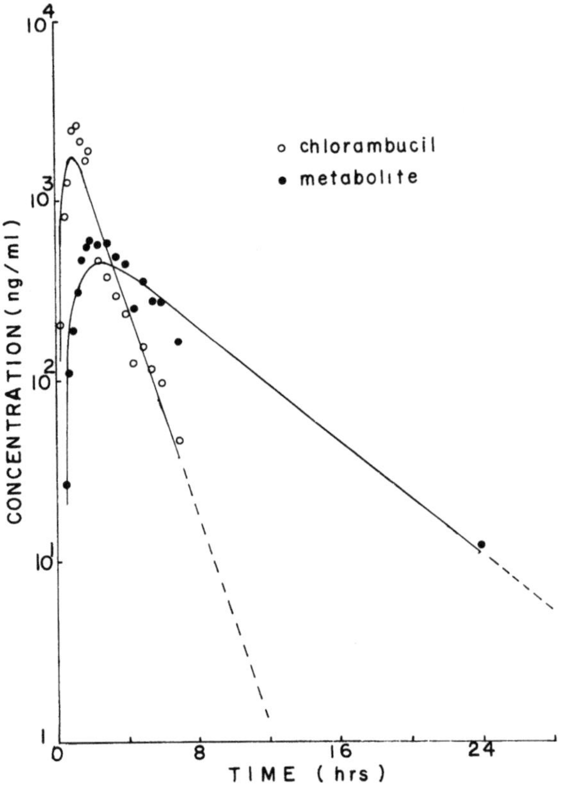

Fig. 2. Plasma disappearance curves for chlorambucil (O——O) and its metabolite, phenylacetic acid mustard (●——●), in a patient who was given 0.6 mg/kg of the parent compound as a bolus oral dose

Table 2. Comparison of melphalan and chlorambucil mean pharmacokinetic parameters after oral administration, 0.6 mg/kg

Drug	Absorption lag time[a] (min)	Peak plasma concentration (μg/ml)	Plasma CXT[b] (μg · min/ml)
Melphalan	59 (0–336)	0.3 ± 0.2	53 ± 33
Chlorambucil	12 (0–42)	1.4 ± 0.8	168 ± 105

[a] Lag time for the appearance of melphalan in the plasma after oral dosing (obtained from curve fitting of plasma concentration · time data)
[b] Plasma concentration · time product

Table 3. Comparison of melphalan and chlorambucil mean pharmacokinetic parameters after oral administration 0.6 mg/kg

Drug	$t_{1/2}^{\beta}$ (min)	Hepatic extraction ratio[a]	24-h Urinary excretion (%)
Melphalan	90 ± 57	–	10.92 ± 4.85
Chlorambucil	86 ± 22	0.22 ± 0.13	0.46 ± 0.23

[a] Calculated using Eq. (1)

tration · time curve (CXT) were 3–4 times greater than those seen in the melphalan-treated patients.

As seen in Table 3, the mean plasma $t^{\beta}_{1/2}s$ for melphalan and chlorambucil patients were similar. The mean hepatic extraction ratio for chlorambucil was 0.22 ± 0.13. Melphalan 24-h urinary excretion averaged $10.9 \pm 4.9\%$, whereas chlorambucil urinary excretion averaged only $0.4 \pm 0.2\%$ of the administered dose. In comparison with chlorambucil pharmacokinetics, phenylacetic acid mustard in five patients had a longer mean plasma $t^{\beta}_{1/2}$ (162 ± 45 min), larger mean plasma concentration · time product (210 ± 94 µg · min/ml), lower mean peak plasma concentration (0.77 ± 0.29 µg/ml), and similar mean 24-h urinary excretion ($0.29 \pm 0.17\%$ of the administered chlorambucil dose).

Discussion

We have compared the in vitro and in vivo disposition kinetics of two clinically important alkylating agents, melphalan and chlorambucil. Chlorambucil proved considerably more stable than melphalan in water and plasma at 37° C. Although melphalan rapidly degrades in these fluids, its stability is enhanced by an acid pH, by taurocholic acid, and chloride ion [5, 6].

Melphalan and chlorambucil have similar plasma half-lives after oral administration in cancer patients. Newell et al. have seen a 1.7-h plasma terminal-phase half-life in six patients treated with low-dose (about 0.15 mg/kg), oral chlorambucil [12]. This is comparable to the approximately 1.5-h half-life observed in our studies of five patients who received 0.6–1.2 mg/kg.

Although chlorambucil appears to have rapid systemic appearance after oral administration, oral melphalan has extremely variable absorption characteristics. In our patients, its lag time to first plasma appearance varied from 15 min to 6 h. Newell et al. have shown that chlorambucil had 67%–100% systemic availability after oral dosing in two patients studied after both oral and IV drug administration [12]. In contrast, our bioavailability studies of melphalan in cancer patients showed that melphalan has variable and, at times, negligible systemic availability [1, 2]. In five patients who received both oral and IV dosing, the ratio of their oral–IV plasma CXTs averaged less than 0.6 [8]. One myeloma patient showed no evidence of melphalan in plasma or urine for up to 24 h after oral dosing. In our chlorambucil studies, the CXT of five patients averaged 3–4 times that of melphalan at identical doses (i.e., 0.6 mg/kg, Table 2).

Tattersall et al. have reported that three patients given oral ^{14}C-melphalan excreted 20%–50% of the radioactive dose in a 6-day period [14]. Thus, one possible explanation for melphalan's variable and low systemic availability is decreased absorption from the gastrointestinal tract in some patients. The formulation of the melphalan tablet is probably not responsible for the drug's eratic bioavailability. Three of our patients were studied after identical doses of tablets and orally administered melphalan solution [1]. There were no significant differences between the plasma CXTs of the tablets or solution in any of these patients.

Chlorambucil's 24-h urinary excretion was less than 0.5% of the administered dose, whereas melphalan had a urinary excretion of greater than 10% (Table 3). Chlorambucil's low urinary excretion is perhaps related to its rapid metabolism. Its in vitro degradation rate is slow, but its major metabolite, phenylacetic acid mustard, appears in plasma soon after chlorambucil's appearance (Fig. 2). The metabolite achieves lower peak plasma levels and larger plasma CXTs than does its parent compound. There is no evidence that melphalan undergoes active metabolism in humans [1, 3]. It degrades rapidly in vitro in human plasma to its monohydroxy and dihydroxy derivatives. We have been unable to identify any other important degradation products or metabolites in the plasma or urine of patients treated with the oral drug. Furthermore, melphalan's disappearance was not significantly enhanced by incubation in rat liver microsomal enzyme preparations or by passage through the isolated, perfused rat liver (T. L. Evans and S. Y. Chang, unpublished work). On a purely pharmacokinetic basis, chlorambucil's greater in vitro stability, its more rapid and predictable systemic availability after oral dosing, and its extremely low urinary excretion make it a more predictable alkylating agent than melphalan, especially for patients with reduced renal function. In clinical trials, chlorambucil has proven equally as effective as melphalan for the treatment of ovarian carcinoma [9]. Unfortunately, little information exists concerning its efficacy in patients with multiple myeloma. These patients, who frequently have impaired renal function, might benefit from chlorambucil's improved disposition characteristics.

References

1 Alberts DS, Chang SY, Chen H-SG, Evans TL, Moon TE (1980) Oral melphalan kinetics. Clin Pharmacol and Ther 26: 737–745

2 Alberts DS, Chang SY, Chen H-SG, Gross JF, Walson PD, Moon TE, Salmon SE (1978) Variability of melphalan absorption in man. Proc Am Assoc Cancer Res and Am Soc Clin Oncol 19: C-112

3 Alberts DS, Chang SY, Chen H-SG, Moon TE, Evans TL, Furner RL, Himmelstein K, Gross JF (1979) Pharmacokinetics of melphalan in man: Intravenous administration. Clin Pharmacol and Ther 26: 73–80

4 Chang SY, Alberts DS, Melnick LR, Walson PD, Salmon SE (1978) High-pressure liquid chromatographic analysis of melphalan in plasma. J Pharm Sci 67: 679–681

5 Chang SY, Evans TL, Alberts DS (1979) The stability of melphalan in the presence of chloride ion. J Pharm Pharmacol 3: 853–854

6 Chang SY, Evans TL, Alberts DS, Sipes IG (1978) The stability of L-phenylalanine mustard in bile. Life Sci 23: 1697–1702

7 Chang SY, Larcom BJ, Alberts DS, Larsen B, Walson PD, Sipes IG (1980) Mass spectrometry of chlorambucil, its degradation products and its metabolite in biological samples. J Pharm Sci 69: 80–84

8 Fisher B, Carbone P, Economou SG, Frelick R, Glass A, Lerner H, Redmond C, Zelen M, Band P, Katrych DL, Wolmark N, Fisher E (1975) L-Phenylalanine mustard (L-PAM) in the management of primary breast cancer. A report of early findings. N Engl J Med 292: 117–122

9 Livingston RB, Carter SK (1970) Single agents in cancer chemotherapy. Plenum, New York, pp 81–111

10 Metzler CM (1969) NONLIN: A computer program for parameter estimation in nonlinear situations. Upjohn Company, Kalamazoo, Michigan, Technical Rep 7292/69/2792/005

11 Moore GE, Bross IDJ, Ausman R, Nadler S, Jones R, Jr, Slack N, Rimm AA (1968) Effects of chlorambucil (NSC 3088) in 374 patients with advanced cancer. Cancer Chemother Rep 52: 661–666

12 Newell DR, Hart LI, Harrap, KR (1979) The estimation of chlorambucil, phenyl acetic mustard and prednimustine in human plasma by high-performance liquid chromatography. Journal of Chromatography 164: 114–119

13 Sedman AJ, Wagner JG (1976) CSTRIP. A Fortran IV computer program for obtaining initial polyexponential parameter estimates. J Pharm Sci 65: 1006–1010

14 Tattersall MHN, Jarman M, Newlands ES, Holyhead L, Milstead RAV, Weinberg A (1978) Pharmacokinetics of melphalan following oral or intravenous administration in patients with malignant diseases. Eur J Cancer 14: 507–513

Clinical Implications of Cisplatin Pharmacology

F. M. Muggia, M. Rozencweig, and J. Penta

Summary

Extensive investigation is taking place to overcome the nephrotoxic manifestations and the gastrointestinal intolerance of cisplatin. Various modes of administration are being explored for this purpose with different schedules, infusion durations, hydration programs, and diuretic regimens. Pharmacokinetic studies suggest that such manipulations may lead to considerable variations in cisplatin excretion and in peak plasma levels of the non-protein-bound species. The clinical impact of these pharmacokinetic alterations is not currently apparent. This should be clarified with additional studies of the behavior of non-protein-bound platinum and its relationship to clinical efficacy and toxicity.

Introduction

Cisplatin, *cis*-diamminedichloroplatinum (II), is the first of the platinum coordination complexes to be used as an antitumor agent in man. Following its introduction into clinical investigation in 1970, extensive studies delineated its spectrum of activity and its toxicologic and pharmacologic properties. These clinical investigations culminated in establishing the therapeutic efficacy of this compound in various malignancies, especially testicular cancer [17, 18]. The drug is presently used in first-line chemotherapy as a single agent or in combination regimens for an increasing number of tumor types [17, 18].

Interpretation of clinical studies is rendered complex by the wide variety of dose schedules that have been employed. In the initial phase II studies, the drug was essentially given by intravenous (IV) push every 3 weeks at doses of 50 mg/m^2 or lower [11] or in a daily for 5 days schedule at doses of 20 mg/m^2/day [10]. The possibility of achieving clinical protection from dose-limiting nephrotoxicity by hydration and forced diuresis was first reported by Hayes and co-workers [8] and led to growing interest in determining optimal modes of administration of the drug. More recently, efforts to overcome gastrointestinal toxicity further stimulated the exploration of new dose schedules, primarily utilizing continuous infusion regimens.

Pharmacologic studies are required to investigate the consequences of such alterations in dose schedules. This paper reviews successively: (a) the experimental effects and relevance of dose schedules, (b) the major clinical toxicities, and (c) the clinical pharmacokinetics. In addition, factors altering drug pharmacology in various clinical situations and their possible applications will be discussed. Knowledge of drug pharmacology may be useful in the recognition and exploitation of interactions with other drugs and radiation, and in the safe exploration of other routes of administration.

Experimental Effects

Cisplatin demonstrates a wide spectrum of activity against rodent tumors [18]. In the L1210 murine leukemia, this effect does not display appreciable schedule dependence [18]. These experiments, however, rely on an IP-IP system and do not properly reproduce the clinical situation. Cytotoxicity of cisplatin has been attributed to its interaction with DNA, in a manner bearing a similarity to bifunctional alkylating agents [17]. The *cis* configuration appears to be important in achieving DNA interstrand cross-linking, the latter correlating with the cytotoxic potency of the *cis* isomer relative to the corresponding *trans* species. Both isomers may also alkylate intracellular proteins, and DNA protein cross-links, which are sensitive to proteinase-K digestion, are recognized by alkaline elution techniques. Serum proteins also interact with cisplatin so that after 24-h incubation at 37° C, only 3%–6% of the drug is capable of passing through an ultrafiltration membrane [7]. Such protein-bound cisplatin in concentrations of 1.0 or 10.0 μ*M* shows no cytotoxicity to L1210 cells during 48-h exposure, whereas saline mixtures at similar concentrations produce a 12% and 67% growth inhibition, respectively, after similar incubation periods. It has also been shown that three components of cisplatin are present in blood: protein-bound, erythrocyte-bound, and free cisplatin [19].

In vitro cytotoxicity of cisplatin to human lymphoma cells has been quantitated by Drewinko and Gottlieb [5]. Cell kill is influenced both by dose and by duration of exposure with a similar 3-log reduction in cell viability being obtained with 50 μg/ml (170 μ*M*) for 1 h or 5 μg/ml (17 μ*M*) for 8 h. The cell kill effect with the latter, however, was obtained with a lower $c \times t$ value, suggesting that prolonged infusions of cisplatin might be advantageous for therapeutic use.

Extensive studies of the pharmacologic disposition of cisplatin in a number of animal species have been published by the Laboratory of Toxicology, National Cancer Institute (Table 1) [13]. Platinum in biologic samples has been mostly determined by flameless atomic absorption spectrometry, which is exceeded in sensitivity only by

Table 1. Distribution and elimination half-lives of cisplatin in several species[a]

Species	$T_{1/2}$ (α)	$T_{1/2}$ (β)	Comment
Mouse	1.5–5 h		Whole body scintillation
Rat	8.6 min	44.9 h	Nontumored
	16.1 min	6.6 day	Tumored
	9.7 min	35.7 h	Control
	12.0 min	22.9 h	Hydrated
Dog	22.0 min	5.0 day	
Shark	71.0 min	17.5 day	

[a] Modified from Litterst et al. [13]

more cumbersome radioactive tracer studies. Pharmacokinetics of platinum in dogs and rats are quite similar and not unlike that in man, showing a rapid distribution phase and a prolonged elimination phase [$t_{1/2}(\beta)$]. The dogfish shark has a very long β half-life (17.5 days), reflecting a lesser renal excretion. Organ distribution in five animal species indicates similar rapid equilibration of platinum in all tissues, and subsequent accumulation to a few selected organs (kidney, liver, muscle, and skin) [13]. Significant levels of platinum are found in kidney, liver, skin, and lung 2–4 weeks after treatment. Prolonged retention in bone has also been reported. High concentrations in the ovary and uterus have been noted in dogs. Only low concentrations of platinum have been localized to the brain or testes in the species studied. Preferential localization in tumor tissues has not been consistently found.

Toxic Effects: Relation to Dose and Schedule

Phase I clinical trials identified dose-dependent nephrotoxicity as the most serious toxic effect of the drug, occurring with increasing frequency in doses greater than 50 mg/m^2 [17]. Dose fractionation was initially used to overcome this problem, but subsequently longer infusion duration and fluid supplementation and forced diuresis with mannitol and furosemide were introduced. These latter measures allow safe increases in dose up to a maximum of 120 mg/m^2 given as a bolus. Above this level, dose-limiting nephrotoxicity and other toxic manifestations become frequent and unpredictable.

Nausea and vomiting are universal at doses above 20 mg/m^2 given as a bolus. For this reason, fractionated schemes have lost their appeal, and attempts at overcoming this toxicity by prolonging the duration of infusion have been introduced [14, 15]. Although such measures have met with variable success, some amelioration seems likely.

Ototoxicity has been reported since the initial trials, often complicating the course of patients also experiencing nephrotoxicity. Myelosuppression, occasionally observed at lower doses, has become more frequent as more intensive regimens have been administered, particularly in patients with extensive prior therapy. Allergic reactions and neurotoxic manifestations, the latter appearing with prolonged treatments, have proven troublesome to some patients. Of more universal significance has been the development of electrolyte abnormalities, particularly hypomagnesemia which is often encountered and occasionally becomes symptomatic. Although a direct toxic effect of the drug on the renal tubules is likely, the diuretic regimen utilized may further contribute to these abnormalities.

Clinical Pharmacokinetics (Table 2)

Initial pharmacokinetic studies were reported by De Conti et al. in 1973 with IV bolus administration of radiolabeled compound [4]. These studies indicated a rapid distribution phase (α half-life: 25–49 min) and a slow elimination phase (β half-life: 58–73 h). The drug was predominantly (> 90%) protein-bound during this latter phase.

Table 2. Comparison of pharmacokinetic parameters in man

Author	Cisplatin dose (mg/m²)	Method, mannitol	Peak plasma level (μ*M*)	$t_{1/2}$ (β)	24-h urinary excretion (% dose)
Gormley et al. [7]	70	1-h Infusion, +	30.4 13.4[a]	67.0 h 40–45 min	23.0
Belt et al. [1]	100	Bolus, +	11.3[a]	58.7 min	16.1
		Bolus, 0	9.1[a]	48.9 min	40.3
		6-h Infusion, +	2.0[a]	26.0 min	14.5
		6-h Infusion, 0	0.8[a]	25.9 min	74.9
Ostrow et al. [16]	100	6-h Infusion, +	13.5	188.0 h	14.6
		6-h Infusion, 0	11.8		17.5[b]
Loo et al. [14]	100	5-day Infusion, 0	1.6–14.3	34.7 h	34.0[c]

[a] Non-protein-bound species
[b] Given furosemide prior to infusion
[c] 8-day collection

Subsequent investigations have extended these observations and have also studied the behavior of non-protein-bound platinum species. Gormley and co-workers [7] studied cisplatin kinetics by flameless atomic absorption spectroscopy in eight patients with ovarian cancer, free of ascites. These patients received 70 mg/m² of the drug infused over 1 h. All were prehydrated for 12 h prior to administration, and infused with 50 g of mannitol as a 10% solution from −1 h to +5 h relative to the start of cisplatin administration. Furosemide (40 mg) was given immediately before cisplatin. Peak *plasma levels* were 30.4 ± 5.9 μ*M* (range: 21.8–36 μ*M*) and followed a biphasic decline with half-lives of 23 min and 67 h for the rapid and slow phases, respectively. A tertiary phase was suggested by the observation of much higher levels than anticipated on day 21. *Urinary excretion* was rapid during and within 4 h after completion of the infusion, with excretion rates of 17 ± 2.7% at 4 h and 23 ± 3.9% at 24 h. Calculation of *renal clearance* of platinum indicated a steady decline from 100% of creatinine clearance at time zero to less than 2% in 5 h. From this relationship, it may be suspected that cisplatin is likely to be primarily excreted by glomerular filtration. Plasma levels of non-protein-bound species showed markedly different clearance kinetics than total platinum. Plasma half-life of this non-protein-bound species was only 8–10 min for the initial phase and 40–45 min for the secondary phase, with a non-protein-bound plasma concentration below 0.5 μ*M* at 4 h.

Belt and associates [1] measured non-protein-bound platinum species in carefully conducted protocols, randomly comparing two different schedules with and without mannitol. All patients received prehydration with 2 l of 5% dextrose and ½ normal saline over 12 h and were maintained on IV fluids for a minimum of 24 h. Kinetics following administration of 100 mg/m² of cisplatin by bolus (15 min) were compared with the same dose given with mannitol. A dose of 12 g of mannitol was administered by bolus before and after cisplatin. Peak plasma levels were 3.39 ± 1.4 μg/ml (11.3 μ*M*) with mannitol, and 2.73 ± 0.29 μg/ml (9.1 μ*M*) without mannitol. The elimination half-life was longer in the presence of mannitol (58.7 ± 4.9 min compared with 48.3 ± 3.2 min) and corresponded to much lower 24-h urinary excretion (16.1 ± 4.1% compared with 40.3 ± 4.1%).

The reduced urinary excretion of filterable platinum observed with mannitol must be pointed out. This effect on platinum retention was even more prominent when the drug was administered as a 6-h infusion. In these infusion studies, peak plasma levels were 0.61 ± 0.10 μg/ml (2 μ*M*) with mannitol and only 0.24 ± 0.02 μg/ml (0.8 μ*M*) without mannitol. Although elimination half-lives were quite comparable (26.0 ± 2.5 min and 25.9 ± 2.1 min), the corresponding cumulative 24-h urinary excretions were strikingly different: 19.5 ± 5.1% vs 74.9 ± 1.6%. it is evident that mannitol exerts a profound effect favoring the retention of platinum, a very unexpected effect. Predictably, with infusions as opposed to bolus administration, peak levels are lower and excretion becomes proportionately greater as non-protein-bound platinum is continuously and efficiently excreted. This may be, however, markedly affected by mannitol. Recent experience reported by Ostrow et al., when compared with the studies made by Belt et al., implies that a similar effect on renal excretion may be observed after furosemide [16]. In fact, an earlier study, in which neither mannitol nor any other diuretic measure was used, shows a greater urinary excretion of platinum [12].

Loo and co-workers [14] have reported on 5-day continuous infusion studies in seven patients receiving a loading dose of 5 mg/m^2 in 30 min followed by 20 mg/m^2/day for 5 days. In four patients, platinum levels were determined by a colorimetric method. Plasma concentrations were between 0.5 and 4.3 mg/l (1.6 and 14.3 μ*M*). The elimination half-life was 34.7 h. The cumulative urinary excretion over 5 days was 22% of the administered dose, and an additional 12% was excreted during the subsequent 3 days. One patient manifested oliguric renal failure during the infusion and had a much lower excretion. Nephrotoxicity (creatinine > 2 mg/dl) was observed in 21% of 61 courses. This relatively high incidence of renal impairment might have resulted from less vigorous hydration programs as compared with those commonly used in shorter-term pharmacokinetic studies.

Other reports have described prolonged retention of filterable platinum in the presence of ascites, and higher levels were obtained in one patient with deranged renal function [1]. Studies following repeated courses have indicated some accumulation of drug in the cerebrospinal fluid [9].

Discussion

The pharmacology of cisplatin has been the subject of several studies, but factors altering pharmacokinetics have been identified only recently. The cytotoxic moiety appears to be the non-protein-bound filterable fraction which is rapidly excreted in the urine by glomerular filtration; it also reacts as hydrated species with plasma proteins to become inactivated [16].

Duration of drug infusion and mannitol administration exert a remarkable effect on peak levels and urinary excretion of platinum. In rats, hydration with normal saline significantly increases the cumulative excretion of platinum in the urine but does not substantially alter plasma levels [13]. Experiments in dogs reported by Cvitkovic et al. [3] indicate greater urinary recovery but lower urinary concentration of platinum in prehydrated dogs than in controls. In contrast, Litterst et al. [13] found that prehydration increased both the excretion and the concentration of platinum in the urine of these dogs. In both studies, mannitol decreased the urinary concentration of platinum. Although protection has been described with these measures in experi-

Table 3. Mode of administration of cisplatin in protocol studies

Protocol	Total dose/ course (mg/m^2)	Schedule	Infusion duration	Mannitol	Furose- mide
NCI	70	d 1 q 3 weeks	1 h	+ inf.[a]	+
CALGB 260	50	d 1 q 3 weeks	1–2 h	+	0
CALGB 0703	70	d 1 q 3 weeks	bolus	+	0
CCSG 071	75	d 1 q 3 weeks	8 h	+	+
SWOG 7730	100	d 1 q 3 weeks	bolus	0 vs +	0
SWOG 7611	75	d 1–5 q 4 weeks	bolus	0	0
SWOG 7629	100	d 1,8 q 4 weeks	bolus	+	0
CALGB 7771	120	d 1,2 q 3 weeks	4 h	+ inf.[a]	(+)[b]
Roswell (Merrin)	60	d 1 q weeks	6 h	+ inf.[a]	0
Stanford (Jacobs)	80	d 1 q 3 weeks	24 h	0	0

[a] Infusion of mannitol spanning cisplatin administration
[b] Specified only if urinary output < 50 ml/h during mannitol administration

mental situations [18], mannitol and particularly furosemide have been found detrimental in overhydrated rats (given 10% of body weight of saline) (D. LEHANE, presented at the Meeting on Combined Modalities, Hilton Head, November 1978).

Clinical studies have incorporated a number of different therapeutic measures, mainly to circumvent nephrotoxicity (Table 3). The need for mannitol and/or furosemide at high-dose regimens is uncertain, and carefully designed clinical trials are required to study the consequences of resulting altered pharmacokinetics.

Other factors may alter cisplatin pharmacology. The presence of ascitic fluid would be expected to be a third space for cisplatin. Elderly patients with a lowered creatinine clearance (CrCl) might be more susceptible to nephrotoxicity and lessened urinary excretion. What effect concomitant therapy may have on cisplatin pharmacology is not known, but interaction with other nephrotoxic drugs is likely.

Pharmacologic monitoring may be of interest in studies employing new routes of administration such as intraarterial or intraperitoneal delivery. In this respect, it is noteworthy that breast carcinoma, which shows little or no sensitivity to IV cisplatin, has been reported to respond favorably to intraarterial administration [2]. Finally, further elucidation of pharmacokinetics and molecular pharmacology will be of assistance in the study of cisplatin analogues, and in drug-radiation interaction.

References

1 Belt RJ, Himmelstein KJ, Patton TF, Bannister SJ, Sternson LA, Repta AJ (1979) Pharmacokinetics of non-protein bound platinum species following administration of cis-diamminedichloroplatinum (II). Cancer Treat Rep 63: 1515–1521

2 Calvo DB, Patt YZ, Wallace S, Chuang VP, Benjamin RS, Pritchard JD, Hersh EN, Bodey GP, Mavligit GM (to be published) Phase I–II trial of percutaneous intraarterial cis-diamminedichloroplatinum (II) for regionally confined malignancy. Cancer

3 Cvitkovic E, Spaulding J, Bethune V, Martin J, Whitmore WF (1977) Improvement of *cis*-dichlorodiammineplatinum (NSC 119875): Therapeutic index in an animal model. Cancer 39: 1357–1361

4 De Conti RC, Toftness BR, Lange RC, Creasey WA (1973) Clinical and pharmacological studies with *cis*-diamminedichloroplatinum (II). Cancer Res 33: 1310–1315

5 Drewinko B, Gottlieb JA (1975) Action of *cis*-dichlorodiammineplatinum (II) (NSC-119875) at the cellular level. Cancer Chemother Rep 59: 665–673

6 Frick GA, Ballentine R, Driever CW, Kramer WG (1979) Renal excretion kinetics of high-dose cis-dichlorodiammineplatinum (II) administered with hydration and mannitol diuresis. Cancer Treat Rep 63: 13–16

7 Gormley PE, Bull JM, LeRoy AF, Cysyk R (1979) Kinetics of cis-dichlorodiammineplatinum. Clin Pharmacol Ther 25: 351–357

8 Hayes DM, Cvitkovic E, Golbey RB, Scheiner E, Helson L, Krakoff IH (1977) High dose cis-platinum diammine dichloride. Amelioration of renal toxicity by mannitol diuresis. Cancer 39: 1372–1381

9 Higby DJ, Buchholtz L, Chary K, Avellaroga A, Henderson ES (1977) Kinetics of cis-platinum (DDP) with intensive diuresis. Proc Am Assoc Cancer Res and Am Soc Clin Oncol 18: 110

10 Higby DJ, Wallace HJ Jr, Albert D, Holland JF (1974) Diamminodichloroplatinum in the chemotherapy of testicular tumors. J Urol 112: 100–104

11 Kovach JS, Moertel CG, Schutt AJ, Reitemeier RG, Hahn RG (1973) Phase II study of *cis*-diamminedichloroplatinum (NSC-119875) in advanced carcinoma of the large bowel. Cancer Chemother Rep 57: 357–359

12 Lange RC, Spencer RP, Harder HC (1973) The antitumor agent cis-pt $(NH_3)_2Cl_2$: Distribution studies and dose calculations from ^{193m}Pt and ^{195m}Pt. J Nucl Med 14: 191–195

13 Litterst CL, LeRoy AF, Guarino AM (1979) The disposition and distribution of platinum following parenteral administration to animals of cis-dichlorodiammine platinum II. Cancer Treat Rep 63: 1485–1492

14 Loo TL, Hall SW, Salem P, Benjamin RS, Lu K (1978) Clinical pharmacologic and toxicological studies of cis-diamminedichloroplatinum (II) by continuous intravenous infusion. Biochimie 60: 957–960

15 Merrin C (1976) A new method to prevent toxicity with high doses of *cis*-diammine platinum (therapeutic efficacy in previously treated widespread and recurrent testicular tumors). Proc Am Assoc Cancer Res and Am Soc Clin Oncol 17: 243

16 Ostrow S, Egorin M, Hahn D, LeRoy A, Markus S, Aisner J, Chang P, Foreman R, Bachur N, Wiernik PH (1979) High dose cis-dichlorodiammine platinum (C-DDP) therapy: Pharmacokinetic analysis and toxicity using furosemide (F) vs mannitol (M) diuresis. Proc Am Assoc Cancer Res and Am Soc Clin Oncol 20: 88

17 Rozencweig M, Von Hoff DD, Abele R, Muggia FM (to be published) Cisplatin. In: Pinedo H (ed) Cancer chemotherapy annuals. Elsevier/North-Holland Biomedical, Amsterdam

18 Rozencweig M, Von Hoff DD, Slavik M, Muggia FM (1977) Cis-diamminedichloroplatinum (II): A new anticancer agent. Ann Intern Med 87: 613–621

19 Wolf W, Cole W, Manaka RC, Odenheimer B (1979) Metabolites of *cis*-dichlorodiamminoplatinum in blood. Its implication for the "active" drug level. Proc Am Assoc Cancer Res and Am Soc Clin Oncol 20: 185

Cisplatinumdiamminodichloride (CPDD) in Chemotherapy of Cancers: A Phase II Therapeutic Trial

M. Hayat, G. Brulé, P. Cappelaere, A. Cattan, J. Chauvergne, B. Clavel, J. Guerrin, J. L. Misset, E. Pommatau, P. Ribaud, F. M. Muggia, M. Rozencweig, and G. Mathé

Summary

We have conducted a phase II trial of cisplatinumdiamminodichloride (CPDD) which not only demonstrated its remarkable activity in embryonic carcinoma of the testes, but also in ovarian carcinoma, in melanoma, and in epidermoid carcinoma, especially of the head and of the uterus cervix. Its toxicity, manifested mainly in the digestive and renal tracts, confines its administration to hospitalized patients only. This compound is now indicated in combination therapy for the above-mentioned tumors.

Introduction

Cisplatinumdiamminodichloride (CPDD) is the first of a series of platinum salts which has been shown to inhibit tumor proliferation in vitro [18–20], and to decrease the growth of different murine tumors in vivo, such as Dunning's leukemia, Walker's tumor [11], sarcoma 180 [21], and DMBA-induced mammary tumor in rats [25]. The cellular target for CPDD's action is DNA [2, 6, 10], to which its molecule is linked.

Experimental toxicologic studies have demonstrated adverse effects of CPDD on digestive, renal, and hematopoietic systems [24]. Early phase I and II clinical trials confirmed these side effects but, at the same time, yielded response rates of up to 80% in testicular cancer, 60% in hematosarcoma, 40% in head and neck cancer, and 40% in cancer of the ovary [4, 8, 12, 15, 22, 26]. CPDD is being used in several chemotherapeutic combinations, in which it seems to contribute significantly to their efficacy [5, 13, 23].

The object of this work was to determine the results of the phase II trial of this drug. The trial revealed the beneficial action of CPDD in some kinds of cancer not emphasized in previous communications, namely, in carcinoma of the uterus cervix and malignant melanoma.

Materials and Methods

The criteria for inclusion of patients in this phase II trial were the same as those defined for the phase II trials conducted by the EORTC, i.e., "search for the sensitivity of major cancers to a new therapeutic agent." Only patients who had advanced cancers not amenable to other therapy were included in the trial, hoping for

Table 1. CPDD Phase II trial

Number of patients included in the trial: 144	
Males:	87
Females:	57
Age range: 5–77 years (median: 53 years)	

Table 2. CPDD Phase II trial: Evaluable patients

Nonevaluable patients	
Major toxicity after 1 or 2 administrations of the drug: 3 cases (2 renal and 1 digestive toxicity)	
Loss of follow-up: 4	
Evaluable for efficacy	137 patients
Evaluable for toxicity	140 patients

some benefit from the new product, based on knowledge obtained from experimental studies and possibly from ongoing clinical trials. The optimal dose for the phase II trial had to be determined by phase I trials which were carried out, in the case of CPDD, by Higby et al. [8]. Thus, included in this trial were 144 patients for whom it was not only ethical, but indicated, to attempt CPDD treatment (Table 1). Table 2 shows that only 137 of these patients were studied. The reasons for the elimination of some patients from the trial are indicated in the table.

The criteria for evaluation are presented in Tables 3 and 4. The object of the phase II trial was to search for and evaluate the effects of an agent in terms of tumor-regression induction. The length of regression was documented only when, for ethical reasons, the administration of the product could be continued. For these same reasons, its administration was discontinued when a result was obtained which led the physician to modify the treatment so that the best therapeutic strategy could be applied to each patient.

We observed complete regressions (CR), partial regressions of more than 50% of the tumor volume (PR > 50%), mild regressions of less than 50% (MR < 50%), stabilizations (no change, NC), or progressions of the diseases (PD). We have not, contrary to certain definitions, considered stabilizations as "responses" to the drug.

The protocol for CPDD administration, shown in Fig. 1, indicates not only the dose, but also the measures recommended by Hayes et al. [7] for securing a sufficient diuresis. The tests to which the patients were submitted are listed in Fig. 1. Patients with the slightest evidence of renal or labyrinthic disorders were considered as ineligible for the trial.

The cycle of administration was repeated every 21 days. For this study, the patients to be evaluated as responders or nonresponders had to have received two or more cycles in case of improvement or stabilization; the patients who had received no more than one cycle were considered as evaluable only if a progression of the disease under therapy was noticeable. All the lesions were assessed and the regressions mentioned above are only those which were measurable and objective.

Table 3. CPDD Phase II trial: Evaluation of the results

	Efficacy
E_4:	Complete regression (CR)
E_3:	Partial regression (PR > 50%)
E_2:	Mild regression (MR < 50%)
E_1:	No change
E_0:	Progression of the disease

Table 4. CPDD Phase II trial: Evaluation of the results

	Toxicity
IT_0:	No toxicity
IT_1:	Minor toxicity or toxicity easily counteracted by symptomatic treatment and/or not necessitating modification of the treatment
IT_2:	Moderate toxicity not responding adequately to symptomatic treatment and/or necessitating an adaptation of the treatment (i.e., reduction and/or modification of dosage frequency) or delayed toxicity (occurring after the end of therapy)
IT_3:	Major toxicity necessitating discontinuation of the drugs
IT_4:	Toxicity that caused death
IT_9:	Toxicity that could not be evaluated

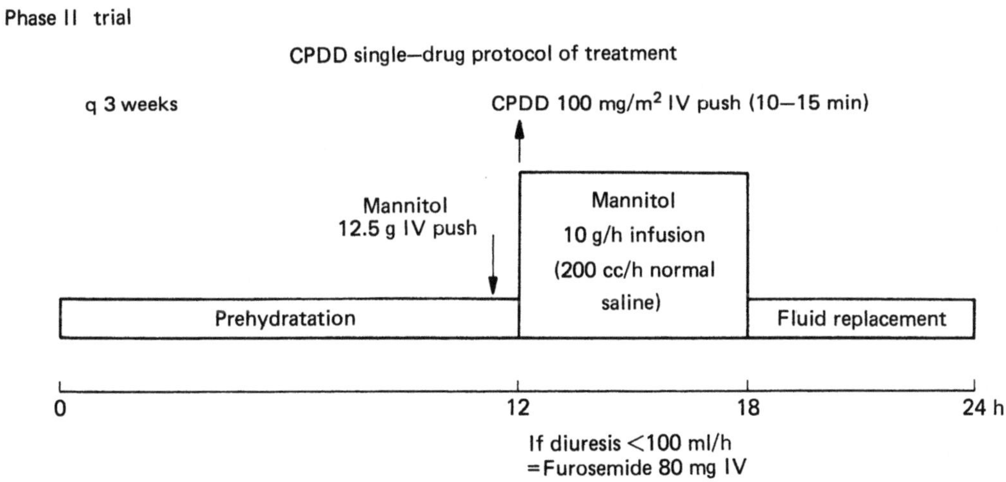

Required examination for entering the trial

- BC (WBC > 3000/mm³ and plat. > 100000/mm³)
- BUN (< 40 mg %) creatinine (< 1.5 mg % and/or clearance > 75 ml/min)
- Urinalysis; uric ac: bilirubin, SGOT, SGPT
- IV urography
- Audiogram

Fig. 1. Protocol and required examination for entering the trial

Table 5. CPDD Phase II trial: Efficacy of CPDD alone in testicular tumors

	Number of patients	Failure	Mild regression < 50%	Partial regression > 50%	Complete regression	Response rate
No prior chemotherapy	8	2	1	1	4	5/8 (62%)
Prior chemotherapy	14	7	4	3	–	3/14 (21%)
Total	22	9	5	4	4	
Response rate	> 50%				−36%	
	Overall			59%		

Table 6. CPDD Phase II trial: Efficacy of CPDD alone in squamous cell carcinoma

Diagnosis	Number of patients	Failure ($E_0 + E_1$)	Mild regression < 50%	Partial regression > 50%	Complete regression
Head and neck	31	23	4	4	
Esophagus	10	4	1	3	2
Lung	4	3		1	
Cervix	15	8	3	3	1
Total	60	38	8	11	3
Response rate	> 50%				23%
	Overall			37%	

Table 7. CPDD Phase II trial: Efficacy of CPDD alone in various tumors

Diagnosis	Number of patients	Failure	Mild regression < 50%	Partial regression > 50%	Complete regression	Response rate
Melanoma	10	5		4	1	5/10 (50%)
Skin	3	2		1		
Breast	10	8	1	1		1/10
Endometrial	4	3	1			
Ovary	8	6	1	1		1/8
Bone	5	5				
Soft-tissue sarcoma	10	10				0/10
Renal	3	3				
Total	53	42	3	7	1	

Table 8. CPDD Phase II trial: Toxicity

Type	Degree				
	No toxicity (IT_0)	Mild (IT_1)	Moderate (IT_2)	Severe (IT_3)	Lethal (IT_4)
Digestive	16	82	38	4	0
Myeloid	97	29	13	1	0
Renal	125	5	5	5	0
Ototoxicity	113	18	7	2	0
General (asthenia; weight loss)	118	17	4	1	0

Other toxicity: seizure: 2 cases; hypocalcemia: 1 case

Results

The overall results are presented in Tables 5–7. The regression rate was 59% in patients with testicular cancer (4 CR, 4 PR > 50%, and 5 MR < 50%). Of 22 patients, 21 had an embryonic type of tumor and one had a disseminated seminoma. The results obtained in patients who had cancer of the uterus cervix were also remarkable. The rate of regression in 15 patients was 46% (1 CR, 3 PR > 50%, and 3 MR < 50%). In head and neck cancer, the response rate was 26% (4 PR and 4 MR in 31 patients). Worth mentioning also are 2 CR, 3 PR and 1 MR in ten cases of carcinoma of the esophagus. We have also recorded 1 CR and 4 PR in ten melanomas.

Even if the number of patients included in this trial is rather low, the results obtained in cancers of the ovary, breast, and endometrium leave us with the hope that these tumors might eventually be sensitive to CDDP. Table 5 shows that the patients who had not been previously treated by chemotherapy were, in general, more often sensitive to CDDP than those who had previously received any of the currently available chemotherapy regimens.

Toxic effects (Table 8), in order of frequency, were mainly digestive tract intolerance (80%), manifested by anorexia, nausea, and vomiting; anemia (29%), always correctable by blood transfusion; vestibulolabyrinthic lesions (19%), which were frequent enough to warrant repeated audiograms; and renal involvement (11%), which was much less frequent, probably due to measures taken concerning diuresis. General side effects, such as malaise and weight loss, did not exceed 24%. We also observed two seizures.

Discussion

CPDD is the product of a new series of oncostatics significantly contributing to the therapy of testicular, ovarian, and head and neck cancers and, as our trial showed, also to the therapy of uterus cervix cancer and melanoma. Its immediate digestive tract toxicity could hardly be avoided in the protocol we used and could not be easily controlled, except in hospitalized patients. It would be of value to conduct the trials with lower doses of the drug, at about 1 mg/kg each week, which reportedly cause less vomiting and could be given to outpatients [14].

Renal toxicity appeared to be lowered by increasing diuresis and by a priori ineligibility for entry to the trial of patients with organic or functional kidney disease. Certainly, the sensitivity of the kidney to CPDD must be considered when including this drug in combination therapy. Some have combined it with cytembena, also a nephrotoxic drug [3], in the treatment of epidermoid cancer [13], in which cytembena was shown to have some efficacy.

CDDP is far from being active in all patients who have the above-mentioned tumors, since they are either primarily or secondarily resistant to the drug. This is a good reason to study other related substances, namely, malonatoplatinum (PHM) which, experimentally, might not present cross-resistance with CPDD, as shown by Burchenal et al. [1], and as suggested clinically by Ribaud et al. [16, 17].

References

1 Burchenal JH, Kalaher K, O'Toole T, Chisholm J (1977) Lack of cross-resistance between certain platinum coordination compounds in mouse leukemia. Cancer Res 37: 3455–3457

2 Butour JL, Macquet JP, Paoletti C (1978) Inhibition of the in vitro growth rate of L1210 leukemic cells by platinum (II) derivatives. In: Satellite Symposium of the Seventh International. Congress of Pharmacology on Coordination chemistry and cancer chemotherapy. Toulouse, July (abstr 25)

3 Clinical Screening Group, EORTC (1977) A phase II clinical trial of cytembena. Biomedicine 26: 392–395

4 DeConti RC, Toftness BR, Lange RC, Creasey WA (1973) Clinical and pharmacological studies with cis-diaminedichloroplatinum (II). Cancer Res 33: 1451–1456

5 Eagan RT, Ingle JN, Frytak S, Rubin J, Kvols LK, Carr DT, Coles DT, O'Fallon JR (1977) Platinum-based polychemotherapy versus dianhydrogalactitol in advanced non-small cell lung cancer. Cancer Treat Rep 61: 1339–1345

6 Harder HC, Rosenberg B (1970) Inhibitory effects on anti-tumor platinum compounds on DNA, RNA and protein synthesis in mammalian cell in vitro. Int J Cancer 6: 207–216

7 Hayes DM, Cvitkovic E, Golbey RB, Scheiner E, Helson L, Krakoff IH (1977) High dose cis-platinum diammine dichloride. Amelioration of renal toxicity by mannitol diuresis. Cancer 39: 1372–1381

8 Higby DJ, Wallace HJ Jr, Holland JF (1973) Cis-diamminodichloroplatinum (NSC-119875): A phase I study. Cancer Chemother Rep 57: 459–463

9 Hill JM, Loeb E, Pardue AS, Khan A, Hill O, King JJ, Hill RW (1977) Platinum coordination compounds in the treatment of acute leukemia and other malignant diseases with particular reference ot malonato 1,2-diaminocyclohexane platinum (II). J Clin Hematol Oncol 7: 681–700

10 Howle JA, Gale GR (1970) Cis-dichlorodiammine platinum (II): Persistent and selective inhibition of deoxyribonucleic acid synthesis in vivo. Biochem Pharmacol 19: 2757–2762

11 Kociba RJ, Sleight SD, Rosenberg B (1970) Inhibition of Dunning ascitic leukemia and Walker 256 carcinosarcoma with cis-diamminedichloro platinum (NSC-119875). Cancer Chemother Rep 54: 325–326

12 Lippman AJ, Helson C, Helson L, Krakoff IH (1973) Clinical trials of cis-diamminedichloroplatinum (NSC 119875). Cancer Chemother Rep 57: 191–200

13 Mathé G, Hayat M, Misset JL, Bayssas M, Gouveia J, De Vassal F, Delgado M, Gil MA, Ribaud P, Machover D, Slioussartchouk V, Dantchev D (1979) Some new chemotherapeutic agents and combinations possibly available for new adjuvant therapies of minimal disease. Recent Results Cancer Res 68: 439–448

14 Merrin CE (1978) Efficacy of cis-diamminedichloroplatinum for the treatment of genitourinary tumors. Experience in 200 patients. In: Satellite Symposium of the Seventh International Congress of Pharmacology on Coordination chemistry and cancer chemotherapy. Toulouse, July (abstr 40)
15 Nitschke R, Starling KA, Vats T, Bryan H (1978) Cis-diamminedichloroplatinum (NSC 119875) in childhood malignancies: A Southwest Oncology Group Study. Med Pediatr Oncol 4: 127–132
16 Ribaud P, Alcock N, Burchenal JH, Young C, Muggia F, Mathé G (1979) Preclinical trial in baboon and phase I–II trial and pharmacokinetics in man of malonato-platinum (MP) (abstr C-186). Proc Am Soc Clin Oncol 20: 336
17 Ribaud P, Kelsen DP, Alcock N, Garcia-Giralt E, Dubouch P, Young CC, Muggia F, Burchenal JH, Mathé G (1980) Preclinical and phase I studies of malonatoplatinum. Recent Results Cancer Res 74: 166–172
18 Rosenberg B, Van Camp L, Krigas T (1965) Inhibition of cell division in *Escherichia coli* by electrolysis products from a platinum electrode. Nature 205: 698–699
19 Rosenberg B, Van Camp L, Grimley EB, Thomson AJ (1967) The inhibition of growth or cell division in *Escherichia coli* by different ionic species of platinum (IV) complexes. J Biol Chem 242: 1347–1352
20 Rosenberg B, Van Camp L, Trosko JE, Mansour VH (1969) Platinum compounds: A new class of potent antitumour agents. Nature 222: 385–386
21 Rosenberg B, Van Camp L (1970) The successful regression of large solid sarcoma 180 tumors by platinum compounds. Cancer Res 30: 1799–1802
22 Rossof AH, Slayton RE, Perlia CP (1972) Preliminary clinical experience with cis-diamminedichloroplatinum (II) (NSC 119875). Cancer 30: 1451–1456
23 Samson MK, Baker LH, Devos JM, Buroker TR, Izbicki RM, Vaitkevicius VK (1976) Phase I clinical trial of combined therapy with vinblastine (NSC-49842), bleomycin (NSC-125066) and cis-dichlorodiammineplatinum (II) (NSC-119875). Cancer Treat Rep 60: 91–97
24 Thompson HS, Gale GR (1971) Cis-dichlorodiammineplatinum (II): Hematopoietic effects in rats. Toxicol Appl Pharmacol 19: 602–609
25 Welsch CW (1971) Effects of cis-platinum diamminedichloride-II on growth of 7,12-dimethylbenzanthracene (DMBA)-induced mammary tumors in female rats (abstr). Proc Am Assoc Cancer Res 12: 25
26 Wiltshaw E, Carr B (1974) Cis-platinum (II) diamminedichloride. Clinical experience of the Royal Marsden Hospital and Institute of Cancer Research in London. Recent Results Cancer Res 48: 178–182

1,2-Diaminocyclohexane Platinum Derivatives of Potential Clinical Value

J. H. Burchenal, G. Irani, K. Kern, L. Lokys, and J. Turkevich*

Introduction

Cisdiamminodichloroplatinum (DDP) has assumed an important role in clinical cancer chemotherapy either alone or, more often, in combination with bleomycin, adriamycin, Cytoxan (cyclophosphamide), vindesine, or the arabinosylcytosine (ara-C) derivatives. With these combinations, many investigators have reported on activity in germ cell tumors of the testis, carcinoma of the head and neck, penis, cervix, bladder, lung, esophagus, and ovary [1, 7]. It has been used much less in the leukemias and lymphomas. Unfortunately, renal toxicity and severe nausea and vomiting have limited its usefulness, and compounds with less toxicity, greater antitumor effectiveness, and a broader spectrum of activity, including the leukemias and lymphomas, are being sought, particularly those lacking cross-resistance to DDP. As previously reported by various investigators [9, 13], the 1,2-diaminocyclohexane platinum derivatives seem to fit these criteria. In the experimental animal renal toxicity does not appear to be limiting [10], and in mouse leukemia there is no cross-resistance to DDP [2, 3]. The dichloro, malonato, and carboxyphthalato derivatives of 1,2-diaminocyclohexane platinum experimentally have shown a high degree of antitumor effectiveness [9, 13], marked synergism with ara-C derivatives, adriamycin, demethylepipodophyllotoxin ethylidene glucoside (VP-16) [2], and with cyclophosphamide, particularly in combination with various ribonucleotide reductase inhibitors such as hydroxyurea, guanazole, and MAIQ-1 [6]. Clinically, the malonato derivative has been reported by Hill et al. [8] to be clinically active in the acute leukemias, and by Ribaud et al. [11] to produce remissions in patients whose disease had become clinically resistant to DDP. Further studies on the dichloro, malonato, and carboxyphthalato derivatives of 1,2-diaminocyclohexane platinum in various mouse leukemia systems are herewith presented.

Materials and Methods

The techniques for evaluating the chemotherapeutic activity of a drug by its ability to prolong the survival time of mice with transplanted leukemia has been reported previously [4]. The experiments described here were done with mouse leukemia L1210, P388, and P815 and their respective sublines resistant to ara-C, methotrexate

* This research was supported by NCI grant CA-18856, ACS grant CH27U, and The Hearst Foundation Grant

(MTX), 5-fluorouracil, or DDP in C57BL/6 × DBA/2F_1 mice. L1210/DDP and P388/DDP are lines of leukemia L1210/0 and P388/0 that were treated with single 8-mg/kg doses of DDP 24 h after inoculation of the leukemias over successive generations until no increase in survival time was seen with any tolerated dose of DDP [3]. In all experiments, 1,000,000 leukemic cells suspended in 0.1 ml of 0.85% NaCl solution were inoculated intraperitoneally (IP) into each animal, producing an ascitic leukemia that later progressed to the generalized disease. The mice were divided into groups of ten animals each, and treatment was initiated 24 h to 6 days after the inoculation of leukemic cells, and continued once every fourth day (days 1, 5, 9, and 13). Compounds were dissolved in 0.85% NaCl solution or sterile H_2O and injected IP.

For cell culture studies, a modification of the technique of Fischer [5, 12] was used. The cells were incubated in McCoy's medium with 15% fetal calf serum. The initial inoculum was 40,000–60,000 leukemic cells/ml. For growth inhibition studies, 0.1 ml of a 50-fold concentration of the drug in question was added to 5 ml of the cell-containing media. The tubes were set up in groups of four, loosely capped, and allowed to incubate in 5% CO_2 at 37° C for 96 h. Growth to approximately 10^6 cells/ml occurred in the control tubes. The contents of each tube were agitated to resuspend the cells and counted on a Coulter counter. The percentage of inhibition of growth and the doses inhibiting 50% of cell growth were calculated. Cell culture experiments were done with lines of mouse leukemia L1210, L1210/DDP, and L5178Y.

Results

As reported previously [3], the only compounds so far showing complete lack of cross-resistance with DDP are the various derivatives of 1,2-diaminocyclohexane platinum and 1,2-diaminocycloheptane platinum (Fig. 1). In vitro these are equally effective against the DDP-sensitive and DDP-resistant lines of L1210, whereas DDP in this same system shows a 20- to 50-fold lack of sensitivity to the resistant line (Table 1). The situation is the same in the two strains of L1210 in vivo with the various 1,2-diaminocyclohexane and 1,2-diaminocycloheptane derivatives being highly active (Table 2). It is of interest that although the saturated cyclic compounds were active against the DDP-resistant L1210, the unsaturated orthophenylenediamine was not.

We have concentrated mainly on the cyclohexane derivatives, particularly the malonato which is in phase I and II clinical trials [11], and the carboxyphthalato which, because of its high solubility in 1% aqueous sodium bicarbonate, is undergoing preclinical toxicology by Philips of our group and should shortly be in phase I clinical trials. We have also studied the dichloro derivative which may be interesting for clinical trial if the solubility problem, which we will discuss later, can be solved, Recently, Gale et al. [6] demonstrated highly synergistic effects with the triple combination of cyclophosphamide and hydroxyurea or other ribonucleotide reductase inhibitors with either the malonato or the carboxyphthalato derivatives. In our studies, the most effective compounds in combination were VP-16, AAFC, and adriamycin. Table 3 shows the markedly increased activity of the malonato derivative in these combinations against advanced P388 leukemia, and Table 4 shows the relative effects of the combination versus the drugs alone using the dichloro and the malonato against advanced L1210 leukemia. Figure 2 shows the synergistic activity of the carboxy-

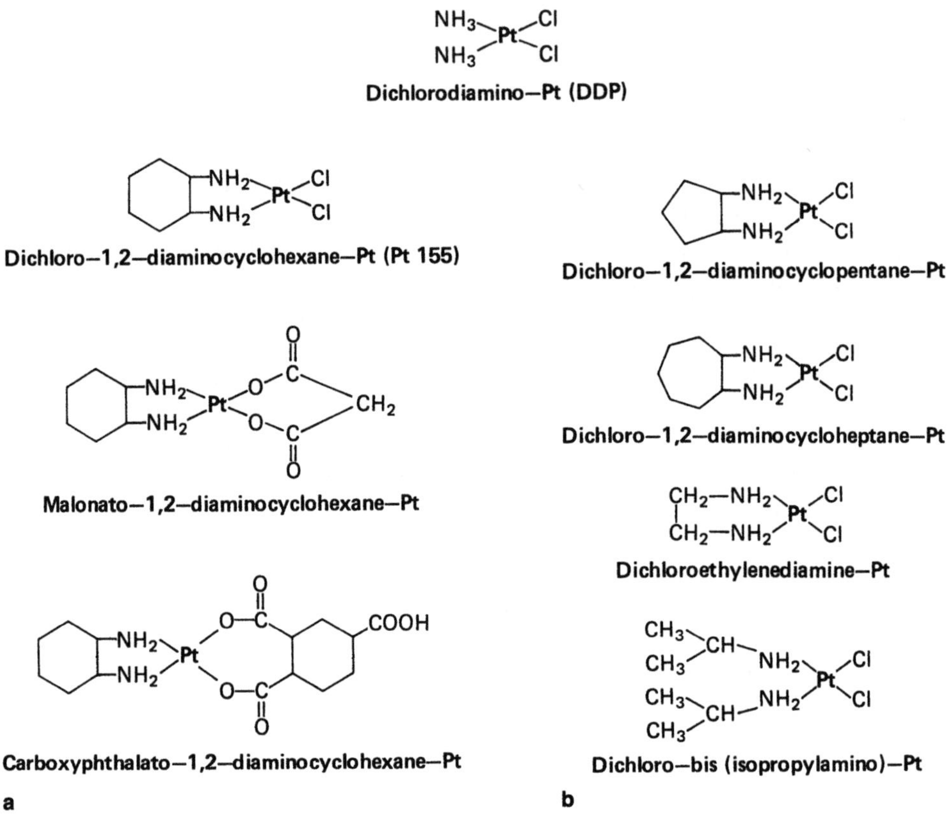

Fig. 1a, b. Various derivatives of 2-diaminocyclohexane platinum

Table 1. In vitro studies of cross-resistance of platinum coordination compounds (PtA_2X_2)

A	X	ID_{50} µg/ml	
		L1210	L1210/DDP
Diammino	Dichloro	0.05	2.50
Diammino	Malonato	0.40	6.50
1,2-Diaminocyclohexane	Malonato	0.25	0.25
1,2-Diaminocyclohexane	Dichloro	0.14	0.14
1,2-Diaminocyclohexane	Sulfato	0.20	0.36
1,2-Diaminocyclohexane	Carboxyphthalato	0.30	0.23
1,2-Diaminocycloheptane	Malonato	0.50	0.09
1,2-Diaminocycloheptane	Dichloro	0.06	0.20
1,2-Diaminocycloheptane	Sulfato	0.30	0.50
1,2-Diaminocyclopentane	Malonato	0.60	5.0
1,2-Diaminocyclopentane	Dichloro	0.30	4.6
1,2-Diaminocyclopentane	Sulfato	0.60	4.9
Ethylenediamine	Dichloro	0.35	29.0
Orthophenylenediamine	Dichloro	0.69	2.4
Bis(isopropylamino)	Dichloro	0.6	4.4
Bis(isopropylamino)	Sulfato	0.6	5.3

Table 2. In vivo studies of cross-resistance in leukemia L1210

Compound	Dose mg/kg days 1, 5, 9, 13	L1210		L1210/DDP		L1210/Pt 155[a]	
		Survival (days)	ILS (%)	Survival (days)	ILS (%)	Survival (days)	ILS (%)
Control	–	8.8	–	12.0	–	12.2	–
Diamminodichloroplatinum	6.7	–	–	12.3	3	18.9	55
Diamminodichloroplatinum	4.5	14.9	69	13.5	13	16.8	38
Dichloro-1,2-Diaminocyclo-hexane Pt	5.0	20.4	132	22.9	90.8	12.3	1
Dichloro-1,2-Diaminocyclo-heptane Pt	5.0	13.2	50	18.9	57.5	14.9	22
Dichloro-1,2-Diaminocyclo-pentane Pt	15.0	12.7	44	18.6	55	12.8	5
Dichloroethylenediammine Pt	20	14.3	63	13.2	10	–	–
Dichloroethylenediammine Pt	13	12.8	45	13.7	14	–	–

[a] Pt 155 is dichloro-1,2-diaminocyclohexane Pt

Table 3. Effect of combinations of malonato-1,2-Diaminocyclohexane platinum (Pt 174) with AAFC, VP = 16, and adriamycin against advanced P388/0 (doses in mg/kg days 4, 8, 12, 16)

Line	Drug	Dose	Mean	ILS (%)	50-day survivors
P388/0	Control	–	11.2	–	0/10
	VP = 16	20	27.1	142	0/10
	AAFC	400	20.5	83	0/10
	Adriamycin	4	13.9	24	0/10
	Pt 174	40	31.3	179	0/10
	Pt 174 VP-16	40 20	44.8	300	8/10
	Pt 174 AAFC	40 400	41.8	273	7/10
	Pt-174 Adriamycin	40 4	36.5	226	2/10
					Exp. 7227

phthalato in these combinations against advanced L1210, and Table 5 shows the synergistic effects of the combinations of AAFC with both the malonato and the carboxyphthalato derivatives, but the lack thereof with DDP in advanced DDP-resistant leukemia (L1210/DDP).

Since the malonato derivative has been difficult to use clinically because of its poor solubility when dissolved in 5% dextrose in water and its instability in the presence of the chloride ion of saline, we have studied other agents which might be useful in

Table 4. Effects of combinations VP-16, AAFC, or MTX with the dichloro- (Pt 155) or malonato- (Pt 174) 1,2-Diaminocyclohexane Pt derivatives on advanced L1210 (doses in mg/kg days 4, 8, 12, 16)

Line	Drug	Dose	Mean	ILS (%)	50-day survivors
L1210/0	Control	–	8.8	–	0/10
	Pt 155	5	15.5	76	0/10
	VP = 16	10	12.8	45	0/10
	AAFC	400	19.5	122	0/10
	MTX	12	15.8	79	0/10
	Pt 155 VP = 16	5 10	30.7	248	1/10
	Pt 155 AAFC	5 400	33.7	283	1/10
	Pt 155 MTX	5 12	28.6	225	0/10
	Pt 174	50	15.3	73	1/10
	Pt 174 VP = 16	50 10	32.3	267	2/10
	Pt 174 AAFC	50 400	35.2	300	2/10
	Pt 174 MTX	50 12	31.0	252	1/10
					Exp. 7274

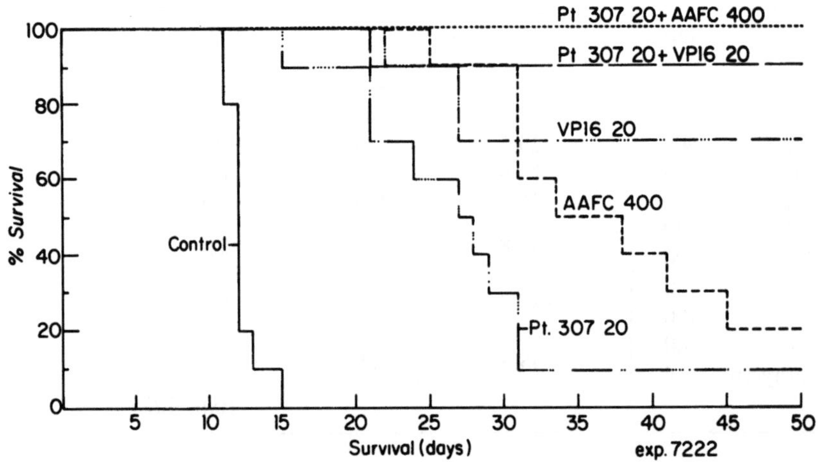

Fig. 2. Effects of carboxyphthalato-1,2-diamino cyclohexane Pt (Pt 307) in combination therapy against leukemia L1210 (dosage mg/kg q 4 d × 4, d 4, 8, 12, 16)

formulating the drug and enabling its administration in a smaller volume of fluid. Preliminary studies in mice in our laboratory have shown that the addition of *N*-methylglucamine (Fig. 3), 2 parts to 1 part of the malonato, has increased the solubility of this compound approximately 40-fold in distilled water. *N*-Methylglucamine (NMG) alone is highly soluble in water, relatively nontoxic, and well-tolerated

Table 5. Effect of the carboxyphthalato-Pt (Pt 307) and malonato-Pt (Pt 174) 1,2-Diaminocyclohexane Pt derivatives and AAFC against the DDP-resistant leukemia L1210/DDP (doses in mg/kg days 4, 8, 12, 16)

Line	Drug	Dose	Mean	ILS (%)	50-day survivors
L1210/DDP	Control	–	10.7	–	0/10
	Pt 307	30	16.2	51	0/10
	Pt 307	20	14.6	36	0/10
	DDP	4	12.4	16	0/10
	Pt 174	40	14.4	34	1/10
	AAFC	400	27.4	156	0/10
	Pt 307 AAFC	20 400	45.4	324	8/10
	DDP AAFC	4 400	25.6	139	0/10
	Pt 174 AAFC	40 400	42.9	300	4/10
					Exp. 7221

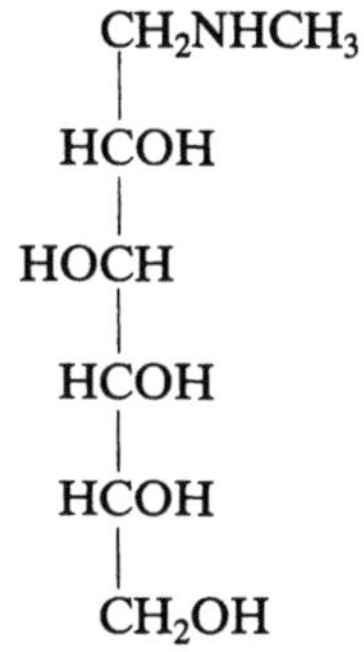

Fig. 3. *N*-Methylglucamine

in doses of 500 mg/kg q 4 d × 4. Surprisingly, however, NMG also renders the compound much more potent so that 3–5 mg/kg of the malonato derivative in the NMG formulation has a toxicity and apparent therapeutic effectiveness equal to 30–50 mg/kg of the malonato in suspension (Table 6). There also appears to be no cross-resistance with DDP (Table 7).

With the dichloro derivative there is at least a 10- to 20-fold increase in solubility, but preliminary studies indicate that the toxicity, therapeutic effectiveness, and lack of cross-resistance are essentially unaltered (Table 8).

Discussion

Compounds containing a 1,2-diaminosaturated cyclic moiety such as cyclohexane or cycloheptane are active against lines of leukemia L1210 and P388 sensitive to and resistant to DDP, whereas unsaturated amines, bis-substituted amines, and ethylenediamine derivatives are inactive. Lines resistant to dichloro-1,2-diaminocyclo-

Table 6. Comparative Activity of Pt 174 and Pt 174 NMG against leukemia L1210 (doses in mg/kg days 1, 5, 8)

	1	2	3	4	5	6	7	8	9	10	11	12	13	14	15	16	17	18	19	20	21	22
Control								**	*	*												
								**	*													
								**	*													
Pt 174 a 45										*							**		**	**		⇉→
Pt 174 a 30										*	**	*	**									
											**		**									
Pt 174 a 20									*	**	**			*								
										**	**											
Pt 174 NMG a 6.7											*	**	*	**			**					→
												*										
Pt 174 NMG a 4.5													*		**		**	*	*	*		→
																	*					
Pt 174 NMG a 3.0													*	*	**		**					⇉→
																	*					

Exp. 7462

Table 7. Comparative activity of malonato-1,2-diaminocyclohexane platinum (Pt 174) in suspension or formulated in solution with *N*-methylglucamine (Pt 174 NMG) (doses in mg/kg days 1, 5, 8)

	1	2	3	4	5	6	7	8	9	10	11	12	13	14	15	16	17	18	19	20	21	22	23	24	25
Control										*	***	**	*			**	*								
DDP a 6									*		***	*****			*										
DDP a 3												*****	***		*					*					
Pt 174 a 45																									→→→→→→→→→→
Pt 174 NMG a 4.5																									→→→→→→→→→→
Pt 174 NMG a 3.0																									→→→→→→→→→→
Pt 174 NMG a 2.0																									→→→→→→→→→→

Table 8. Comparative activity of Pt-155, Pt-155 (NMG), and DDP in leukemia L1210/DDP (doses in mg/kg days 1, 5, 9)

	1	2	3	4	5	6	7	8	9	10	11	12	13	14	15	16	17	18	19	20	21	22	23	24	25
Control												*****		*	*		**	*							
DDP a 6											**	****	**		**										
DDP a 4												******	*		*					**					
Pt-155 a 6.7																						****			→→→→→→
Pt-155 (NMG) a 10														*			*	*				*			→→→→→→
Pt-155 (NMG) a 6.7																						*			→→→→→→→→→

Exp. 7459

hexane platinum (Pt 155) still retain sensitivity to high doses of DDP. Substitutions on the anionic side may alter solubility, but have so far had no effect on the cross-resistance or lack thereof.

The problem of the solubility of the 1,2-diaminocyclohexane platinum derivatives is particularly acute with the dichloro and malonato. The carboxyphthalato, however, is stable in the dry form and is soluble in 1% aqueous sodium bicarbonate. This solution is stable enough for clinical use, but should be utilized within 2 h of reconstitution and is at present undergoing preclinical toxicology. Studies done elsewhere have shown that at the ID_{50}, both the malonato and the carboxyphthalato derivatives do not cause nephrotoxicity, whereas DDP causes severe nephrotoxicity at a comparable dose [10]. The malonato derivatives have been difficult to solubilize in the presence of chloride since the compound will rapidly degrade to the dichloro form, which is markedly more toxic. Solubilization of both the dichloro and malonato compounds can be effected by using 2 parts of *N*-methylglucamine to 1 part of the compound and the mixture dissolved in distilled water. As previously mentioned, with the dichloro compound there appears to be no marked change in therapeutic activity or toxicity. With the malonato derivative, on the contrary, there is a five- to tenfold increase in activity both in toxicity and in therapeutic effectiveness so that 3–5 mg/kg of the compound formulated with NMG is the equivalent of 30–50 mg/kg of the compound suspended in 5% carboxymethylcellulose in water when both are given IP every fourth day for 3–4 doses.

These studies are extremely preliminary and two possibilities have been entertained. One is a biochemical change in which the malonato group is substituted for by two *N*-methylglucamine moieties. It is thought, however, that this is likely to give a polar compound, and polar platinum compounds have so far generally not been effective in antitumor tests. Also, studies against mouse leukemia L1210 and L1210/DDP cells in culture show ID_{50}s for the malonato NMG of 0.3 and 0.5, respectively, which are not significantly different from those of the malonato in water alone of 0.2 and 0.25, respectively. Another possiblity is that solution in *N*-methylglucamine markedly increases the bioavailability of the compound so that, in effect, the suspended malonato derivative is a depot form of platinum, whereas the solubilized form is active immediately. This postulate is under test at present, giving larger doses of the suspended malonato and the NMG-formulated malonato as a single dose on day 1. This should demonstrate whether the rapid availability (and presumably shorter half-life) of the NMG formulation is still as effective in a much lower dose as the depotlike activity of the suspended compound. These studies obviously are very preliminary and further chemical and biologic studies are in progress to delineate and explain this difference in activity.

If the solubility of these 1,2-diaminocyclohexane compounds can be enhanced without any loss of the therapeutic index, as appears probable, these platinum complexes with antitumor activity but without cross-resistance to DDP might be of value to patients whose disease has developed resistance to DDP.

References

1 Burchenal JH (1978) A clinical overview of dichloro diammino platinum. Biochimie 60:915–923

2 Burchenal JH, Kalaher K, Dew L, Lokys L, Gale GR (1978) Studies of cross-resistance, synergistic combination and blocking of activity of platinum derivatives. Biochimie 60: 961–965

3 Burchenal JH, Kalaher K, O'Toole T, Chisholm J (1977) Lack of cross-resistance between certain platinum coordination compounds in mouse leukemia. Cancer Res 37: 3455–3457

4 Burchenal JH, O'Toole T, Kalaher K, Chisholm J (1977) Synergistic effects of the combination of cis-platinum diamminodichloride and 2,2'-anhydro-1-β-D-arabinofuranosyl-5-fluorocytosine in transplanted mouse leukemias. Cancer Res 37: 4098–4100

5 Fischer GA (1958) Studies on the culture of leukemic cells in vitro. Ann NY Acad Sci 76: 673–680

6 Gale GR, Atkins LM, Meischen SJ, Schwartz P (1978) Schedule-dependency assessments of ribonucleoside diphosphate reductase inhibitors when used in combination with platinum compounds plus cyclophosphamide in the treatment of advanced L1210 leukemia. Cancer Treat Rep 63: 449–456

7 Gottlieb JA, Drewinko B (1975) Review of the current clinical status of platinum coordination complexes in cancer chemotherapy. Cancer Chemother Rep 59: 621–628

8 Hill JM, Loeb E, Pardue AS, Khan A, Hill NO, King JJ, Hill RW (1977) Platinum coordination compounds in the treatment of acute leukemia and other malignant diseases with particular reference to malonato 1,2-diaminocyclohexane platinum (II). J Clin Hematol Oncol 7: 681–700

9 Meischen SJ, Gale GR, Lake LM, Frangakis CJ, Rosenblum MG, Walker EM, Jr, Atkins LM, Smith AB (1976) Antileukemic properties of organoplatinum complexes. J Nat Cancer Inst 57: 841–845

10 Prestayko A, Bradner W, Haftalen J, Rose W, Schurig JE, Cleary MJ, Hydes PC, Crooke ST (1979) Antileukemia (L1210) activity and toxicity of cis-platinum (CDDP II) analogs. Cancer Treat Rep 63: 1503–1508

11 Ribaud P, Alcock N, Burchenal JH, Young CW, Muggia F, Mathe G (1979) Preclinical trial in baboon and phase I-II trial and pharmacokinetics in man of malonato platinum (MP). Proc Am Soc Clin Oncol 20: 336, abstr #C-186

12 Schindler RS, Day SM, Fischer GA (1958) Culture of neoplastic mast cells and their 5-hydroxytryptamine and histamine content in vitro. Fed Proc 17: 1617

13 Schwartz P, Meischen SJ, Gale GR, Atkins LM, Smith AB, Walker EM Jr (1977) Preparation and antitumor evaluation of water-soluble derivatives of dichloro (1,2-diaminocyclohexane) platinum (II). Cancer Treat Rep 61: 1519–1525

Preclinical and Phase I Studies of Malonatoplatinum

P. Ribaud, D. P. Kelsen, N. Alcock, E. Garcia-Giralt, P. Dubouch,
C. C. Young, F. M. Muggia, J. H. Burchenal, and G. Mathé

Summary

After a preclinical toxicologic study in baboons, we are conducting a phase I trial of malonatoplatinum, starting with 3 mg/kg and now reaching 16 mg/kg. Toxicity, mainly hematologic, was mild and our study was mainly limited by poor solubility. Regressions, which have been rare in the advanced-tumor patients, have been observed in three patients considered as clinically resistant to cisdichlorodiammino-platinum (DDP). Malonatoplatinum pharmacokinetics appeared similar to those of DDP as far as total platinum is concerned.

Introduction

Cisdichlorodiamminoplatinum (DDP) has been extensively used in cancer clinical therapeutics and is now known to have induced substantial improvement in several types of tumors, especially testes, ovary [6], and probably most epidermoid carcinomas [4]. There are still primary resistant neoplasias, however, and secondary resistance may appear in patients even if they have had an initial strong response.

Since we were interested in the experimental observation made by Burchenal et al. [2], in which a cisplatinum-resistant L1210 leukemia may have been sensitive to malonato (1,2-diamminocyclohexane) platinum, we conducted a clinical study to determine whether DDP-nonresistant and DDP-resistant tumors are sensitive to malonatoplatinum. Although Hill et al. [5] had already used this compound in patients, administering doses of up to 16 mg/kg, we conducted a preclinical toxicologic study and a phase I trial in man, due to the difficulty we had in solubilizing the compound.

Preclinical Toxicology in Baboons

Malonatoplatinum solubilized in water with 5% glucose, at doses varying from 6–16 mg/kg, was administered to baboons. Since the solubilizing process needs a huge quantity of fluid for the high dose, we tried to enhance it with a solution of the compound heated at 70° C in water with 5% glucose, 10% propylene glycol, and 0.2% sodium chloride, under magnetic stirring. The main parameters followed were fever,

blood pressure, urine volume, and behavior, as well as renal and liver functions.
Neither clinical nor biologic toxicity was observed for the small doses nor for 16 mg/kg injected in glucose solution prepared according to the first procedure. On the contrary, the other preparation which heated the solution to reduce the administered volume was lethally toxic, inducing renal failure due to tubular necrosis. This toxicity was probably due to the conversion of malonatoplatinum into another very toxic platinum derivative.

Phase I Trial in Man

We started a phase I trial in man; 35 patients were studied, and the administered doses ranged from 3 to 16 mg/kg (Table 1). The methods of administration were the same as for DDP, i.e., fluid loading, mannitol diuresis, and fluid replacement (Fig. 1). We observed gastrointestinal (GI) toxicity: universal nausea, frequent vomiting, and occasional diarrhea. No renal abnormalities were seen as reflected by BUN and creatinine values. Bone marrow toxicity was indicated by neutropenia in six of 32 courses, and by thrombocytopenia in nine of 31 courses. This toxicity was most often mild, not dose-related, and not cumulative (Table 2).
Of the 30 patients who received 10 or 16 mg/kg/course and had a measurable disease, 21 were evaluable (Table 3). Six patients had acute myeloid leukemia (AML), one had acute lymphoid leukemia (ALL), and none had received DDP previously; four were evaluable. Eight of 17 evaluable patients who had solid tumors were considered as

Table 1. Patients submitted to the phase I trial

Doses	Number of patients
3 mg/kg	1
6 mg/kg	1
8 mg/kg	1
10 mg/kg	15
16 mg/kg	17

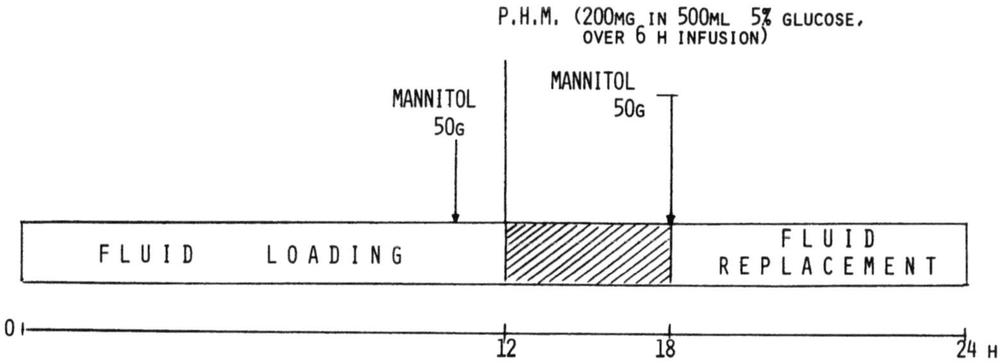

Fig. 1. Protocol of the phase I trial

Table 2. Toxicity

Toxicity	< 10 mg/kg no. courses		10 mg/kg no. courses		16 mg/kg no. courses		
GI toxicity	2/3		10/12		20/25		Almost universal vomiting Occasional diarrhea
Ototoxicity	0/3		0/10		0/25		
Renal toxicity	0/3		0/10		0/25		
Hematologic PMN[a]	 1/3	1***	3/9	2**	2/20	1***	Mild, not dose-related, not cumulative
Platelets[b]	2/3	2*	4/8	2*** 2*	3/20	2* 1**	(maximum, 3 courses)
Other	0		0		0		

[a] PMN 1,500–1,000*; 999–500**; < 500***
[b] Platelets, 100,000–50,000*; 49,000–20,000**; < 20,000***

Table 3. Stratification parameters

Number of patients submitted to trial				30
Number of evaluable patients				21
Sex F: 12	Age	F	Mean 39.5	(13–55)
M: 18		M	Mean 40	(12–69)
Prior treatment				
Chemotherapy only				21
Radiation therapy only				0
Radiation therapy and chemotherapy				8
No prior treatment				1

Table 4. Patients and diseases

Diagnosis	Total number	Evaluable	Non evaluable	Resistance to DDP		
				Yes	No	Uncertain
AML	6	3	2 Early deaths 1 Own discharge	–	3	–
ALL	1	1	–	–	1	–
Teratoma	7	7	–	5	–	2
Ovarian carcinoma	3	2	1 Under study	2	–	–
Squamous cell carcinoma						
Lung	5	2	3 Under study	–	2	–
Cervix uteri	2	2	–	1	–	1
Miscellaneous	6	4	1 Under study 1 Lost to follow-up	–	4	–
Total	30	21	9	8	10	3

Table 5. Results

Diagnosis	Total number	Responses					Resistance to DDP		
		Complete response	Partial response	Minor response	No change	Progressive disease	Yes	No	Uncertain
AML	3	–	–	–	–	3	–	3	–
ALL	1	–	–	–	–	1	–	1	–
Teratoma	7	–	1	1	1	4	5	–	2
Ovary carcinoma	2	–	–	1	–	1	2	–	–
Squamous cell carcinoma									
Lung	2	–	–	–	–	2	–	2	–
Cervix uteri	2	–	–	–	–	2	1	–	1
Miscellaneous	4	–	–	–	–	4	–	4	–
Total	21	–	1	2	1	17	8	10	3

Table 6. Details on responders

Patient	Diagnosis	No. of courses	DDP resistance	Response	Duration of response	Evaluation parameters
ERM	Embryonal testes carcinoma	10 mg/kg, 2 courses	Yes	Partial	9 Weeks	Pain, lumbo-aortic tumor, liver functions tests
HIG	Embryonal mediastinal carcinoma	16 mg/kg, 3 courses	Yes	Minor	8 Weeks	Vena cava superior obstruction, marker (α foetoprotein)
CROM	Ovary carcinoma	16 mg/kg, 1 course	Yes	Minor	Non-evaluable	Intestinal obstruction

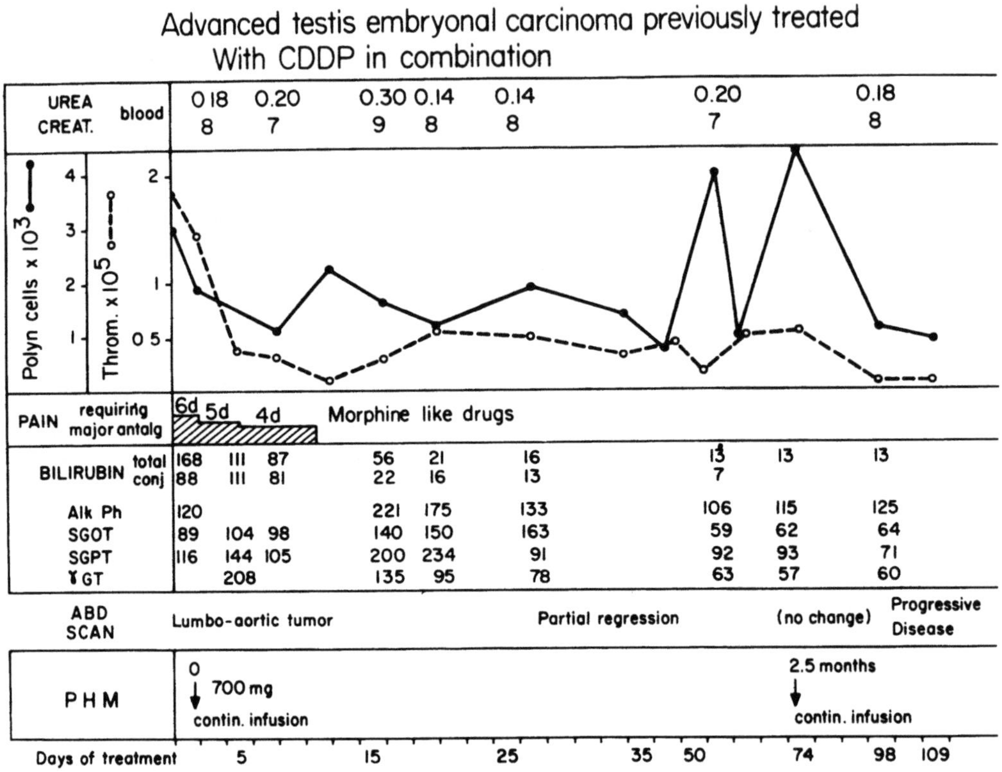

Fig. 2. Patient ERM: details of response

clinically resistant to DDP given alone or in combination (see details in Table 4).

No response was seen in acute leukemia patients. Responses were observed in only three patients who had solid tumors (Tables 5 and 6). The tumors included (a) an ovary carcinoma, the measurable parameter being an intestinal obstruction; (b) a mediastinal embryonal carcinoma, the measurable parameter being a vena cava superior syndrome; and (c) a testis embryonal carcinoma (Fig. 2). The results showed a decrease in the demande of morphinelike drugs. Other results included the normalization of hepatic tests altered by liver metastasis, and the decrease of a lumbo-aortic tumor mass indicated by two interval abdominal tomodensitometries.

Pharmacokinetics Study in Man

A pharmacokinetics study was initiated. The total platinum concentrations in urine and plasma were measured by flameless atomic-absorption spectrophotometry. The samples were collected in France and airmailed to New York, and the measurements were performed in Dr. Alcock's laboratory. Seven patients were studied, with dosage levels ranging from 3–16 mg/kg.

The results are shown on Figs. 3 and 4. The peak level was reached at the end of the infusion and there was a prolonged excretion phase. The higher the dose, the higher is

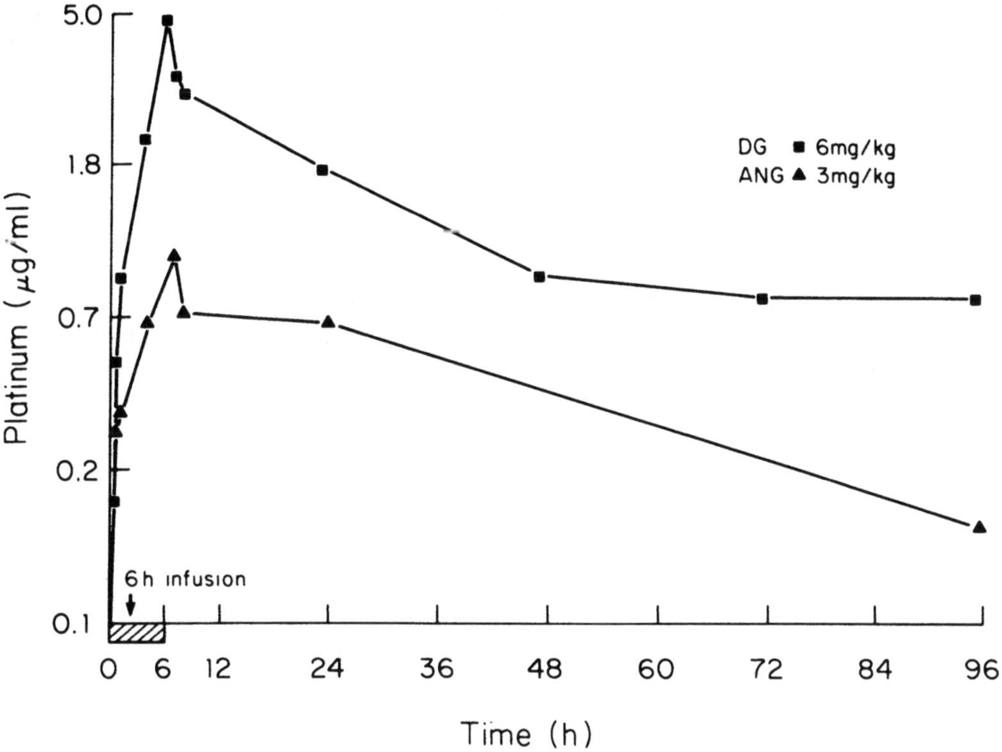

Fig. 3. Malonatoplatinum: plasma platinum concentrations after 3 and 6 mg/kg

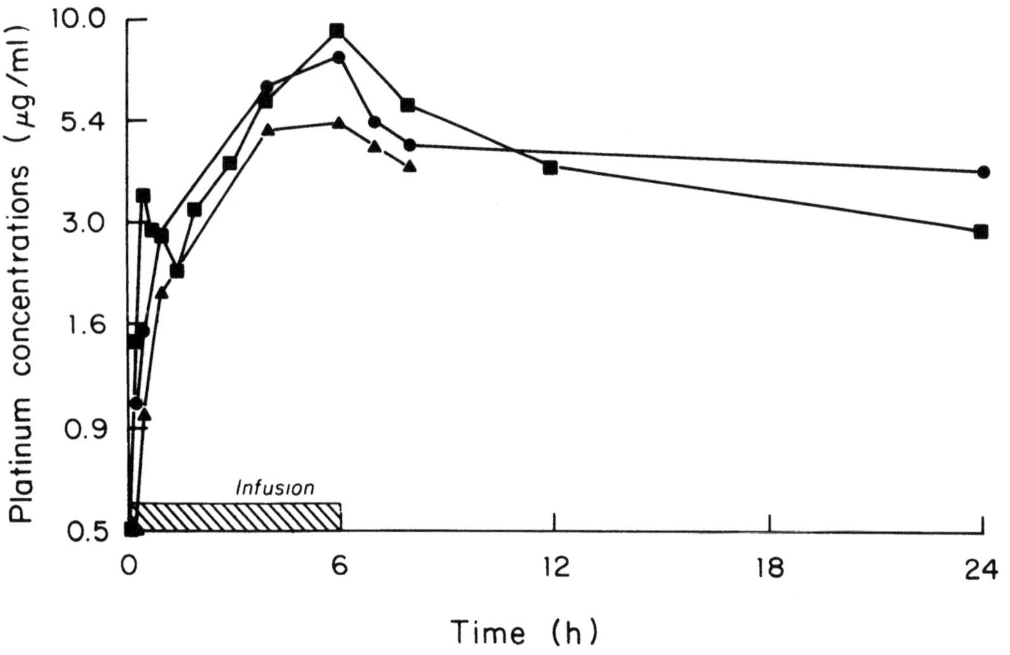

Fig. 4. Malonatoplatinum: platinum plasma concentrations (16 mg/kg; 3 patients)

the peak: 1.1 μg/ml for a dose of 3 mg/kg, 4.9 μg/ml for 6 mg/kg, 5.6 and 6 μg/ml for 10 mg/kg, and 5.5–9.4 μg/ml for 16 mg/kg. The excretion phase has a $t_{1/2}\beta$ value of 42–92 h (mean 63.5 h). Urinary excretion was measured in one patient receiving 16 mg/kg malonatoplatinum: 37.5% of the total administered dose was recovered in the urine within 96 h of the beginning of the infusion.

Conclusion

1) The poor solubility limited our phase I study of malonatoplatinum. Escalation of dosage yielded an inconvenient increase in the duration of the infusion. However, a new approach to the solubilization problem has been proposed by Burchenal [1].
2) Hematologic and GI toxicities were usually mild. No other toxicity was seen.
3) Actually, these are the early results of the phase I trial. As the dose-limiting toxicity has not yet been achieved, additional therapeutic results might be expected while increasing the dosage (we recently gave 20 mg/kg to two patients and 24 mg/kg to two other patients without seeing any more intense acute toxicity). Malonatoplatinum may induce (although up to now, it has been rare in this study) responses in patients considered as clinically resistant to DDP, which suggests that, in man, there might be no clinical cross-resistance between two analogues of platinum, as previously observed in murine leukemia.
4) Malonatoplatinum kinetics are similar to those of cisdichlorodiamminoplatinum (DDP) [3] as far as total platinum is concerned. We now intend to include measurements of total and filterable platinum concentrations in plasma and to make additional urine recoveries.

References

1 Burchenal JH, Irani G, Kern K, Lokys L, Turkevich J (1980) 1,2-Diaminocyclohexane platinum derivatives of potential clinical value. Recent Results Cancer Res 74: 156–165
2 Burchenal JH, Kalaher K, O'Toole T, Chisholm J (1977) Lack of cross-resistance between certain platinum coordination compounds in mouse leukemia. Cancer Res 37: 3455–3457
3 DeConti RC, Toftness BR, Lange RC, Creasey WA (1973) Clinial and pharmacological studies with cis-diamminedichloroplatinum (II). Cancer Res 33: 1310–1315
4 Hayat M, Brulé G, Cappelaere P, Cattan A, Chauvergne J, Clavel B, Guerrin J, Misset JL, Pommatau E, Ribaud P, Muggia FM, Rozencweig M, Mathé G (1980) Cisplatinumdiamminodichloride (CPDD) in chemotherapy of cancers: A phase II therapeutic trial. Recent Results Cancer Res 74: 149–155
5 Hill JM, Loeb E, Pardue AS, Khan A, Hill NO, King JJ, Hill RW (1977) Platinum coordination compounds in the treatment of acute leukemia and other malignant diseases with particular reference to malonato-1,2-diaminocyclohexane platinum (II). J Clin Hematol Oncol 7: 681–700
6 Prestayko AW, D'Aoust JC, Issell BF, Crooke ST (1979) Cisplatin (cis-diamminedichloroplatinum II). Cancer Treat Rev 6: 17–39

A Review of Clinical Studies of Pepleomycin

S. Oka

Summary

Pulmonary toxicity was less frequent in pepleomycin treatment of squamous cell carcinoma than in bleomycin treatment. The tumor-regressing effect appeared at about day 10 of pepleomycin treatment, and at about day 21 of bleomycin treatment. The cumulative dose of pepleomycin to complete remission was smaller than that of bleomycin. Pepleomycin is effective against bleomycin-sensitive malignancies: squamous cell carcinoma and Hodgkin's disease. It is more effective than bleomycin against lymph node metastases. Pepleomycin may have a broader antitumor spectrum: prostatic carcinoma responded.

Introduction

Pepleomycin was screened out of about 200 bleomycin analogues by testing their pulmonary toxicity in aged mice. This method of testing pulmonary toxicity has been

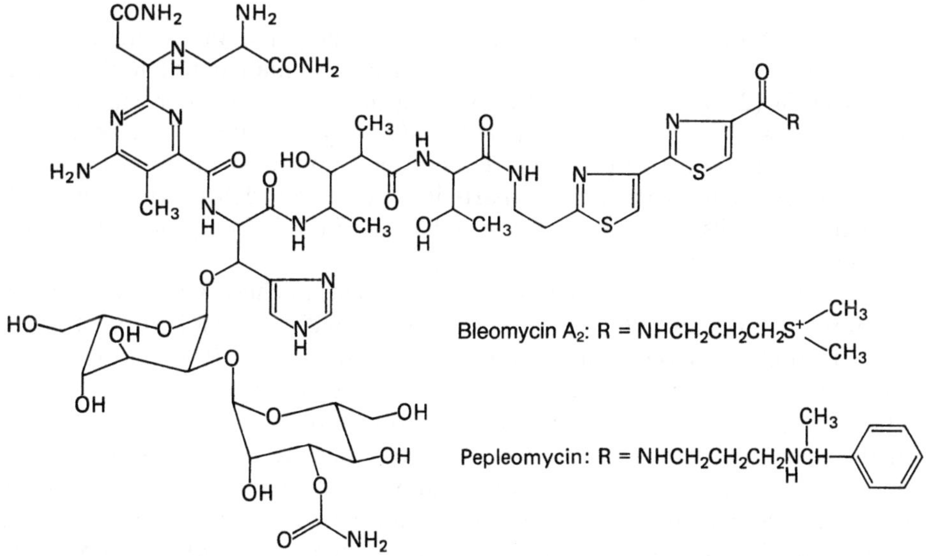

Fig. 1. Structures of pepleomycin and bleomycin. 1) Low pulmonary toxicity: lower in mice, rats, and dogs than bleomycin by intraperitoneal and intratracheal routes. 2) Wider antitumor spectrum: only pepleomycin is effective against MNNG rat gastric carcinoma

developed by MATSUDA et al. [8] and UMEZAWA [15]; and with the pulmonary toxicity index of the present bleomycin as 1.0, the index of pepleomycin was 0.25. The lower pulmonary toxicity of pepleomycin has also been shown by other methods giving a test material intratracheally. This was also shown by the pulmonary toxicity test in dogs.

Pepleomycin, as shown in Fig. 1, contains 3-[(S)-1-phenylamino]-propylamine as the terminal amine moiety of its structure. The phase I studies of pepleomycin were, as reported by MATSUDA et al. [8] and TANAKA [13], made from August 1976 through February 1977. The phase II studies have been carried out by doctors at 27 institutions throughout Japan since March 1977 [1, 2, 4–7, 9–12, 16]. The present review is mainly concerned with studies of pepleomycin in bleomycin-responsive tumors.

Pepleomycin in Bleomycin-Sensitive Tumors

In the studies were entered 65 patients with skin cancer, 345 with head and neck cancer, and 28 with malignant lymphoma. Of these patients, 298 were male and 140 were female, aged from 17 to 87, most of them from 40 to 79 years old.

Dose Schedule. Of these patients, 329 were given pepleomycin alone: 164 were treated intravenously; 126 intramuscularly, and 20 intraarterially. Most of them were given 10 mg of pepleomycin twice or three times a week, to a total dosage of about 200 mg, and there have been no signs of toxicity so far. The other 109 patients were given pepleomycin in combination with other antitumor agents and/or radiotherapy, but the combination chemotherapy with pepleomycin will be presented elsewhere.

Results

Toxicity (Table 1). Of the 329 patients who received pepleomycin alone, including the patients with head and neck cancer, skin cancer, and malignant lymphoma, fever was found in 74 (22.5%), nausea and vomiting in 27 (8.2%), anorexia in 85 (25.8%), lassitude in 43 (13%), stomatitis in 44 (13.4%), pigmentation of the skin in 33 (10%), sclerosis of the skin in 38 (11.6%), redness and exanthema chiefly over the trunk and on the lateral side of the flexible parts in 34 (10.3%), deformity, pigmentation and thickening of nails in 35 (10.6%), loss of hair in 93 (28.3%), dyspnea in seven (2.1%), and pulmonary fibrosis in three (1.0%).

Of the 329 patients, 43 were examined for changes in chest X-ray, VC, and PaO_2; 51 for those in X-ray and VC; 28 for those in X-ray and PaO_2; and 207 for those in X-ray only. Definite pulmonary toxicity was found in three (1.0%) of the 329 patients, indicating the lower pulmonary toxicity of pepleomycin.

The three patients with pulmonary toxicity were: a 68-year-old woman with carcinoma of the mandible, who was given pepleomycin despite the appearance of fever and dyspnea; a 79-year-old woman with squamous cell carcinoma of the tongue who had bronchial asthma; and a 77-year-old woman with squamous cell carcinoma of the cheek who had a history of coronary insufficiency. Therefore, pepleomycin was thought to produce pulmonary toxicity, though infrequently, in older patients with an underlying lung disease or cardiovascular disease.

Of 87 patients who died, 16 were autopsied, but none were found to have pulmonary fibrosis by pathologic examination.

Table 1. Toxicities of pepleomycin in 329 cancer patients

Toxicity	Cumulative dose (mg)							
	1–50	51–100	101–150	151–200	201–250	251–300	301–400	Total
Fever	5 (12.8)[a]	19 (18.3)	19 (30.1)	26 (24.5)	5 (50.0)			74 (22.5)
Nausea and vomiting	3 (7.7)	7 (6.7)	5 (7.9)	7 (6.6)	5 (50.0)			27 (8.2)
Anorexia	9 (23.0)	14 (13.5)	20 (31.7)	35 (33.0)	6 (60.0)	1 (16.7)		85 (25.8)
Lassitude	6 (15.4)	13 (12.5)	13 (20.6)	11 (10.4)				43 (13.0)
Stomatitis	1 (2.6)	5 (4.8)	9 (14.3)	23 (21.7)	4 (40.0)	1 (16.7)	1	44 (13.4)
Pigmentation of the skin		2 (2.0)	8 (12.7)	16 (15.1)	5 (50.0)	1 (16.7)	1	33 (10.0)
Sclerosis of the skin	1 (2.6)	7 (6.7)	6 (9.5)	16 (15.1)	5 (50.0)	2 (33.3)	1	38 (11.6)
Redness, eczema, and exanthema	4 (10.3)	10 (9.6)	8 (12.7)	12 (11.3)				34 (10.3)
Change of nails	1 (2.6)	1 (1.0)	7 (11.1)	17 (16.0)	6 (60.0)	2 (33.3)	1	35 (10.6)
Loss of hair		17 (16.3)	16 (25.4)	51 (48.1)	6 (60.0)	2 (33.3)	1	93 (28.3)
Dyspnea	1 (2.6)	3 (2.9)		3 (2.8)				7 (2.1)
Definite pulmonary toxicity		1 (1.0)		1 (1.0)	1 (10.0)			3 (1.0)
No toxicity	26 (66.7)	51 (49.0)	21 (33.3)	20 (18.9)	2 (20.0)	3 (50.0)		123 (37.4)
Number of patients	39	104	63	106	10	6	1	329

[a] The figures in parentheses ( ) denote percents

Laboratory Findings. A decrease in the number of erythrocytes to less than 350 × 10^4 cells/mm^3 was found in five patients (2.8%), and that of leukocytes to less than 4000 cells/mm^3 in five patients (2.8%), indicating slight or no bone marrow suppression of pepleomycin. Elevation of SGOT was found in four patients (2,7%); that of SGPT in five patients (3.4%), and that of BUN in only two patients (1.8%), showing slight or no hepatic or renal impairments attributable to pepleomycin. A decrease of sodium in the blood serum was found in one patient, and that of chlorine also in one. Pepleomycin was thus found to have slight or no bone marrow toxicities nor any renal or hepatic toxicities.

Table 2. Responses of skin cancer to pepleomycin (single use in 46 cases)

	Number of evaluable cases	Response			
		Markedly effective[a]	Moderately effective[b]	Slightly effective[c]	Not effective
Without previous treatment					
Squamous cell carcinoma	27	17 (63)[d]	5 (18)	3 (11)	2 (7)
Others	11	4 (36)	2 (18)	1 (9)	4 (36)
With previous treatment					
Squamous cell carcinoma	7	2 (29)	1 (14)	3 (43)	1 (14)
Others					
Total	45	23 (51)	8 (18)	7 (16)	7 (16)
			31 (69)		

[a] More than 90% regression of tumor
[b] More than 50% regression of tumor
[c] Less than 50% regression of tumor
[d] The figures in parentheses ( ) denote percents

Table 3. Responses of head and neck cancer to pepleomycin

	Number of evaluable cases	Response			
		Markedly effective[a]	Moderately effective[b]	Slightly effective[c]	Not effective
Without previous treatment					
Squamous cell carcinoma	162	39 (24)[d]	57 (35)	35 (22)	31 (19)
Others	6		1 (17)	3 (50)	2 (33)
With previous treatment					
Squamous cell carcinoma	65	5 (8)	12 (19)	22 (34)	26 (40)
Others	2			1 (50)	1 (50)
Total	235	44 (19)	70 (30)	61 (26)	60 (26)
			114 (49)		

[a] More than 90% regression of tumor
[b] More than 50% regression of tumor
[c] Less than 50% regression of tumor
[d] The figures in parentheses ( ) denote percents

Response. A response by more than 50% regression of tumor was found in 31 (69%) of 45 patients with skin cancer on whom the effect of pepleomycin was evaluable (Table 2). This response was also noted in 114 (49%) of 235 patients with head and neck cancer on whom the effect of the drug was likewise evaluable (Table 3). A more than 50% regression of tumor was observed in 72 (60%) of 123 patients with tumor of the

Table 4. Responses of head and neck cancer to pepleomycin (at different sites)

Site	Number of evaluable cases	Response				
		Markedly effective[a]	Moderately effective[b]	Slightly effective[c]	Not effective	Total
Oral cavity						
Lips	4	3 (75)[d]	1 (25)			
Tongue	57	13 (23)	21 (37)	10 (17)	13 (23)	57 (100)
Others	62	10 (16)	24 (39)	15 (24)	13 (21)	62 (100)
Total	123	26 (21)	46 (37)	25 (20)	26 (21)	123 (100)
		72 (60)				
Pharynx	28	5 (18)	5 (18)	7 (25)	11 (40)	28 (100)
		10 (38)				
Larynx	48	4 (8)	11 (23)	20 (42)	13 (27)	48 (100)
		15 (31)				
Maxilla	34	8 (23)	8 (23)	8 (23)	10 (30)	34 (100)
		16 (47)				
Others	2	1 (50)		1 (50)		2 (100)
Total	235	44 (19)	70 (30)	61 (26)	60 (25)	235 (100)

[a] More than 90% regression of tumor
[b] More than 50% regression of tumor
[c] Less than 50% regression of tumor
[d] The figures in parentheses ( ) denote percents

Table 5. Responses of malignant lymphoma to pepleomycin

	Number of evaluable cases	Response		
		Complete remission	Partial remission	No response
Without previous treatment				
Hodgkin's disease	2	1	1	
Reticulum cell sarcoma	8	5	2	1
Lymphosarcoma	2	1	1	
Others	4	4		
With previous treatment				
Hodgkin's disease	1	1		
Reticulum cell sarcoma	2	1	1	
Lymphosarcoma	1	1		
Total (%)	21 (100)	15 (71.4)	5 (23.8)	1 (4.8)

oral cavity, 10 (38%) of 28 with tumors of the pharynx, 15 (31%) of 48 with tumors of the larynx, and 16 (47%) of 34 with tumors of the maxilla, on all of whom the effect of pepleomycin also was evaluable (Table 4). Of the 28 patients with malignant lymphomas, the effect of pepleomycin was evaluable on 21; 15 showed a complete remission, and 5 (24%), a partial remission. Thus, the patients with malignant lymphomas responded well to the treatment (Table 5).

Pepleomycin in Bleomycin-Resistant Tumors

The antitumor spectra of pepleomycin against bleomycin-resistant prostatic cancer and metastatic lymph nodes were also included in this study.

Effect Against Prostatic Cancer. Patients with prostatic cancer are now being treated with pepleomycin alone. Some patients showed the category I response of Karnofsky's criteria, or had symptomatic improvements, suggesting an efficacy of pepleomycin against prostatic cancer which usually is refractory to the conventional chemotherapy. The findings on the treatment are scheduled to be reported in the near future. However, a single modality treatment for prostatic cancer is now not promising, so it *did* indicate the potential values of studies on combination therapy with pepleomycin.

Effect Against Metastatic Lymph Nodes (Table 6). Metastatic lymph nodes have been considered refractory to bleomycin. Therefore, 41 metastatic lymph nodes from cancers of the head and neck and those of the skin were studied in the treatment with pepleomycin. Of the 41 lymph nodes, two became completely impalpable, four were reduced in size by more than 50%, and five showed histologic responses when an average cumulative dose of 103 mg had been given.

Discussion

The response of the skin cancer and of the head and neck cancer group to the pepleomycin treatment in no statistically significant way differed from that to bleomycin treatment. However, skin cancer began to regress with an average cumulative dose of 41 mg, head and neck cancer with 58 mg, and malignant lymphomas with 25 mg, indicating a rapid regression of tumor (Fig. 2). Moreover, the average total cumulative dosage of pepleomycin to the responders of the skin cancer group was 131 mg, and that to the responders of the head and neck cancer group 169 mg, while that of bleomycin was, as reported in many papers, about 330 mg. The total cumulative dosage of pepleomycin to the responders of the malignant lymphoma group was 123 mg, while that of bleomycin was, also as reported in many papers, about 255 mg, showing pepleomycin's more potent antitumor activity.
In the study by Ikeda et al. [5] in testing the effect against skin squamous cell carcinoma after pepleomycin treatment, all cases were operated on and, in most of them, bestatin immunotherapy was also performed. In these cases, relapses hardly occurred during the following year, and the cases were under continued observation. It is often said that the duration of partial or complete remission after bleomycin

Table 6. Response of regional lymph nodes to pepleomycin treatment (average dose 103 mg)

Age and sex	Cancer by primary sites		Regional lymph nodes: Status	Sites		Response: Turned impalpable	Diminished in size	Histologically effective
59 Years (average)	Tongue	8	N_1 27	Cervical	8	2 (N_1, N_3)[a]	3 (N_3, N_2, N_2)	–
	Oral cavity	6	N_2 5	Submaxillary	27	1 (N_1)	1 (N_1)	2 (N_1, N_1)
Male 26	Pharynx	9	N_3 9	Inguinal	4	0	0	2 (N_1, N_2)
Female 15	Larynx	2		Axillary	2	0	0	1 (N_1)
	Sinus	1						
	Gingiva	1						
	Lip	1						
	Tonsil	5						
	–							
	Skin	7						
	Unknown	1						
Total (%)		41					12 (30%)	

[a] The entries in parentheses ( ) denote status of lymph nodes before treatment

treatment is relatively short. As described above, in study reported by IKEDA et al., all cases were operated on and bestatin treatment was continued.

It cannot be concluded, therefore, whether the effect of pepleomycin lasts longer than that of bleomycin. In this connection, it may be necessary to remember that the repetition of bleomycin treatment alone at intervals of 1–2 months, as reported by ICHIKAWA [3], has produced a complete cure of squamous cell carcinoma.

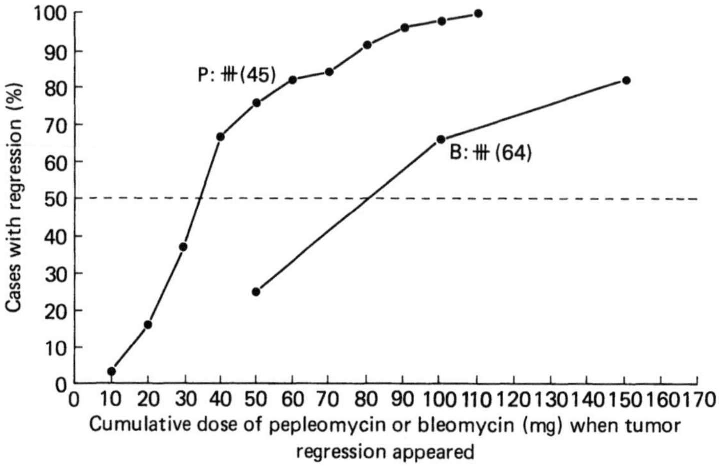

Fig. 2. Regression of head and neck tumors. *P*, pepleomycin; *B*, bleomycin UENO et al. [14]. ⧺, more than 90% regression of tumor. ( ), Number of cases

Prostatic cancer seemed to respond to pepleomycin, suggesting its broader antitumor spectrum. Therefore, further studies are needed to confirm the possible broader antitumor spectrum of this drug.

The incidence and pattern of toxicity of pepleomycin were found to be similar to those of bleomycin. That is, anorexia, loss of hair, fever, stomatitis, nausea, and vomiting were the more frequent side effects. Pulmonary toxicity, however, was found only in 1% of the 329 patients, including the patients with skin cancer, head and neck cancer, and malignant lymphoma. However, the definition of pulmonary toxicity which was considered attributable to the drug varied from investigator to investigator.

Definite pulmonary toxicity as meant in this paper was defined as a condition which showed a development of pneumonialike shadows or a diffuse interstitial pattern of fibrosis on the chest roentgenogram, accompanied by impaired pulmonary functions, when these signs were considered to be due to pepleomycin administration. Suspected or subclinical pulmonary toxicity was excluded from this paper, because the causes in such cases so far surveyed were not determined to be due to the administration of the drug. However, pepleomycin should be given carefully to aged patients or those with an underlying lung disease, although pepleomycin has less pulmonary toxicity, and the serial measurements of VC and $AaDO_2$ need to be conducted to prevent the occurrence of pulmonary toxicity in patients with cancer of any organ.

References

1 Hashimoto K, Shioda S, Amagasa T, Shimizu M, Sato O, Ito H, Fujibayashi T, Soda T (1979) Clinical experience with pepleomycin (NK631). Jpn J Antibiot 32: 451–462

2 Hayashida K, Watanabe H, Ito M, Nakashima T, Toriya Y, Hiroto I, Jingu K, Hayabuchi N (1979) Clinical application of NK631 in the treatment of cancer of the tongue and floor of the mouth. Jpn J Antibiot 32: 509–515

3 Ichikawa T (1976) Studies of bleomycin; discovery of its clinical effect, combination treatment with bleomycin and radiotherapy, side effects, and long-term survival. GANN Monogr Cancer 19: 99–115

4 Iida T, Matsumoto K, Komiyama H, Okano H, Inaba O, Ogawa F, Takeda G, Takasu J (1978) Clinical experience with NK-631 in the case of oral cancer. Jpn J Oral Surg 24: 983–992
5 Ikeda S, Miyasato H, Nakayama H, Kobayashi Y, Tajima K (1979) Clinical trial of pepleomycin for the malignant skin tumors. Jpn Cancer Clin 25: 677–687
6 Inuyama Y, Murakami Y, Kohno N, Mashino S, Asaoka K, Nakajima Y, Ozu R, Horiuchi M (1978) Clinical effect of NK-631 (pepleomycin) for head and neck cancer. Practica Otologica (Kyoto) 71: 1517–1527
7 Majima H, Oguro M, Takagi T (1979) Preclinical trial of NK631 of malignant lymphoma. Cancer Chemother 6: 401–404
8 Matsuda A, Yoshioka O, Yamashita T, Ebihara K, Umezawa H, Takeuchi T, Miura T, Katayama K, Yokoyama M, Nagai S (1978) Fundamental and clinical studies on new bleomycin analogs. Recent Results Cancer 63: 191–210
9 Miura T, Katayama K, Wada T (1979) Phase I and phase II studies of a new bleomycin (pepleomycin). Jpn J Antibiot 32: 265–277
10 Nobe O, Kubo H, Yoshii K, Tashiro M (1979) Clinical experience with NK631 in malignant tumors of skin. Jpn J Antibiot 32: 463–469
11 Sekiya T, Kawabe Y, Ito A, Kaneda T, Suzuki T, Shiraishi T (1979) A joint study of NK631 treatment of head and neck cancers. Cancer Chemother 6: 777–784
12 Takata K, Honda T (1979) Primary effect of NK631 against head-and-neck cancers. Jpn J Antibiot 32: 106–114
13 Tanaka W (1977) Development of new bleomycins with potential clinical utility. Jpn J Antibiot [suppl] 30: 41–48
14 Ueno T, Shimizu M, Michi K, Ishibashi K, Kohama G (1973) Klinische Erfahrungen über die Behandlung mit Bleomycin von 551 Fällen der Mundhöhlenkarzinome in Japan. Bull Tokyo Med Dent Univ 62: 117–126
15 Umezawa H (1976) Bleomycin; discovery, chemistry, and action. GANN Monogr Cancer Res 19: 3–36
16 Yokoyama M, Sato K, Wakui A, Saito T (1979) Phase I and phase II study of new bleomycin analogs – NK5033 and NK631. Cancer Chemother 6: 749–758

Experimental and Clinical Activity of a New Anthracycline Derivative: Detorubicin (14-Diethoxyacetoxydaunorubicin)

R. Maral, D. Heusse, F. Lavelle, G. Cueille, M. Marlard, C. Jacquillat, J. Maral, M.-F. Auclerc, M. Weil, G. Auclerc, and J. Bernard*

Summary

This report concerns the experimental activity and the preliminary clinical results obtained with detorubicin, an anthracycline. Experimentally, in comparison with doxorubicin, detorubicin is less toxic, less immunodepressive, and less mutagenic, its experimental antitumor activity is equal or superior, and differences are found in pharmacokinetics. Its most interesting activities in clinical cancer therapy are found in non-Hodgkin lymphomas, in carcinomas, and in soft-tissue sarcomas.

Introduction

The anthracycline derivatives are intercalating drugs of major importance in the treatment of leukemias and in the management of solid tumors. The aim of the research in the anthracycline field is to find new agents or derivatives which have less toxicity, few or no adverse side effects, which have a good activity when compared with the parent compounds (daunorubicin or doxorubicin). This report concerns our present experience with a new derivative: 14-diethoxyacetoxydaunorubicin or detorubicin (Fig. 1) [4, 6]. When compared with doxorubicin, this semisynthetic derivative fulfills some of the objectives mentioned above: it is less toxic, less immunodepressant and mutagenic, and has an equal or superior experimental antitumor activity. These differences may be explained by pharmacokinetics (blood and cellular levels, metabolism, fixation in the tissues).

Experimental Studies

Cytotoxicity (Table 1)

We used KB cells in tissue culture flasks (10^5 cells/ml nutritive medium). Beginning of the culture: day 0.

---

* This research was supported by a grant from Institut National pour la Santé et la Recherche Médicale (INSERM Commission 8), USPHS grant 5-R 10 CA 13239-05 from the National Cancer Institute, French and American Cooperative Cancer Program (INSERM and NCI)

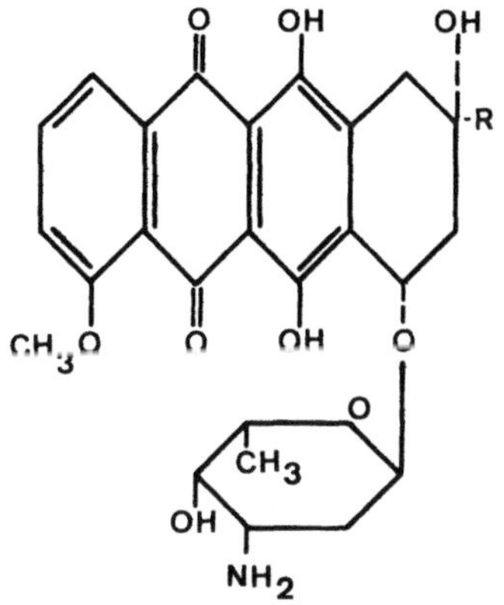

Compound	-R	Molecular weight	M W ratio
Detorubicin NSC 292 652	$COCH_2OCOCH(OC_2H_5)_2$	673.6	1.23
Doxorubicin (Adriamycin) NSC 123 127	$COCH_2OH$	543.5	

Fig. 1

Table 1a. On day 2, the compound was added at different concentrations in the culture medium. On day 4, the remaining living cells were counted: the IC_{50} is the concentration of the drug which inhibits 50% of the cell population. Detorubicin is less toxic than doxorubicin (on a molar concentration basis, the detorubicin–doxorubicin toxicity ratio is about 1.4).

Table 1b. The compound was added on day 2; 4 h later tritiated thymidine was added to the culture medium. After 5 h of pulse, the cell incorporation of the precursor was measured (liquid scintillation count): the IC_{50} is the concentration of the drug which inhibits 50% of the precursor incorporation in the cells. Detorubicin is less toxic than doxorubicin (on a molar concentration basis, the detorubicin–doxorubicin toxicity ratio is about 2.2).

Subacute and Acute Toxicity in Mice (Table 2)

Subacute toxicity (treatments: 5 days; route of treatment: intraperitoneal, IP, or intravenous, IV) and acute toxicity (route: IV) were evaluated in mice (LD_{50}, LD_0, and maximal tolerated dose or MTD: dose which induced no death and no weight loss). No significant difference was observed with the IP route, but the IV toxicity of detorubicin was clearly lower (about 50% less) than that of doxorubicin.

Table 1a and b. Cytotoxic activity (KB cells)

a Inhibition of the number of cells in culture (Coulter counter)

0 1 2 3 4 d

Culture KB — Compound — Cell counting

Compound	IC_{50}	
	µg/ml	nmol/ml
Detorubicin	0.26	0.38
Doxorubicin	0.15	0.27

b Inhibition of DNA synthesis

0 1 2 d

Culture KB — Compound

– 4 h

^{3}H-thymidine 5 h

CPM

Compound	IC_{50}	
	µg/ml	nmol/ml
Detorubicin	0.79	1.17
Doxorubicin	0.29	0.53

Table 2. Subacute and acute toxicity in mice: LD_{50}–LD_0 and MTD (mg/kg)

Number of treatments	Route of treatment	Compound	LD_{50}	LD_0	MTD
5	IP	Detorubicin	3.50 (3.1–3.7)	1.25	1.20
		Doxorubicin	3.00	1.50	0.70
	IV	Detorubicin	7.00 (6.10–7.80)	5.00	2.50
		Doxorubicin	4.50 (4.00–5.00)	2.50	1.20
I	IV	Detorubicin	27.50	20.00	15.00
		Doxorubicin	19.00	12.50	5.00–8.00

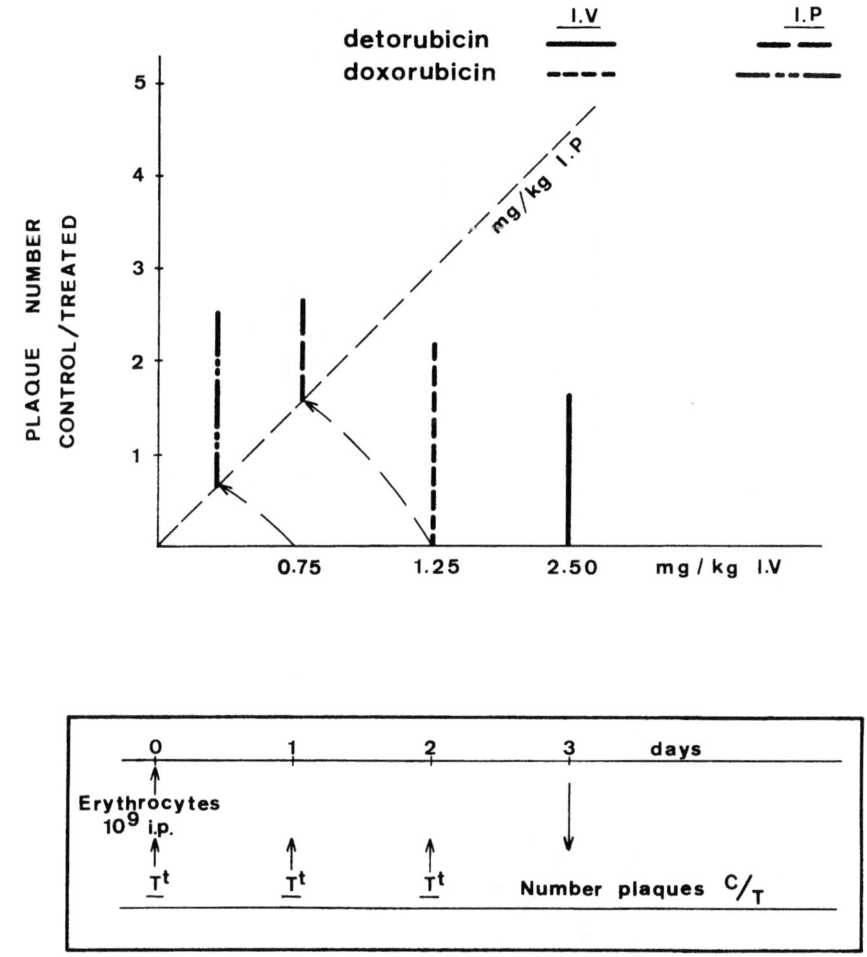

Fig. 2. Spleen cell plaques of hemolysis in gel (Jerne's technique)

Immunodepressive Activity

Activity on Spleen Cell Plaques of Hemolysis in Gel (Fig. 2). According to the Jerne-Nordin's technique [5], mice were injected IP with 10^9 sheep red blood cells on day 0; the drug was administered IV or IP on days 0, 1, and 2. Gel plaque was assayed on day 3 (count of the number of plaques/spleen). We determined the ratio of the number of plaques control/treated (the more depressive the compound, the higher the ratio). Even at lower doses IP or IV, detorubicin was less depressive than doxorubicin.

Activity on Macrophages. Using a mouse peritoneal macrophage culture in a flask and counting the remaining adherent cells at different times (4, 12, and 18 days), detorubicin (0.09 nmol/ml) was less toxic than doxorubicin (0.07 nmol/ml) (Fig. 3). With the same cell type, but according to another experimental system (Fig. 4), we studied the inhibiting activity of detorubicin on the phagocytic activity: it was lower than that of doxorubicin (IC_{50}: detorubicin 0.59 nmol/ml; doxorubicin: 0.40 nmol/ml; detorubicin–doxorubicin ratio 1.47).

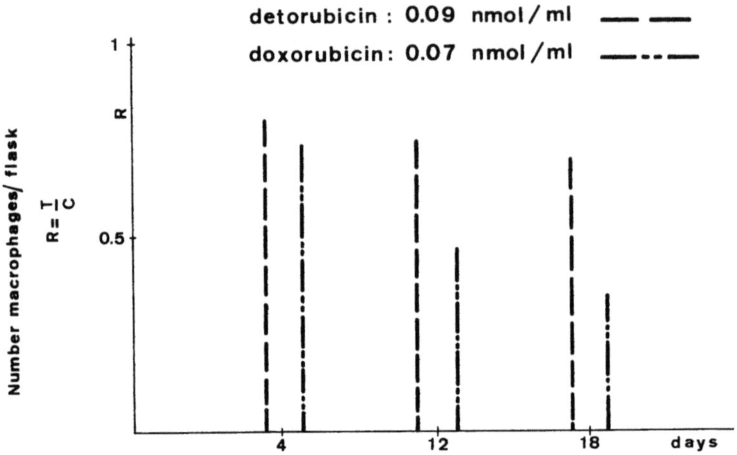

Fig. 3. Mouse macrophage cytotoxicity: n = number macrophages per flask T/C

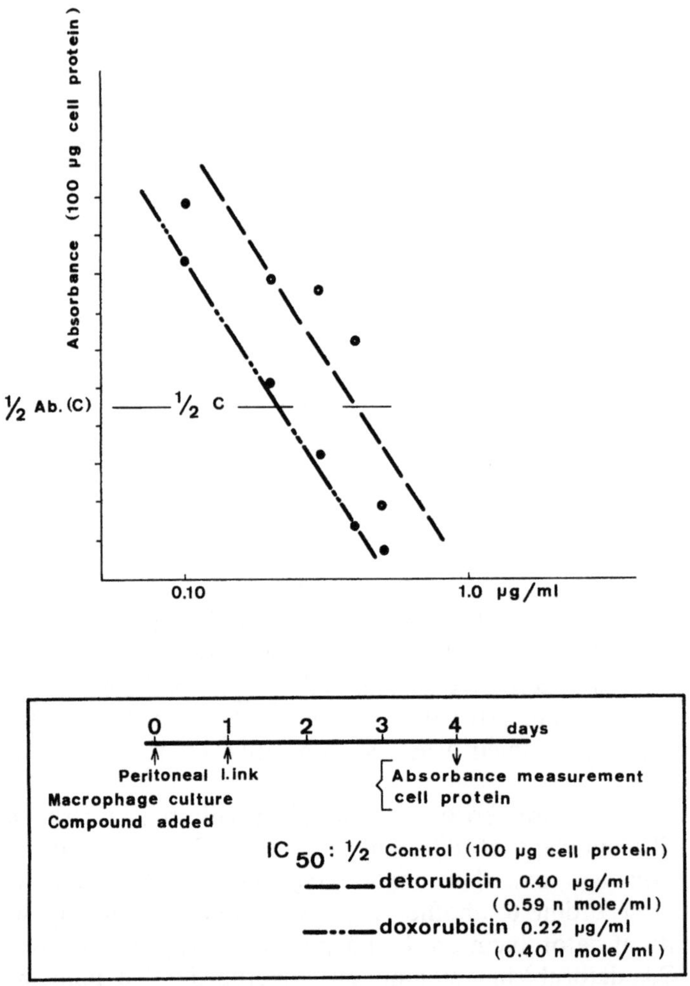

Fig. 4. IC_{50} macrophage inhibition (Indian-ink phagocytosis test)

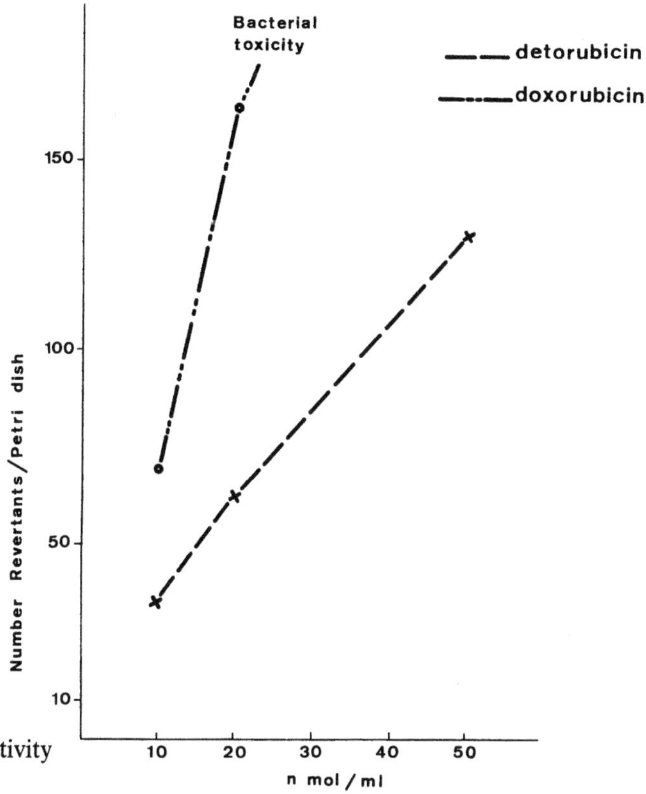

Fig. 5. Ames test: mutagenic activity *S. typhimurium* TA 98

Mutagenic Activity (Fig. 5)

According to the Ames technique [1] with *Salmonella typhimurium* strain TA 98, on a molar basis, the mutagenic activity (number of revertants/Petri dish) was lower with detorubicin than with doxorubicin.

Antitumoral Activity

As far as experimental antitumor activity is concerned, detorubicin is superior or equal to doxorubicin.

Table 3. L1210 leukemia. The chemotherapeutic index of detorubicin is better.

Table 4. Leukemia AKR(S): treatments IV. The number of survivors is considered; better activity with detorubicin.

Table 5. Sarcoma 180, mammary carcinoma RIII, lung carcinoma C57Bl, melanocarcinoma B16: treatments IV at the optimal dosage. Better activity with detorubicin.

Table 6. Lewis lung carcinoma: treatments IV. Better activity with detorubicin, principally on lung metastases.

Table 3. Leukemia L1210[a]

Compound	LD_{50} (mg/kg IP)	AD_{150} (mg/kg IP)	Chemotherapeutic index LD_{50}/AD_{150}
Detorubicin	3.5–3.7	0.2	17.5–18.5
Doxorubicin	2.8–3.0	0.2	14.0–15.0

[a] $B_6D_2F_1$ mice. Day 0: graft (10^3 cells IP. Treatments IP, days 0, 1, 2, 3, and 4

Table 4. Leukemia AKR (S)[a]

Compound	mg/kg IV	Day 40 Survivors (9 mice/group)
Detorubicin	15.0	+ (Toxicity)
Doxorubicin	7.5	+ (Toxicity)
Detorubicin	10.0	———
Doxorubicin	5.0	+ (Toxicity)
Detorubicin	7.5	———
Doxorubicin	3.7	———
Detorubicin	5.0	———
Doxorubicin	2.5	———
Detorubicin	3.75	+ (No activity)
Doxorubicin	1.75	+ (No activity)

[a] AKR mice. Day 0: graft (10^5 cells IP. Treatments IV, days 0, 1, 2, 3, and 4

Table 5. Sarcoma 180, mammary carcinoma RIII–lung carcinoma C57Bl

Compound	Days of treatment	mg/kg IV	TW 0.25 0.50 0.75 100
Detorubicin	0, 1, 2, 3, and 4	2.50	———
Doxorubicin		1.25	Sarcoma 180 (tumor weight T/C)
Detorubicin	0, 1, 2, 3, and 4	2.50	———
Doxorubicin			
Detorubicin	0, 1, 2, and 3	1.25	———
Doxorubicin		0.62	———
Detorubicin	3 and 8	2.50	———
Doxorubicin		1.25	———
			Mammary carcinoma RIII (tumor weight T/C)
Detorubicin	1, 4, and 7	2.50	———
Doxorubicin		1.25	———
			Lung carcinoma C57Bl (tumor weight T/C)
Melanocarcinoma B16			ILS 1.25 1.50 1.75 200
Detorubicin	1, 4, 7, and 10	2.50	———
Doxorubicin		1.25	———
			Melanocarcinoma B16 (ILS)

Table 6. Lewis lung carcinoma[a]

Compound	mg/kg IV	Tumor weight T/C	No. metastases T/C
Detorubicin	7.50	0.00	0.00
Doxorubicin	3.75	0.04	0.00
Detorubicin	5.00	0.11	0.00
Doxorubicin	2.50	0.34	0.01
Detorubicin	2.50	0.77	3.13
Doxorubicin	1.25	0.70	0.33

[a] C_{57} Bl mice. Day 0: graft (5×10^6 cells) SC. Treatments IV, days 1, 4, 7, 11, 14, and 18

Clinical Activity

This report concerns our preliminary clinical experience in 139 patients with detorubicin.

Materials and Methods

The good experimental activity of detorubicin prompted our study of it in man. Table 7 shows the distribution of malignant diseases for the 139 patients who were given this drug at the Hospital Saint-Louis since September 1977. All had advanced diseases deserving phase 1 and phase 2 therapeutic trials.

Detorubicin was administered alone by IV infusion in saline. Doses and schedules of administration varied according to the type of malignancy. In acute leukemias, all 35 patients had had relapses resistant to previous treatments. Detorubicin was given 2 mg/kg daily × 5 or 6, and the mean total dose was 12 mg/kg. Aplasia of the bone marrow was usually noted after day 10. During aplasia, antibiotic treatment was essential; 30 patients also received platelet transfusions and 25 patients were given white cell transfusions from donors with chronic myeloid leukemia. Mucous toxicity (oral ulceration, vomiting, diarrhea) was very severe in those patients, and all subsequent patients with acute leukemias were given intermittent schedules (6 mg/kg in one dose).

In non-Hodgkin lymphomas (NHL), all patients (21) had diffuse lymphomas at a disseminated stage and all relapses were resistant to the usual combination of cyclophosphamide, prednisone and doxorubicin. Detorubicin was given 2 mg/kg day × 2 every 2 weeks, or 3 mg/kg every 3 weeks. In solid tumors, detorubicin was given either weekly as a single dose of 1 mg/kg, or every 3 weeks as a single dose of 2 mg/kg.

The toxicity of detorubicin is summarized in Table 8. As already stated, toxicity for daily administration was prohibitive, but it was tolerable for intermediate and intermittent schedules. Alopecia was observed in all patients. Nausea and vomiting were observed in half of the patients.

In solid tumors and NHL, the median nadir of WBC was $1500/mm^3$, and that of platelets was $80{,}000/mm^3$. ECG was performed before and after each cure. A cardiac failure appeared after 32 mg/kg given within 6 months in only one patient.

Table 7. Number of patients treated by detorubicin

Disease	Number of patients treated
ALL	26
AML	9
APL	3
Acute monoblastic leukemia	4
CML acutisation	5
Non-Hodgkin lymphoma	25
Soft-tissue sarcoma	4
Hodgkin	4
Epithelioma	28
Malignant melanoma	16
Mesothelioma	1
Osteosarcoma	3
Ewing sarcoma	1
Parker and Jackson sarcoma	2
Fungoid mycosis	8
Total	139

Table 8. Detorubicin toxicity

Schedule of administration	Disease	Number of patients	Hematologic[a]		Mucous[a]	
			1.2	3.4	1.2	3.4
Daily schedules	Acute leukemias	42		35	11	17
Intermediate	NHL	25	8	12	6	4
Intermittent	Solid tumors	72	13	8	10	1

[a] Toxicity: 1.2 = mild-moderate; 3.4 = severe

Results

In acute leukemias, response to treatment was evaluated by using the criteria of the Acute Leukemia Cooperative Group B [3], and the results of treatment are summarized in Table 9. In acute lymphoblastic leukemias (ALL), 13 (50%) of the 26 patients had complete remission. Of the 16 patients in their first relapse, ten (62%) achieved complete remission. Of the eight patients in their second relapse, three achieved complete remission. Eight patients were resistant to detorubicin. Three deaths occurred during induction treatment in the phase of bone marrow aplasia caused by the first course of the drug. Complete remission was brief (median: 20 days). In a child with Burkitt cell leukemia resistant to the combination of prednisone, vincristine, Cytoxan (cyclophosphamide), and daunorubicin, a single dose of detorubicin 6 mg/kg achieved a complete hematologic remission.

In acute granulocytic leukemias, 5 (33%) of 15 patients achieved complete remission: one of the eight patients with acute myeloblastic leukemia, two of the four patients

Table 9. Results of detorubicin treatment in acute leukemia

	ALL	AML	Acute monoblastic leukemia	Acute promyelytic leukemia
Complete remission	13 (50%)	1	2	2
Partial remission	2	–	–	1
Failure	8	6	1	–
Death in aplasia	3	1	1	–
Total	26	8	4	3

Table 10. Results of detorubicin treatment in non-Hodgkin lymphomas

	Remission (CR + PR)	Failure	Total
First attack without prior treatment	4	–	4
Prior treatment[a]	13[b]	8	21
Total	17 (68%)	8	25

[a] Patients resistant to CHOP (prednisone, cyclophosphamide, vincristine, and doxorubicin)
[b] Four patients with skin involvement

with acute monoblastic leukemia, and one of the two patients with acute promyelocytic leukemia. One of the patients with acute monoblastic leukemia in complete hematologic remission had a skin relapse which was assessed histologically, and two skin nodules disappeared after a total dose of 4 mg/kg.

The complete remissions, however, were brief and mucous toxicity (oral ulcerations) was severe in these patients.

In non-Hodgkin lymphoma patients, the results have been especially encouraging (Table 10); remission was obtained in 17 (68%) of the 25 patients. The activity of detorubicin on skin involvement appeared especially striking. In these advanced patients, remissions were brief, but the achievement of remission after one or two doses of detorubicin in these rapidly progressive diseases resistant to all other drugs emphasizes the major activity of this new derivative and suggests the need for randomized studies with doxorubicin vs detorubicin in non-Hodgkin lymphomas [4].

A complete remission was obtained in one child who had *rhabdomyosarcoma* with bone marrow involvement, and with bone, liver, and pulmonary localizations. The complete remission lasted 6 months.

Of eight patients with *fungoid mycosis,* low-dose detorubicin (1 mg/kg/week) achieved more than 50% regression of this resistant disease in seven patients. A striking skrinkage of an abdominal liposarcoma was also observed and surgery was made possible by treatment with detorubicin. A complete remission was observed in one case of peritoneal mesothelioma resistant to radiotherapy.

Five patients with *bone sarcoma* received detorubicin. A complete remission was achieved in a patient with PARKER and JACKSON sarcoma resistant to previous treatment (i.e., doxorubicin, actinomycin, etc.). In two patients with osteosarcoma, who

Table 11. Results of detorubicin treatment in carcinomas

Primary tumor type	Number of patients	Regression 50%	Regression 50%	Failure
Breast	5	1	3	1
Thyroid	3	2	1	
Kidney	2	1		1
Ovary	3		2	1
Primary unknown	6	1	3	2
Miscellaneous	9		1	8[a]
Total	28	5	10	13

[a] One patient death in aplasia

received one dose of detorubicin before amputation, bone pain disappeared completely.

In carcinomas, results of treatment by detorubicin are summarized in Table 11. Among 28 patients, we observed 15 good results: more than 50% regression in three patients (one with node metastasis from a thyroid carcinoma, one with skin metastasis from renal carcinoma, and the other with bone metastasis).

In 11 patients with *disseminated malignant melanoma* resistant to chemotherapy, one complete remission lasting 7 months and three partial regressions were noted.

In short, these clinical results show that detorubicin has a wide range of activity in malignant diseases. In acute leukemias its daily administration proved active, but too toxic. In non-Hodgkin lymphomas, intermittent administration led to 71% CR, even in advanced disseminated disease with poor histologic prognosis. Skin involvement proved to be especially sensitive to this drug. At low doses, detorubicin may be useful in advanced stages of mycosis fungoides. Its activity is striking in soft-tissue sarcomas and still encouraging in melanomas. It may improve treatment of various other types of cancers.

Discussion and Conclusion

Pharmacokinetic studies of this compound are presently in progress. We can mention already the study of Deprez-de Campeneere et al. [2] on the pharmacokinetic, toxicologic, and chemotherapeutic properties of detorubicin in mice (a comparative study with daunorubicin and doxorubicin); the tissue distribution of the drugs and the metabolites after injection of detorubicin differs significantly from that obtained after administration of doxorubicin.

By autoradiography in mice, we studied comparatively the tissue distribution of [^{14}C]-labeled detorubicin (at the carbonyl of the diethoxyacetate radical) 4 mg/kg IV; and [^{14}C]-diethoxyacetic acid (at equivalent doses).

The unchanged detorubicin was detected in the blood and in different tissues during the first hours. Differences in tissue distribution were observed between the two labeled compounds (Fig. 6): with detorubicin, the decreasing order of affinity was for the kidneys, the lungs, the heart, the skin, the bone marrow, and the spleen; with diethoxyacetic acid, the decreasing order was for the liver, the kidneys, and the lungs.

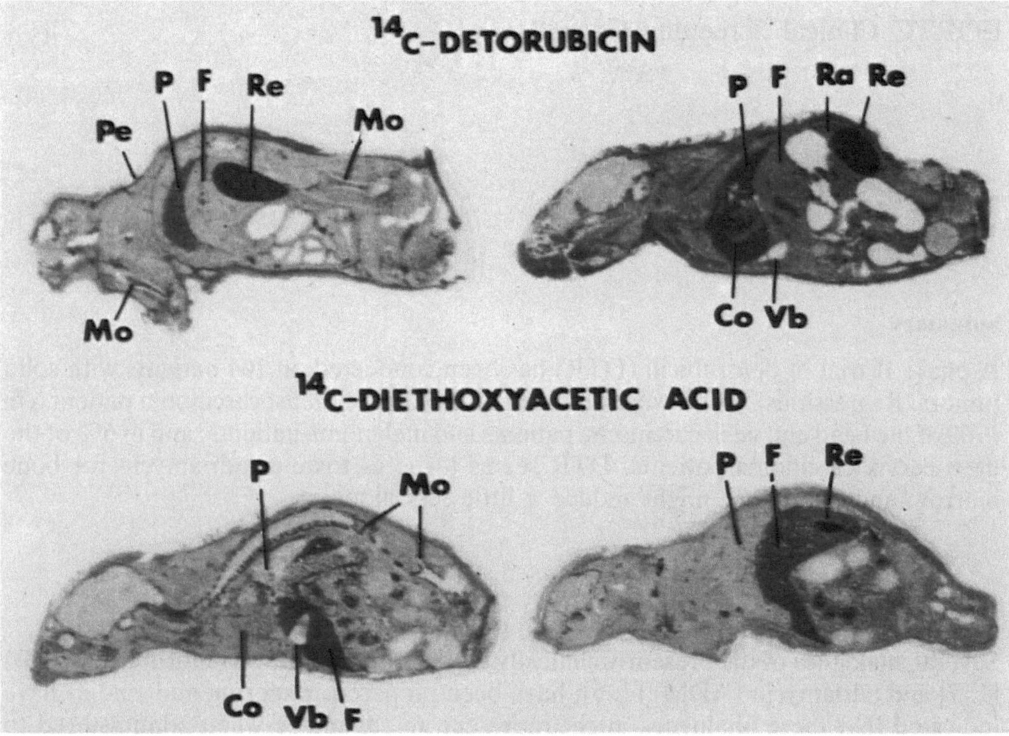

Fig. 6. Autoradiogram of mice 10 min after iv injection of ^{14}C-detorubicin or ^{14}C-diethoxyacetic acid: *Pe* skin, *P* lung, *F* liver, *Re* kidney, *Mo* bone marrow, *Ra* spleen, *Co* heart, *Vb* gall bladder

The experimental activities, the clinical results, and the above-mentioned data show clearly that detorubicin is an interesting derivative of the anthracycline family; this compound deserves further study.

References

1 Ames BN, McCann J, Yamasaki E (1975) Methods for detecting carcinogens and mutagens with the *Salmonella*/mammalian-microsome mutagenicity test. Mutat Res 31: 347–364

2 Deprez-de Campeneere D, Baurain R, Trouet A (1979) Pharmacokinetic, toxicologic and chemotherapeutic properties in mice of detorubicin: A comparative study with daunorubicin and doxorubicin. Cancer Treat Rep 63: 861–867

3 Ellison RR, Holland JF, Weil M, Jacquillat C, Boiron M, Bernard J, Sanitsky A, Rosner F, Gussof B, Silman R, Karanas A, Cuttner J, Spurr C, Hayes D, Bloom J, Leone L, Hernani F, Kyle R, Hutchinson J, Porcier L, Moon J (1968) Arabinosyl cytosine: An useful agent in the treatment of acute leukemia in adults. Blood 4: 507–523

4 Jacquillat C, Weil M, Auclerc MF, Maral J, Schaison G, Boiron M, Bernard J (1979) A survey of the anthracycline derivatives in hematology. Cancer Chemother Pharmacol 2: 53–59

5 Jerne NK, Nordin AA (1963) Plaque formation in agar by single antibody-producing cells. Science 140: 405

6 Maral R, Ducep JB, Farge D, Ponsinet G, Reisdorf D (1978) Préparation et activité antitumorale expérimentale d'un nouvel antibiotique semi-synthétique: la diéthoxyacétoxy-14 daunorubicin (33 921 R.P.). CR Acad Sci [D] (Paris) 286: 443–446

Clinical Study of Detorubicin

EORTC Clinical Screening Group*

Summary

A phase II trial of detorubicin (DTR) has been conducted on 164 patients with solid tumors. Regressions ≥ 50% were obtained in 23% of the breast carcinoma patients, in 17% of the head and neck carcinoma patients and melanoma patients, and in 6% of the uteri cervix carcinoma patients. DTR seems to be as toxic as adriamycin for bone marrow and heart, but might induce a little less alopecia.

Introduction

Several analogues of the presently clinically used anthracyclines, daunorubicin (DRB) [1, 7] and adriamycin (ADM) [4, 5], have been prepared. Experimental studies have indicated that these analogues might represent an advantage when administered to patients, since they may induce less cardiac toxicity and less alopecia than DRB and ADM. These analogues are the French detorubicin (DTR) [8, 10, 11], the Italian 4′-epi-adriamycin (EAD) [3], the American AD-32 [2], and the Japanese aclacinomycin A (ACM) [12–14]. This paper reports the results of a phase II trial on DTR conducted by our group.

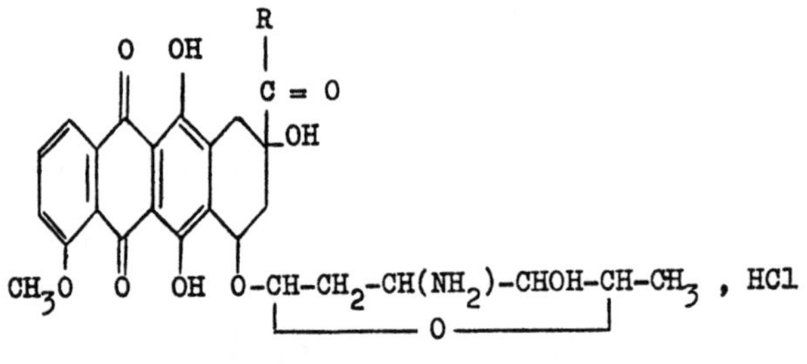

Fig. 1. Formula of [amino-3-tridesoxy-2,3,6-L-lysohexosyloxy] -7-[(diethoxyacetoxy)-2-acetyl-9] trihydroxy-6,9,11-methoxy-4-tetra-hydro-7,8,9,10-naphtacenequinone-5,12⁻ or detorubicin (DTR)

* *Chairman:* E. Pommatau; *Councillor:* G. Mathé; *Secretary:* M. Hayat; *Members:* S. Schraub, A. Monnier (Besancon); J. Chauvergne, J. Reboul, L. Traissac, M. Caudry (Bordeaux); J. Guerrin (Dijon); P. Cappelaere (Lille); E. Pommatau, F. Cheix, N. Bonnafous (Lyon); J. Gary-Bobo (Montpellier); O. Godin (Nantes); M. Schneider (Nice); A. Cattan, Ch. Pourny (Reims); H. Piquet, C. Jeanne, P. Bastit (Rouen); P. Serpantié (Saint-Etienne); J. M. Lang, R. Keiling, T. Klein (Strasbourg); B. Clavel, J. Berlié (Saint-Cloud); G. Mathé, M. Hayat, F. de Vassal (Hôpital Paul-Brousse and ICIG, Villejuif); G. Brulé, F. May-Levin (IGR, Lagrange); C. Cauchie, R. Maurus (Bruxelles); T. J. Kuipers (Rotterdam); C. Oliveira (Coimbra)

Materials and Methods

The chemical structure of DTR [11], [amino-3-tridesoxy-2,3,6-L-lyxohexosyl-oxy] - 7 - [(diethoxy-acetoxy)-acetyl-9]trihydroxy-6,9,11-methoxy-4-tetrahydro-7,8,9,10-naphtacinequinone-5,12, or dietoxyacetoxy-14-daunorubicin, is shown in Fig. 1. In 22 conventional experimental models, the activity of DTR has been demonstrated and compared with that of ADM at their respective maximally efficient doses. The activity of DTR was more efficient than that of ADM in eight models, and less efficient in only two [11]. No difference between DTR and ADM was detected, however, in our electron-microscopic study of myocardium toxicity and light-microscopic study of the skin in golden hamsters [6]. Thus, only the higher incidence of the oncostatic effect of DTR compared with that of ADM on experimental tumors [11] led us to conduct this clinical (phase II) screening trial.

The compound was administered as a rapid intravenous (IV) bolus every 21 days at an initial dose of 120 mg/m^2; the doses of the following cycles were adapted to the blood counts obtained during therapy, as indicated in Table 1.

The criteria for a patient's eligibility for the trial were those defined by the EORTC: the patient must have had "nothing to loose and something to hope" from the application of the tested compound. This ethical rule obviously tends to underestimate the effect of the compound, as the patients have previously been submitted to most cancer treatments, especially to the drugs available through chemotherapy, and, often, to radiotherapy. The question is not the proportion of the patients responding to the tested compound, but whether some tumors respond or are sensitive enough to the drug to justify further trials.

Eligible patients included those who had histologic confirmation of a malignancy for which no therapy had a proven clinical benefit, or who had demonstrated disease progression while on other therapies. Only ambulatory patients with an estimated survival in excess of 2 months and who had objectively measurable disease were entered.

Toxicity and efficacity were recorded according to the codes used by our group; these are summarized in Table 2. Treatment was continued until there was objective evidence of tumor progression or until the patient experienced unacceptable toxicity. An adequate therapeutic trial was defined as a minimum of three courses of DTR, unless objective tumor progression occurred after one or two courses.

A total of 164 patients were entered into this phase II study. Of the 135 evaluable patients (79 females and 56 males; median age, 48 years), 60 had previously received chemotherapy and 75 had not been given prior chemotherapy.

Table 1. Phase II trial of detorubicin: Adaptation of doses of DTR to the hemograms[a]

Minimal figures reached for neutrophil granulocytes	Minimum figures reached for platelets	Modification of the following dose
> 3,000	> 150,000	↗ 50%
> 2,000 but < 3,000 and/or	> 100,000 but < 150,000	↗ 25%
> 1,000 but < 2,000 and/or	> 15,000 but < 100,000	None
< 1,000 and/or	< 75,000	↘ 25%
Morbidity (infection, hemorrhage)		↘ 50%

[a] Protocol of treatment: 120 mg/m^2/day, q 3 weeks, IV push (maximum total tolerated dose: 2,120 mg)

Table 2. Codes for evaluation of toxicity and efficacy

Evaluation of intolerance and toxicity (IT)[a]

IT_0: Absence of any evidence to toxicity

IT_1: Minor toxicity or toxicity easily countered by symptomatic treatment and/or not necessitating modification of the treatment

IT_2: Toxicity not responding adequately to symptomatic treatment and/or necessitating adaptation of the treatment (e.g., reduction and/or modification of dosage frequency) or delayed toxicity (occurring after the end of therapy)

IT_3: Major toxicity necessitating discontinuation of the drug

IT_4: Toxicity having produced death

IT_5: Toxicity that could not be evaluated

Evaluation of efficacy

Efficacy is evaluated by taking into account the subjective, symptomatic, and objective signs

Subjective and symptomatic responses (S)

Only symptoms related to the treated malignant disease are to be taken in account:

S_0: Aggravation, status quo, or slight improvement

S_1: Definite improvement

S_2: Normalization of all symptoms

S_3: Nonassessable effect

Objective effect

The only effect (E) to be considered is that observed in lesions that can be assessed clinically or through X-rays at the end of the course of therapy, regardless of its duration

E_0: Aggravation

E_1: Checking of progression of lesions or regression up to 20%

E_2: Regression $<$ 50% of the volume of the tumor

E_3: Regression $>$ 50% but incomplete

E_4: Complete regression (disappearance of all lesions)

[a] The abbreviation IT was adopted because it adequately describes the reactions observed and to avoid confusion between the letter I and number 1, and also between the letter T (toxicity) and that used to represent tumoral extension in the TNM system

Table 3. Phase II trial of detorubicin: Patients nonevaluable for efficacy

Lost to follow-up within the first 2 weeks of treatment	5
Primary tumor unknown	11 (6)
Protocol violation (drug not single or one cycle only)	9
Incomplete data	1
Major toxicity after one or two cycles	3
Total	29/164 = 18%

Results

Efficacy

Of the 164 patients in the study, 29 were not fully evaluable for response: Table 3 indicates the reasons for their exclusion from the trial for the evaluation of tumor response.

Table 4 indicates the types of the tumors treated and the incidence of responses corresponding to a regression $\geqslant$ 50% of the tumor volume. Of the 135 evaluable patients, 17 had an objective response: 5 with E_4 and 13 with E_3. DTR induced 23% of such regressions in 26 breast carcinoma patients, 17% in 12 patients with melanoma, 17% in 24 patients with head and neck tumors, and only 6% in 16 patients with cervix carcinoma. Responses were obtained in one of four patients with ovarian carcinoma, one of three with bladder cancer, one of two with esophagal carcinoma, and one in a patient with Hodgkin's disease.

Table 5 shows the characteristics of the patient population who responded to DTR, including those with only minor response or E_2: tumor type, age, sex, previous chemotherapy, localization of measurable lesions in which the response was obtained, total dose administered, efficacy, and duration of the response. The doses given to responders ranged from 395 mg to 2120 mg (mean: 950 mg, about five cycles), and their duration, varying from 1–8 months (mean: 3.4 months). Table 6 shows that the incidence of response was higher in patients not previously submitted (32%) than in those previously submitted to chemotherapy (20%), but these percentages were not significantly different.

Toxicity

Toxicity data is presented in Tables 5 and 7. Of the 164 patients in the study, four were not fully evaluable for toxicity. The overall digestive toxicity was 52% and hematologic toxicity was 36%. Asthenia was seen in 44% of the patients and must be considered as a side effect; 50% of the treated patients had alopecia. Among 34 patients, cardiac toxicity (21%) consisted of cardiac rythm abnormalities (13 cases), ECG modifications (23 cases: T-wave alterations), or both (eight cases). Blood pressure fell in 26% of these patients; thoracic pain occurred in 9% and thrombophlebitis in 6%. The appearance of the cardiovascular manifestations also cannot be correlated with the previous administration of adriamycin, because only a few patients had received it.

Table 4. Phase II trial of detorubicin: Results[a]

Diagnosis	Total no. of cases	No. of evaluable patients	Efficacy					Response rate	
			Apparently complete regression	Partial regression	Minor response	No change	Progressive disease	> 50%	Overall
Head and neck	26	24	1	3	1	9	10	17%	21%
Esophagus	5	2	–	1	–	–	1	1/2	
Large bowel	3	2	–	–	–	–	2		
Rectum	5	3	–	–	–	–	3		
Pancreas	1	1	–	–	–	–	1		
Bronchus	14	13	–	–	3	3	7		3/13 (23%)
Bones	4	4	–	–	2	–	2		2/4
Soft tissue	8	8	–	–	1	1	6		1/8
Melanomas	13	12	–	2	–	1	9	2/12 (17%)	
Skin	1	1	–	–	–	1	–		
Breast	32	26	2	4	6	5	9	23%	46%
Cervix uteri	18	16	–	1	3	2	10	1/16 (6%)	25%
Endometrium uteri	5	4			1	2	1		1/4
Ovarian	6	4	1	–	–	1	2	1/4	
Vagina	1	1	–	–	–	–	1		
Testis	3	2	–	–	–	2	–		
Penis	1	1	–	–	–	–	1		
Bladder	3	3	–	1	–	–	2	1/3	
Kidney	7	6	–	–	2	1	3		2/6
Thyroid	1	1	–	–	–	1	–		
Hodgkin's disease	1	1	1	–	–	–	–	1/1	
	164	135	5	12	19	27	72		
			4%	9%	14%	20%	53%		
			13% (complete + partial)						
			27% (complete + partial + minor)			73% (no change + progressive)			

[a] Total number of patients in the trial: 164; total number of evaluable patients: 135

Table 5. Characteristics of responders to detorubicin

Tumor	Age	Sex	Previous chemotherapy		Localization	Total dose	Efficacy			Duration (months)	Toxicity				
			No	Yes			E_4	E_3	E_2		Digestive	Hematologic	Cardiac	Alopecia	Other
Head an neck	67	M	+		Lung	780		+		3	1	0	0	1	2
	57	M		+	Lung, skin	600		+		2	1	1	0	0	1
	40	M	+		Lung, nodes	800		+		3	1	0	0	1	0
	43	M	+		Lung	540		+		2	1	0	0	0	0
	50	M	+		Sternum	680	+			5	0	0	0	1	0
Esophagus	73	M	+		Tumor	2120		+		2+	0	0	1	1	0
Lung	57	M	+		Nodes, skin	740			+	4	0	0	2	1	0
	49	F	+		Nodes	1800			+	6	1	0	1	0	1
	67	M	+		Liver, mediastinal	530			+	2	1	0	0	1	1
Bone	18	F		+	Lung	1020			+	1	0	0	0	0	0
	50	M	+		Lung	870			+	3	0	1	0	1	0
Soft tissue	52	F		+	Lung	700			+	3	2	0	1	0	2
Melanoma	63	F	+		Lung, skin	1760		+		7	1	0	1	1	0
	34	M	+		Nodes, bone	1200		+		4	1	0	0	1	0
Breast	43	F		+	Nodes, skin, bone	1200			+	3	1	1	0	0	1
	59	F	+		Nodes	540			+	4	0	0	0	0	0
	64	F		+	Nodes, lung	1235			+	3	1	2	0	1	1
	47	F		+	Liver, bone	450			+	2	1	2	0	–	2
	39	F		+	Lung, nodes	1500			+	2	1	1	0	1	0
	47	F	+		Liver, brain, bone	450			+	3	1	1	0	1	1
	47	F		+	Liver, bone	840		+		3	0	1	1	0	0
	56	F	+		Lung	1540		+		5	0	0	0	1	0
	60	F		+	Bone, lung, skin	1060		+		8	2	2	0	0	0
	55	F	+		Lung	1140	+			3	0	0	0	1	0
	70	F	+		Lung	690	+			5	1	1	1	1	1
	75	F	+		Skin, bone	400		+		3	1	4	0	1	1
Cervix uteri	40	F	+		Nodes, vulva	800		+		3	1	0	0	0	2
	69	F		+	Tumor, nodes, vulva	920			+	3	2	0	0	0	2
	50	F	+		Tumor	1440			+	8	0	1	0	1	0
	64	F	+		Tumor, nodes	600			+	2	1	1	0	1	1
Endometrium uteri	55	F	+		Tumor, lung	395			+	2	1	0	0	1	1
Ovary	56	F		+	Tumor, nodes	600	+			1+	0	0	1	1	2
Bladder	51	M	+		Lung	740		+		3	1	1	0	0	2
Kidney	65	M	+		Lung, nodes	400			+	1	2	0	0	1	1
	58	M	+		Skin	1390			+	5	2	2	1	0	2
Hodgkin's disease	36	F		+	Nodes	1760	+			5	1	1	0	0	0
Total	(n=36)	M: 13 F: 23	24	12			5	13	18	m=3.4	21	15	10	19	18

Table 6. Phase II trial of detorubicin: Responses related to previous treatment

Diagnosis	No.	Previous chemotherapy	
		Yes	No
Head and neck	24	1/9	4/15
Esophagus	2	0/1	1/1
Large bowel	2	0/1	0/1
Rectum	3	0/1	0/2
Pancreas	1	0/1	–
Bronchus	13	–	3/13
Bone	4	1/3	1/1
Soft tissue	8	1/5	0/3
Melanoma	12	0/8	2/4
Skin	1	0/1	–
Breast	26	6/20	6/6
Cervix uteri	16	1/3	3/13
Endometrium	4	0/1	1/3
Ovary	4	1/4	–
Vagina	1	–	0/1
Testis	2	0/1	0/1
Penis	1	0/1	–
Bladder	3	0/1	1/2
Kidney	6	0/1	2/5
Thyroid	1	–	0/1
Hodgkin's disease	1	1/1	–
Total	135	12/60 (20%)	24/75 (32%)

Table 7. Summary of toxicity of detorubicin

	IT_0 (%)	IT_1 (%)	IT_2 (%)	IT_3 (%)	IT_4 (%)
Digestive	77 (48)	60 (37)	22 (14)	1 (1)	
Hematologic	102 (64)	33 (21)	18 (11)	5 (3)	2 (1.2)
Cardiac	126 (79)	20 (12.5)	7 (5)	6 (4)	1 (0.6)
Alopecia	79 (50)	80 (50)			
Others (asthenia)	90 (56)	38 (26)	31 (21)		
Total				12 (7)	3 (2)

The appearance of these cardiac side effects did not correlate with the number of cycles given (one cycle in three patients). Treatment was discontinued in six cases because of cardiotoxicity. Efficacy did not correlate with any type of toxicity (Tables 5 and 6).

Three patients died: two with bone marrow aplasia (a 75-year-old woman with breast cancer, brain and bone complications, and no previous chemotherapy: 3-month treatment at a dose of 400 mg with E_3 efficacy; and a 52-year-old woman with breast cancer and previous radiochemotherapy: at a dose of 200 mg); and one with myocardial lesions (a 70-year-old woman with breast cancer, lung metastases, and previous radiochemotherapy: at a dose of 210 mg, with tachyarythmia).

Discussion

In conclusion, our phase II trial shows that DTR is an efficient oncostatic in solid tumors, just as Jacquillat [10] observed its efficiency in leukemias. In our trial on solid tumors, DTR seems to be frequently efficient in breast carcinoma, in head and neck tumors, and in melanoma. Its toxicity, like that of ADM, appears in the bone marrow and the heart. Alopecia appeared in 50% of the patients, and may be a little less frequent than that produced by ADM. Myocardial and hair toxicities correlate with the prediction of electron- and light-microscopic studies of the heart and of the skin of golden hamsters reported by Dantchev et al. [6].

References

1 Bernard J, Jacquillat C, Weil M, Boiron M, Tanzer J (1970) Present results in daunorubicin (rubidomycin, daunomycin). In: Mathé G (ed) Advances in the treatment of acute (blastic) leukemias. Springer, Heidelberg New York, pp 3–8

2 Blum RH, Garnick MB, Israel M, Canellos GP, Henderson IC, Frei E III (1979) Initial clinical evaluation of N-trifluoroacetyladriamycin-14-valerate (AD-32) an adriamycin analog. Cancer Treat Rep 63: 919–923

3 Bonfante V, Bonadonna G, Villani F, Di Fronzo G, Martini A, Casazza AM (1979) Preliminary phase I study of 4'-epi-adriamycin. Cancer Treat Rep 63: 915–918

4 Carter SK, Di Marco A, Ghione M, Krakoff IH, Mathé G (eds) (1972) Adriamycin. Springer, Heidelberg New York

5 Clarysse A, Kenis Y, Mathé G (1976) Cancer chemotherapy. Its role in the treatment strategy of hematologic malignancies and solid tumors. Springer, Heidelberg New York

6 Dantchev D, Slioussartchouk V, Paintrand M, Hayat M, Bourut C, Mathé G (1979) Electron microscopy of the heart and light microscopy of the skin after treatment of golden hamsters with adriamycin, detorubicin, AD 32 and aclacinomycin. Cancer Treat Rep 63: 875–888

7 EORTC Leukemia and Hematosarcoma Cooperative Group (1970) Rubidomycin (or daunomycin): A clinical evaluation. In: Mathé G (ed) Advances in the treatment of acute (blastic) leukemias. Springer, Heidelberg New York, pp 9–13

8 EORTC Clinical Screening Group (1978) Detorubicin: Preliminary results of a phase II trial in solid tumors (abstr 37). Med Oncol 4: 10

9 Hori S, Shirai M, Hirano S, Oki T (to be published) Antitumor activity of new anthracycline antibiotics, aclacinomycin A (NSC 208734) and its analogues, and their toxicity. Gann

10 Jacquillat Cl, Auclerc MF, Weil M, Maral J, Degos L, Auclerc G, Tobelem G, Schaison G, Bernard J (1979) Clinical activity of detorubicin : a new anthracycline derivative. Cancer Treat Rep 63: 889–893

11 Maral R, Ducep JB, Farge D, Ponsinet G, Reisdord D (1978) Préparation et activité antitumorale, expérimentale d'un nouvel antibiotique semi synthétique: 1a (diétoxyacé-toxy)-14-daunorubicine (33921 RP). CR Acad Sci (Parais) [D] 286: 443–446

12 Mathé G, Bayssas M, Gouveia J, Dantchev D, Ribaud P, Machover D, Misset JL, Schwarzenberg L, Jasmin C, Hayat M (1978) Preliminary results of a phase II trial of aclacinomycine in acute leukaemia and lymphosarcoma. An oncostatic anthracycline that is rarely cardiotoxic and induces no alopecia. Cancer Chemother Pharmacol 1: 259–262

13 Ogawa M, Inagaki J, Horikoshi N, Inoue K, Chinen T, Ueoka H, Nagura E (1979) Clinical study of Aclacinomycin A. Cancer Treat Rep 63: 931–934

14 Oki T, Matsuzawa Y, Yoshimoto A, Numata K, Kimatura I, Ori S, Takamatsu A, Umezawa H, Ishizuka M, Naganawa H, Suda H, Hamada M, Takeuchi T (1975) New antitumor antibiotics, aclacinomycins A and B. J Antiobiot (Tokyo) 28: 830–834

Preliminary Clinical Experience with 4'-Epidoxorubicin in Advanced Human Neoplasia

V. Bonfante, G. Bonadonna, F. Villani, and A. Martini*

Summary

4'-Epidoxorubicin (epi-DXR) was tested in 56 patients with various types of advanced malignancies. The pattern of acute toxicity was similar to that of doxorubicin (DXR), but epi-DXR produced a lower incidence of vomiting, stomatitis, alopecia, and myelosuppression. The study of cardiac toxicity, utilizing only noninvasive methods, indicated that epi-DXR also is cardiotoxic. The increase in the systolic time intervals after the first dose as well as after cumulative doses was slightly lower compared with that observed after DXR. Antitumor activity occurred in a variety of tumors including malignant melanoma, renal cancer, and rectal cancer, which are refractory to DXR. Present results suggest that further studies with epi-DXR are indicated.

Introduction

4'-Epidoxorubicin (epi-DXR) is one of the adriamycin (doxorubicin, DXR) analogues currently being tested in various forms of human neoplasia by the Istituto Nazionale Tumori of Milan [3]. Chemically, epi-DXR is a stereoisomer of DXR, with a different absolute configuration at position 4 of the sugar moiety. Its molecular weight is identical to that of DXR (Fig. 1). In experimental tumors, the antitumor activity of epi-DXR was shown to be equal to that of DXR. General toxicity and cardiac toxicity were lower compared with those of DXR when epi-DXR was tested in mice and

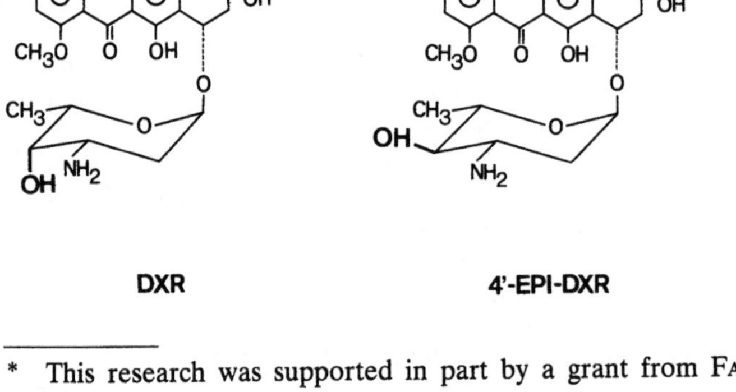

DXR   4'-EPI-DXR

Fig. 1. Structural formulas af doxorubicin (*left*) and 4'-epidoxorubicin (*right*)

* This research was supported in part by a grant from Farmitalia-Carlo Erba, SpA

rabbits during acute and chronic toxicity studies [5, 6]. Therefore, epi-DXR showed an increased therapeutic ratio and was considered a compound worthy of clinical trial.

Materials and Methods

Epi-DXR was supplied by FARMITALIA-Carlo Erba, Milan, Italy, as a red powder in 10-mg vials. The drug was reconstituted with twice distilled water and administered by rapid intravenous (IV) injection every 3 weeks. The starting dose level was 10 mg/m^2. Progressive dose escalation was carried out according to the Fibonacci scheme up to the dose of 50 mg/m^2.

Subsequently, we selected doses (60, 75, and 90 mg/m^2) which could be comparable to therapeutically effective doses of DXR. Table 1 presents the total number of patients treated and the number of cycles administered at each dose level. Doses higher than 50 mg/m^2 were rarely escalated in individual patients who received multiple courses. Therapy was discontinued if there were definite signs of tumor progression or when the total dose of epi-DXR (including, in eight patients, that of prior DXR) neared 550 mg/m^2. The highest dose administered in the present series was 555 mg/m^2.

Adult patients with documented advanced malignancy were included in this phase I–II study. Each patient had a performance status $\geq$ 50 (Karnofsky scale) and an estimated survival of at least 8 weeks. No patient had received chemotherapy and/or radiotherapy during the preceding 3 weeks. Of the 56 patients in the study, 41 had been previously treated with chemotherapy. In particular, eight patients had also received DXR to a mean total dose of 200 mg/m^2. Fifteen patients had not been previously treated. In this group were ten patients for whom there was no proven effective therapy for their advanced disease: renal carcinoma, two cases; lung

Table 1. Doses of 4′-epidoxorubicin

mg/m^2 q 3 weeks	No. of patients (total 56)	No. of cycles (total 173)
10	3	3
20	4	4
30	5	7
50	6	15
60	17	32
75	18	57
90	21	55

Table 2. Patient characteristics

Total	56 (31 men, 25 women)
Median age	45 years (18–71 years)
Prior treatment	41 (73%)
No prior treatment	15 (27%)
Prior DXR	8 (14%) mean total dose 200 mg/m^2 (60–320)

carcinoma, two cases; bladder carcinoma, two cases; chondrosarcoma, two cases; thyroid carcinoma, one case; and adenocarcinoma of unknown origin, one case. There were also two patients with chronic leukemia, and three with non-Hodgkin lymphoma. In this latter group, 1–2 doses of epi-DXR were given to test the therapeutic activity of the drug before starting conventional treatment (Table 2).

Parameters of Evaluation

Pretreatment evaluation consisted of complete history and physical examination with radiologic documentation of the extent of disease. Liver and bone scans were performed only when indicated by the clinical situation. Blood tests included complete hemogram, blood sugar, blood urea nitrogen (BUN), serum creatinine, uric acid, electrolytes, bilirubin, total proteins and albumin, alkaline phosphatase, and transaminases (SGOT, SGPT). All patients had an initial leukocyte (WBC) count ≥ 4000/mm^3 and platelet (PLT) count ≥ 110,000/mm^3, as well as adequate liver and renal function tests (e.g., bilirubin < 1.5 mg/100 ml, creatinine < 1.5 mg/100 ml). Hemograms were repeated at least once a week and chemistry was repeated prior to each course. Patients were followed closely for any evidence of toxicity, and appropriate roentgenographic studies were repeated prior to every course to document drug response.

Arterial blood pressure, pulse rate, electrocardiogram (ECG), and left ventricular systolic time interval were recorded 30 min before each drug administration while patients were fasting and resting for about 20–30 min. The same parameters were repeated 1 h after injection of epi-DXR. Systolic time intervals were determined according to the method described by Weissler et al. [8].

Results

Toxicity

A total of 56 patients (31 men and 25 women) with a median age of 45 years (18–71 years) were entered into the study as of April 1, 1979; 50 patients were evaluable for toxicity through 167 cycles of epi-DXR, and six patients were unevaluable because of early death due to progressive cancer, which prevented the collection of sufficient data for the present investigation.

No side effects were detected after single doses of 10, 20, and 30 mg/m^2. Table 3 shows the percent of toxic manifestations observed after various doses with 50, 60, 75, and 90 mg/m^2. The pattern of acute toxicity was similar to that observed after comparable doses of DXR [2–4], but a lower incidence of some side effects such as vomiting, stomatitis, alopecia, and myelosuppression was noted after epi-DXR. The nadir of leukocyte and platelet counts for all patients and courses occurred between days 8 and 15 after drug administration (Table 4). Leukopenia was observed more frequently than thrombocytopenia. Myelotoxicity did not appear to be dose related and tended to be moderate, with complete marrow recovery by the third week in almost all instances. A severe degree of myelosuppression was encountered in only three patients, who had been previously treated with chemotherapy. In the first patient the level of leukocytes fell to 800/mm^3, while in the other two patients the level of platelets dropped to

Table 3. Percent toxic manifestations

Toxicity	Dose (mg/m^2)			
	50	60	75	90
	No. of patients			
	6	15	16	19
Nausea	66	73	56	73
Vomiting	33	60	50	47
Stomatitis	0	0	6	5
Diarrhea	0	0	0	10
Fever[a]	0	0	12	5
Hair loss	50	40	37	42
Alopecia	16	20	50	52
Leukopenia[b]	66	60	62	52
Thrombocytopenia[c]	50	13	12	0
Renal or hepatic	0	0	0	0

[a] > 38° C
[b] WBC < 4,000/mm^3
[c] PLT < 110,000/mm^3

Table 4. Nadir of leukocyte and platelet fall

Dose (mg/m^2)	WBC[a]			PLT[a]		
	Median	Range	Median day	Median	Range	Median day
50	2.3	(1.7–4.3)	15	85	(45–200)	11
60	3.7	(1.4–5.5)	14	260	(120–400)	12
75	2.6	(1.7–5.9)	12	176	(55–350)	8
90	3.9	(0.8–7.3)	12	230	(120–410)	10

[a] Cells × 10^3/mm^3

45,000/mm^3 and 55,000/mm^3, respectively. Also in these patients the hematologic recovery occurred without complications. A decrease in the hemoglobin level of about 10% from the basal values occurred in most patients between days 7 and 14, but it was completely reversible by the third week of treatment.

The electrocardiographic abnormalities recorded during treatment with epi-DXR are presented in Table 5. These changes were transient and occurred at doses exceeding 30 mg/m^2. They were similar to those observed after DXR, but the incidence was not comparable to that reported after DXR because of the different frequency of ECG monitoring. Figure 2 shows the time course of PEP/LVET ratio after a single dose of epi-DXR. The systolic time interval sharply increased within 1 h after drug injection, followed by prompt return to near normal values 24 h after injection. This observation indicates that, as already observed with DXR, left ventricular dysfunction is transient

Table 5. ECG changes in 54 patients during 4′-epidoxorubicin

ECG changes	No. of patients	%
Tachycardia	4	7.4
Arrhythmias		
Coronary sinus rhythm	1	1.8
Atrial premature beats	3	5.5
Ventricular premature beats	6	11.1
ST-T segment		
ST-T segment depression	2	3.7
Flattening of T wave	11	20.0
Inversion of T wave	2	3.7
Combination of ECG changes	4	7.4
Total	29/54	54.0

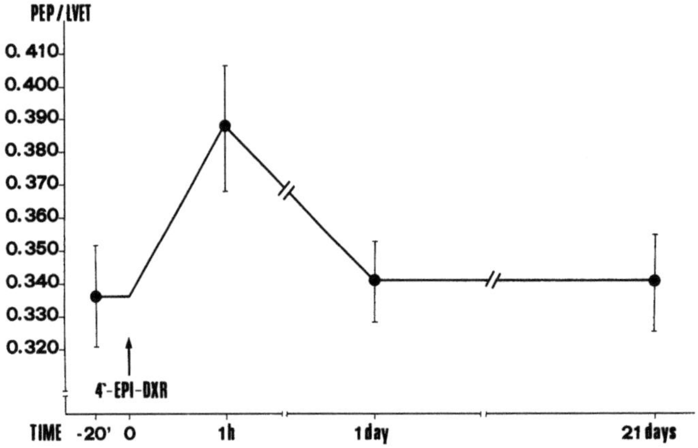

Fig.2. Time course of PEP/LVET ratio after a single IV dose (90 mg/m^2) of epi-DXR (mean ± SE of 11 patients)

and completely reversible after low doses of epi-DXR [7]. Figure 3 illustrates the variation of PEP/LVET ratio, expressed as a percent change $+\Delta$ % from basal values, produced by the first dose of epi-DXR. The values were compared with those obtained after equal doses of DXR administered in a previous investigation. There was a dose-dependent effect for both drugs on myocardial contractility [1]. However, the increase in PEP/LVET ratio produced by epi-DXR was lower than that observed in patients treated with DXR, although the difference was not statistically significant.

Figure 4 shows the changes in the systolic time interval recorded after different cumulative doses in eight patients who had received a total dose of epi-DXR near 550 mg/m^2. There was a linear regression relationship between PEP/LVET ratio and cumulative doses of epi-DXR. Mean PEP/LVET ratio values recorded after 50 mg/m^2 of epi-DXR were compared with those obtained in a previous investigation after the same cumulative doses of DXR. In patients treated with epi-DXR, mean PEP/LVET ratio values were lower compared with those observed after DXR, but the difference was not statistically significant (Table 6).

In the present study, no patient developed clinical signs or symptoms of congestive heart failure.

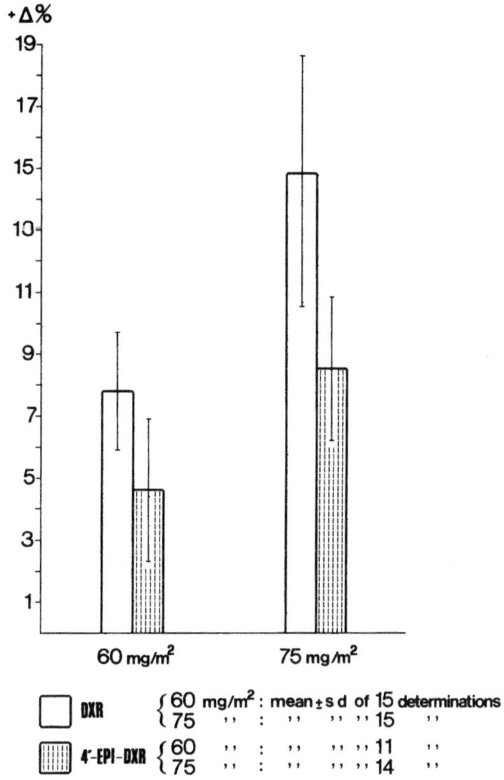

Fig. 3. Percentage change of PEP/LVET ratio after the first dose of epi-DXR: comparison with DXR

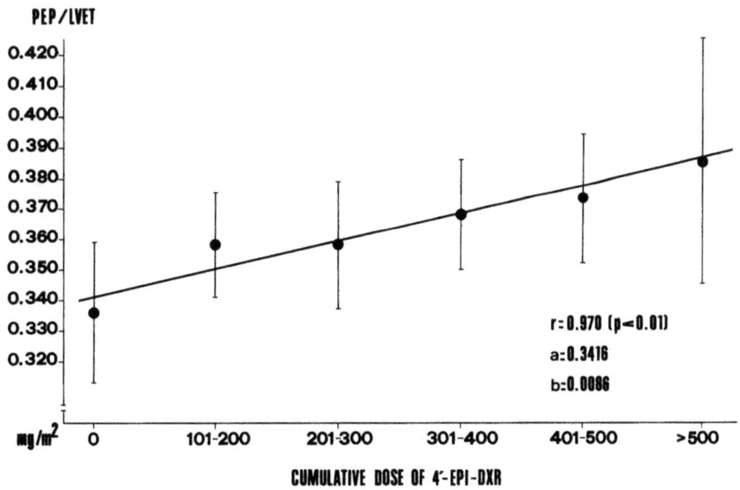

Fig . 4. Serial PEP/LVET ratio (mean ± SE) in 8 patients after various cumulative doses of epi-DXR

Table 6. Mean PEP/LVET ratio after 500 mg/m² of 4′-epidoxorubicin and doxorubicin

Epi-DXR (mean of 8 patients)	0.385 ± 0.040	$P > 0.05$
DXR (mean of 20 patients)	0.394 ± 0.013	

Table 7. Therapeutic activity of 4′-epidoxorubicin

Tumor	No. of patients	CR	PR	Improvement	Duration of response (weeks)
Melanoma	6			2	4–6
Renal cancer	6	1	1		14^{+}–52^{+}
Lung cancer	5				
Breast cancer	5		1	2	6–6^{+}–12^{+}
Head and neck cancer	4				
Bladder cancer	3				
Ovarian cancer	2				
Rectal cancer	3		1		15^{+}
Gastric cancer	1				
Soft tissue sarcoma	4				
Kaposi sarcoma	1		1		26
Thyroid cancer	2		1		30^{+}
Testicular cancer	1				
Non-Hodgkin lymphoma	3	1	2		Not evaluable
Polycythemia	1		1		Not evaluable
CLL	1		1		Not evaluable
CML	1		1		Not evaluable
Site unknown	1				

Therapeutic Results

The various types of malignant disease and their responses to epi-DXR are indicated in Table 7. Antitumor activity was documented in 16 (32%) of 50 evaluable patients after doses of 60, 75, and 90 mg/m^2. Eight responsive patients had not been previously treated with chemotherapy. Response in melanoma was minimal. In renal carcinoma, complete response (CR) was documented at the level of recurrent pleuropulmonary disease. The three patients with breast carcinoma had advanced local-regional disease, and tumor regression occurred in primary disease and in regional adenopathy. One patient with rectal carcinoma had shrinkage of a subcutaneous metastasis associated with normalization of a previously abnormal liver scan. In Kaposi sarcoma, response was obtained at the level of cutaneous lesions while in thyroid carcinoma this was observed at the level of pulmonary metastases. In non-Hodgkin lymphomas, CR was observed in one patient with Waldeyer's ring involvement, and partial response (PR) in two patients with retroperitoneal lymphadenopathy. PR was also documented in three patients with polycythemia vera, chronic lymphocytic, and chronic myelogenous leukemia in terms of decreased level of abnormal cells in the peripheral blood, reduced adenopathy, and hepatosplenomegaly. The latter six patients received only 1–2 doses of epi-DXR and were then treated according to a conventional therapeutic program. Therefore, the duration of response as well as the actual degree of tumor regression could not be evaluated.

Conclusion

4′-Epi-DXR has been the first DXR analogue tested at the Istituto Nazionale Tumori. The data regarding general toxicity indicated that the pattern of side effects was similar to that of DXR. However, epi-DXR showed less acute toxicity, as suggested by the lower incidence of vomiting, stomatitis, alopecia, and myelosuppression. Studies to assess cardiac toxicity showed that, like DXR, epi-DXR produced cumulative myocardial damage, although the mean PEP/LVET values after the first dose as well as after cumulative doses were slightly lower than those observed after the same doses of DXR. Although a significant difference was not observed between epi-DXR and DXR, present data, including the fact that no patient developed cardiac symptoms, suggests a higher threshold limit for epi-DXR cardiac toxicity. This hypothesis should be confirmed in a larger series of patients treated with high cumulative doses and after longer follow-up observation after the end of treatment. Therapeutic results indicated that epi-DXR may have a broader spectrum of antitumor activity than DXR if positive results on melanoma as well as on renal and colorectal carcinoma are confirmed in a larger group of patients.

References

1 Al Ismail SAD, Whittaker JA (1979) Systolic time interval as index of schedule-dependent doxorubicin cardiotoxicity in patients with acute myelogenous leukemia. Br Med J 1: 1392–1395

2 Bonadonna G, Beretta G, Tancini G, Brambilla C, Bajetta E, De Palo GM, De Lena M, Fossati Bellani F, Gasparini M, Valagussa P, Veronesi U Adriamycin (NSC-123127) studies at the Istituto Nazionale Tumori, Milan. Cancer Chemother Rep (part 3) 6: 231–245

3 Bonfante V, Bonadonna G, Villani F, Di Fronzo G, Martini A, Casazza AM (1979) Preliminary phase I study of 4′-epi-adriamycin. Cancer Treat Rep 63: 915–918

4 Blum RH, Carter SK (1974) Adriamycin, a new anticancer drug with significant clinical activity. Ann Intern Med 80: 249–259

5 Casazza AM, Di Marco A, Bertazzoli C, Formelli F, Giuiliani F, Pratesi G (1978) Antitumor activity, toxicity and pharmacological properties of 4′-epi-adriamycin. Curr Chemother 2: 1257–1260

6 Di Marco A, Casazza AM, Dasdia T, Necco A, Pratesi G, Rivolta P, Velcich A, Zaccara A, Zunino F (1977) Changes of activity of daunorubicin, adriamycin and stereo-isomers following the introduction or removal of hydroxyl groups in the amino sugar moiety. Chem Biol Interact 19: 291–302

7 Rinehart JJ, Lewis RP, Balcerzak SP (1974) Adriamycin cardiotoxicity in man. Ann Intern Med 81: 475–478

8 Weissler AM, Harris WS, Schoenfeld CD (1969) Bedside technics for the evaluation of ventricular function in man. Am J Cardiol 23: 577–583

Quelamycin: A Summary of Phase I Clinical Trials

H. Cortés-Funes, A. Brugarolas, and M. Gosálvez

Summary

Quelamycin is triferric doxorubicin, a metallic derivative of adriamycin which, in experimental studies, has been found to have a better therapeutic index than adriamycin and no cardiotoxicity. In Spain, phase I clinical trials carried out in 96 patients with advanced cancer have shown that the drug has low toxicity and considerable antitumor activity, while it is not cardiotoxic, even at cumulative doses of nearly 3 g.

Introduction

Quelamycin is triferric doxorubicin, a metallic derivative of adriamycin made by chelating three atoms of ferric iron in each molecule of adriamycin (Fig. 1). Quelamycin was discovered by MARIO GOSÁLVEZ in 1976 [7] and was introduced in the clinics as a possible noncardiotoxic derivative of adriamycin [10]. GOSÁLVEZ et al. [8, 9, 11, 12] found that adriamycin inhibited, at very low concentrations, the enzyme Na-K ATPase of the plasma membrane and postulated that the cardiotoxicity of adriamycin was a digitalislike cardiotoxicity. As the effect of the enzyme was counteracted by calcium and adriamycin was known to form metallic complexes, GOSÁLVEZ developed a triferric complex which was inactive in the Na-K ATPase and was noncardiotoxic in the rat [10]. Quelamycin had, on the other hand, the same potency as adriamycin in inhibiting DNA synthesis and in inhibiting the growth of ascites tumors in mice, while

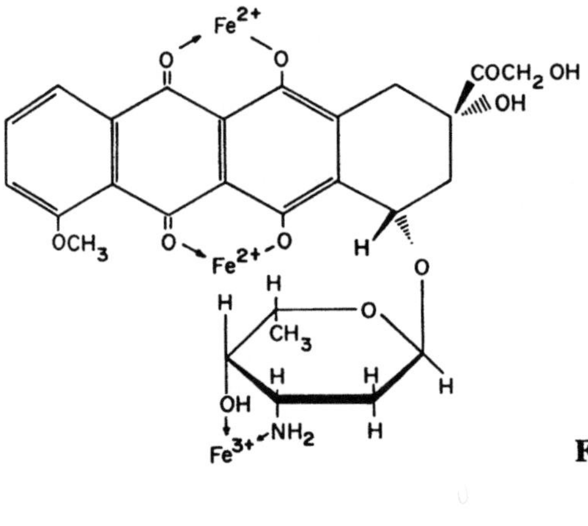

Fig. 1. Chemical structure of quelamycin

Table 1. Content of iron and adriamycin in several quelamycin lots

Lot	Adriamycin (mg)	Fe^{+++} (mg)	Theoretical % adriamycin	Theoretic % Fe^{+++}	Free iron in excess (mg)
K-1	24	10.6	96	153	3.69
K-2	23	9.75	92	146	3.31
L 1	25.5	11.40	102	155	4.02
M-2A	24.0	10.60	96	153.4	3.69
M-3	26.01	8.85	104	118.85	1.36
N-1	22.45	6.24	90	96.29	none

it was much less toxic [10]. This improvement in therapeutic index was accompanied by other advantages such as oral absorption and the ability of the drug to cross the blood-brain barrier. These possible advantages of using quelamycin prompted phase I clinical trials with the drug in Spain [1, 3–6].

Although the experimental studies by Gosálvez and his group were done with freshly made quelamycin devoid of free iron, the first pharmaceutical formulations carried an excess of free iron (Table 1), which was responsible for the acute and chronic iron toxicity encountered by Brugarolas et al. in the first clinical trial of quelamycin [1, 3, 4]. Quelamycin is presently available devoid of free iron.

In what follows we summarize the results of the phase I clinical trials with quelamycin carried out in Spain during 1977, 1978, and 1979 [1, 3–6].

Materials and Methods

The 96 patients entered into the study had histologic evidence of solid malignant tumors for which no therapy of proven clinical benefit was available. Selection criteria also included a life expectancy of > 8 weeks, Karnofsky performance status of > 30%, and no chemotherapy of radiotherapy in the past 12 weeks. Five patients had received previously adriamycin until the limiting dose. All patients had normal cardiac (clinical and ECG) functions, > 5,000 WBC, > 100,000 platelets, serum creatinine > 2 mg/100 ml, SGOT > 100,000 U, and bilirubin > 2.5 mg/100 ml. Blood cell counts were repeated every other day in hospitalized patients and weekly in outpatients. Physical examination, ECG, chest X-ray, performance status, and tumor measurements were recorded before each cycle. Quelamycin was supplied and manufactured by Dr. Gosálvez at Montedison Farmaceutic (Barcelona) in vials containing a black lipophylized powder of 25-mg equivalent of quelamycin. Each vial of quelamycin was reconstituted with 10 ml of bid stilled water for intravenous (IV) injection. Quelamycin was administered as a slow IV infusion for at least 1 h every 3 weeks [5, 6], as a rapid IV injection every 3 weeks [3], as three consecutive daily injections every 3 weeks [4], or as a single rapid injection every 3 weeks, followed by administration of the iron-chelator deferoxamine [1]. Doses of quelamycin every 3 weeks ranged from 75–175 mg/m^2. A minimum WBC of 3,000/mm^3 required before giving the next course. The dose was reduced if the patient tolerance or toxicity was severe.

Objective response to therapy was defined as a decrease by 50% or more in the growth of the two largest perpendicular diameters of measurable lesions. Stable disease corresponded to a decrease by < 50% or by unchanged lesions. Progression was defined by any increase in the size of lesions or the appearance of new lesions.

Results

Toxicity was different with the different methods of administration. It is necessary to distinguish between the toxicity of quelamycin and the toxicity of the free iron accompanying the drug. By comparising the toxicity of lot *N*-1 with that of the other lots, it was concluded that the toxicity of quelamycin consists of mild nausea and vomiting, leukopenia, and alopecia. Iron toxicity was characterized by fever and chills, and the sympatomimetic crisis described by Brugarolas et al. [3]. The dose-limiting toxicity of quelamycin was identified as hematologic. Leukocyte and platelet count nadirs occurred on day 13 after single-dose quelamycin administration, and recovery was observed by day 19 after treatment. Maximum recommended dose for intermittent single-dose schedule was 125–150 mg/m^2 every 3 weeks. Alopecia was a common side effect. Hair growth occurred during therapy in several patients. No local toxicity after extravasation of the drug was noticed. Regional vein thrombosis was observed in a small proportion of patients receiving quelamycin, and hyperpigmentation of the skin was frequent.

The most remarkable finding concerning the toxicity of quelamycin is that chronic cardiotoxicity was not documented in patients who had received large cumulative doses. Repeated ECG studies in patients receiving high cumulative quelamycin doses showed no alterations in voltage or repolarization. Systolic time interval measured in several patients appeared to be within normal limits. No clinical signs of heart toxicity were demonstrated. Cumulative quelamycin doses reached in long-term treatment are shown in Table 2. Eight patients have received cumulative quelamycin doses in excess of 1 g/m^2. One patient received 2.8 g/m^2 quelamycin.

In view of these results, several patients who reached the total limiting dose of adriamycin while maintaining a clinical response were transferred to quelamycin therapy. Table 3 demonstrated the cumulative doses of adriamycin and quelamycin administered to a group of such patients.

Two patients with breast cancer and anthracycline heart toxicity were of special interest. One patient was a 57-year-old woman with a widely disseminated breast cancer previously treated by bilateral adrenalectomy who had failed to respond to combination chemotherapy with cyclophosphamide, methotrexate, fluorouracil, and vincristine (CMFV).

She was treated with adriamycin upon progression of the disease, and presented subjective decrease of pain and stabilization of bony lesions for 1 year. Total adriamycin dose was 880 mg/m^2 when she developed several episodes of congestive heart failure which required repeated hospitalization and vigorous treatment with digitalis, diuretics, and salt restriction. Adriamycin therapy was discontinued, and a steady state was maintained with exertional dyspnea and tachycardia not sensitive to digitalis. Quelamycin was initiated after clinical recurrence of pain and significant deterioration in her general condition. There was an improvement in her tumor symptoms and no subsequent deterioration in the heart condition. The cumulative quelamycin dose at the time of this report was 620 mg/m^2.

Another patient aged 54 years had a diagnosis of metastatic breast cancer who failed to respond to previous bilateral adrenalectomy and CMFV therapy. She showed an

Table 2. Analysis of long-term treatment with quelamycin

Patient	Quelamycin total dose (mg/m²)	Cardiotoxicity		
		Clinical	ECG	Heart biopsy
BSA	2850	None	None	Pending
JMV	1700	None	None	Negative
MBV	1607	None	None	Negative
MBG	1500	None	None	Pending
JMGV	1396	None	None	Not done
JSP	1244	None	None	–
MACG	1080	None	None	Not done
CSD	1050	None	None	–
SFF	933	None	None	Not done

Table 3. Analysis of quelamycin treatment after adriamycin limiting dose

Patient	Tumor type	Adriamycin total dose (mg/m²)	Quelamycin total dose (mg/m²)	Heart toxicity
JMFH	Bone sarcoma	700	1158	None
AFA	Breast cancer	880	620	None
JRFG	Bone sarcoma	525	600	None
MAGR	Bone sarcoma	650	500	None
LMM	Breast cancer	550	375	None

objective response to adriamycin and presented ECG changes consistent with a decrease in the QRS voltage, ST segment changes, and tachycardia nonsensitive to digitalis after adriamycin total dose of 550 mg/m^2. She had an episode of heart failure before quelamycin therapy was initiated. Total quelamycin dose given was 375 mg/m^2, which was tolerated without cardiac side effects of further deterioration in the symptoms.

Lastly, a 16-year-old boy who received chest irradiation after incomplete pulmonary resection of metastatic osteosarcoma resistant to adriamycin received a total quelamycin dose of 1150 mg/m^2. His previous cumulative adriamycin dose was 700 mg/m^2. No heart toxicity was noticed despite mediastinal irradiation, dose-limiting adriamycin therapy, and subsequent high-dose quelamycin treatment.

These results indicated that long-term quelamycin could be given up to the extent of the presently reported levels without an increase in overt cardiotoxicity. Patients with adriamycin cardiotoxicity appeared to tolerate quelamycin without significant deterioration in the heart function for the periods of time noted.

Concerning antitumor activity, objective responses were obtained in carcinoma of the lung, breast, stomach, colon, ovary, and in soft-tissue and bone sarcomas (Table 4). Cross-resistance with adriamycin was not clearly established. Patients with tumors resistant to adriamycin were resistant to quelamycin as well, except for two patients with osteogenic sarcoma. On the other hand, there was a limited experience with

Table 4. Response to quelamycin therapy

Tumor type	Patients	Objective responses[a]	% Responses
Lung carcinoma	58	11	18.9
Breast carcinoma	8	4[a,b]	
Stomach carcinoma	6	1	
Soft-tissue sarcoma	9	1[a,c]	
Osteogenic sarcoma	5	5[a,c]	
Renal carcinoma	2	0	
Lymphoma (NHL)	2[d]	0	
Colon carcinoma	1	1	
Ovary carcinoma	1	1	
Other tumors	4	0	
Overall	96	22	22.9

[a] 50% or more decrease in tumor size unless otherwise stated
[b] Stable disease
[c] One patient maintained an objective response previously induced with adriamycin
[d] Indicates prior adriamycin treatment

Table 5. Analysis of the responses obtained in bronchogenic carcinoma with quelamycin

Cell type	Patients	Objective responses	Duration of response	% Responses
Epidermoid carcinoma	18	2	15 + months 8 months	11.1
Adenocarcinoma	7	1	8 + months	14.2
Anaplastic large cell carcinoma	18	5	14 + months 14 + months 7 + months 5 + months 5 months	27.7
Overall results	43	8		18.6

patients who received quelamycin after a limiting dose of adriamycin while maintaining a clinical response to it. These patients maintained the remission. Non-small cell bronchogenic carcinoma was the only tumor category with an evaluable number of patients. In Table 5, the results obtained in one series are shown. Overall response rate was 18.6% with a median duration of response of 8 months. This was probably consistent with the expected activity of adriamycin in this tumor type.

Discussion

Quelamycin has several remarkable features. First, it was designed according to a rationale as a drug which would not affect the major mechanism of adriamycin cardiotoxicity. Secondly, biochemical and experimental animal models predicted a decrease in cardiotoxicity as compared with adriamycin. Finally, these data have been confirmed by the results of the initial clinical studies. Long-term quelamycin as single anthracycline therapy after dose-limiting adriamycin treatment was not associated with an increase in cardiotoxicity. Assessment of heart damage by means of endomyocardial biopsy electron-microscopic studies is currently under way.

Several other findings appeared of interest. The pharmacokinetics of quelamycin [2, 5] offers as possible advantages the prolonged circulation time and the ability to cross the brain-blood barrier. Oral absorption and prolonged hepatic exposure to high-dose quelamycin due to enterohepatic circulation [2] is another interesting aspect because it might enable some form of selective treatment of hepatic tumors.

Finally, quelamycin appeared to be active in a wide spectrum of tumors, which was consistent with adriamycin activity. Responses were obtained at 75 mg/m^2 while the dose-limiting hematologic toxicity was 150 mg/m^2, suggesting a good therapeutic index which could be important in case the drug moves into combination chemotherapy studies.

Based on the reported data, continuation of clinical studies is recommended for obvious reasons. The immediate fields of investigation appeared to be pharmacokinetics and metabolism of quelamycin, confirmation of a decreased cardiotoxicity by endomyocardial biopsies, schedule modification and oral quelamycin administration, and phase II clinical trials focusing on a complete range of tumors including those nonsensitive to adriamycin.

Two especially attractive clinical uses of quelamycin treatment appeared at this time: follow-up therapy in patients with clinical response to adriamycin who reached the limiting toxic dose, and metastatic liver disease from gastrointestinal cancer and hepatoma.

In summary, the initial reports on quelamycin appeared negative because of its acute and chronic iron toxicity. As quelamycin is now pharmaceutically formulable without accompanying free iron, these side effects have been prevented and the clinical interest in this drug is now very clear: low hematologic toxicity at therapeutic doses, low cardiotoxicity, oral absorption, and antitumor activity.

In view of these reasons, expansion of investigation is encouraged and obviously expected to occur in the near future. If the promising features just uncovered in the early clinical testing of this drug are confirmed, quelamycin deserves an important role in cancer chemotherapy.

References

1 Brugarolas A, Gracia Marco M, García Miralles MT, Ribas A, Valle M, Izarguzaga I (to be published) Prevention of long term iron associated toxicity of quelamycin by deferoxamine. Cancer Treat Rep

2 Brugarolas A, Lacave AJ, Gracia Marco M, Buesa JM, Cortés H, Gosálvez M (to be published) Quelamycin. Cancer Chemother Rev

3 Brugarolas A, Pachón N, Pérez-Llanderal JA, Lacave AJ, Buesa JM, Gracia Marco M (1978) Phase I clinical trial of quelamycin. Cancer Treat Rep 62: 1527–1534
4 Brugarolas A, Pérez Llanderal JA, García Miralles MT, Lacave AJ, Gracia Marco M, Izquierdo JM, Rodríguez Lloviran AL, Ribas A (1979) Iron toxicity studies of quelamycin. Cancer Treat Rep 63: 909–913
5 Cortés-Funes H, Gosálvez M, Moyano A, Mañas A, Mendiola C (1979) Early trial clinical with quelamycin. Cancer Treat Rep 63: 903–908
6 Cortés-Funes H, Vicente J, Baena L, Otero J, Gosálvez M (1978) Preliminary evaluation of a phase I clinical study of quelamycin. Eur J Cancer 14: 1359–1361
7 Gosálvez M (1976) Triferric adriamycin, a possible noncardiotoxic derivative with antitumor activity equal to adriamycin. In: Proceedings of the tenth International Congress of Biochemistry. Edited by the International Union of Biochemistry. Published by Brönners Druckerei Breidenstein KG. Hamburg, July 25, 1976
8 Gosálvez M, Blanco MF (1975) Inhibition of Na-K ATPase by the antitumor antibiotic adriamycin. In: Proceedings of the 5th International Biophysic Congress. Edited by the International Union for pure and applied Biophysics. Printed in Denmark by Villedsen and Christensen. Copenhagen, August, 1975
9 Gosálvez M, Blanco MF (1978) Requirements for the inhibition of sodium and potassium ion transporting adenosine triphosphatase by adriamycin. Biochem Soc Trans 6: 945–947
10 Gosálvez M, Blanco MF, Vivero C, Vallés F (1978) Quelamycin, a new derivative of adriamycin with several possible therapeutic advantages. Eur J Cancer 14: 1185–1190
11 Gosálvez M, Rossum GDV van, Blanco MF (1979) Inhibition of sodium-potassium activated adenosine-5-triphosphatase and ion transport by adriamycin. Cancer Res 39: 257–261
12 Rossum GDV van, Gosálvez M (1976) Inhibition of ion transport by the antitumor antibiotic adriamycin. Fed Proc 35: 3201

Current Status of Japanese Studies with the New Anthracycline Antibiotic Aclacinomycin A

T. Oki, T. Takeuchi, S. Oka, and H. Umezawa

Summary

Fundamental and clinical studies on a new yellow anthracycline antibiotic aclacinomycin A are reviewed. Favorable responses were seen in patients with acute leukemia refractory to daunomycin and adriamycin, malignant lymphoma, and breast, ovarian, lung, gastric, intestinal, and urinary bladder cancers by intravenous and intraperitoneal infusions or bladder instillation of aclacinomycin A alone in the phase II study.

Introduction

Aclacinomycin A (ACM) is a yellow anthracycline antibiotic which was isolated from a culture broth of *Streptomyces galilaeus* [10]. Although related to the clinically used adriamycin by having the planar, tetracyclic ring structure common to anthracyclines (Fig. 1), the structures are dissimilar enough to expect differences in biologic activities; in fact, ACM is characteristic of (a) oral activity on various experimental tumors, (b) preferential inhibition of RNA synthesis; (c) nonmutagenicity, whereas adriamycin is known to be highly mutagenic; (d) reduced cardiotoxicity; (e) high tissue distribution in the lungs, spleen, and lymph nodes; (f) resistance to NADPH-cytochrome P450 reductase. Clinical testing using ACM hydrochloride was initiated in mid-1976 and a phase II study is proceeding at 35 institutions throughout Japan.

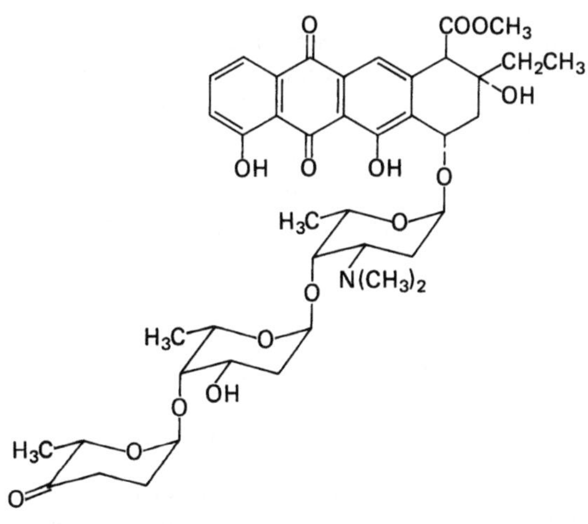

Fig. 1. Structure of aclacinomycin A

Antitumoral Activity

ACM has a broad spectrum of activity against ascites and solid transplantable tumors [3]. ACM was highly active on L1210 and P388 leukemias, sarcoma 180 solid tumor, CD mammary carcinoma, colon 38, and some of the human xenografts. Even greater increases in survival were noted for several ascitic hepatoma lines in rats. A moderate effect has been shown against Lewis lung carcinoma and B16 melanoma. In general, the activities against various transplantable tumors were approximately the same as for daunomycin, but somewhat less than for adriamycin. The optimal dose of ACM was about twice that of ADM and DM, and the activity of ACM against intraperitoneally (IP) inoculated L1210 leukemia was schedule-dependent for multiple dosing. Unlike adriamycin and daunomycin, ACM was orally active against L1210 and P388 leukemias, sarcoma 180, and colon 26 solid tumor, as shown in Table 1. ACM in combination with cyclophosphamide and vincristine was therapeutically synergistic in a P388 leukemia system (in vivo).

The effect of various anthracyclines on nucleic acid synthesis of L1210 cells was examined by determining the incorporation of ^{14}C-TdR and ^{14}C-UR into acid-in soluble fractions of the cells. The concentrations required to inhibit synthesis by 50% (IC_{50}) of DNA and RNA were plotted, as shown in Fig. 2. ACM was a more potent inhibitor of RNA synthesis than were DM and ADM [8].

The IC_{50} of ACM for RNA synthesis was one-tenth that of DNA synthesis. In contrast, the IC_{50} of ADM for RNA synthesis was only one-third that of DNA synthesis. Recently, Crooke et al. [1] found that class II anthracyclines, including ACM, inhibit nucleolar RNA synthesis of Novikoff hepatoma cells at a 170-fold lower concentration than is necessary to inhibit DNA synthesis.

Mutagenicity

Mutagenicity of ACM was determined by the Ames' test using *Salmonella typhimirium,* and the results in Table 2 show that ACM was confirmed to have no mutagenic activity.

Table 1. Oral activity of aclacinomycin A

Tumor	Schedule (day)	Optimal dose (mg/kg/day)	ILS (%)	Inh. (%)
Ascites				
L1210	1–9	10	69	
P388	1–9	8	58	
Rat hepatoma AH44	3–12	2	200	
Solid				
Sarcoma 180	1–9	10		62
Lewis lung[a]	1–9, q2d	5	19	
Colon 26[a]	2–22, q2d	8	100	
Colon 38[a]	1–37, q4d	5	42	

ILS (%): Increase in median lifespan
Inh. (%): Inhibition of tumor growth (weight)
[a] Turuo et al. [12]

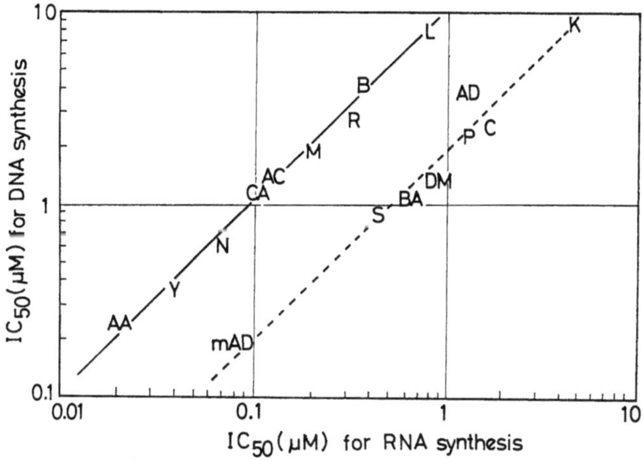

Fig. 2. Inhibitory effect of anthracycline antibiotics on DNA and RNA syntheses in cultured L1210 cells. Aclacinomycin type: (———) *AC*, aclacinomycin A; *L*, MA144 L1; *B*, aclacinomycin B; *R*, roseorubicin A; *M*, MA144 M1; *CA*, cinerubin A; *N*, MA144 N1; *Y*, aclacinomycin Y; *AA*, 4‴-NH_2-ACM. Adriamycin type: (– – –) *AD*, adriamycin; *K*, *N*-didemethyl-ACM; *C*, carminomycin; *P*, pyrromycin; *DM*, daunomycin; *BA*, baumycin A1; *S*, MA144 S1; *mAD*, *N*-dimethyl-ADM

Table 2. Mutagenicity of aclacinomycin A (Ames test)[a]

Concentration of ACM (nmol/plate)	Strain	No. of his⁺ revertants/plate					
		TA98	TA100	TA92	TA94	TA1535	TA1538
0		61	106	42	15	10	22
1		57	–	38	17	11	20
2		40	108	37	19	11	15
3		33	–	–	–	–	–
5		45	82	47	20	13	15
10		39	68	50	13	13	31
20		34	83	42	15	8	17
30		24	48	43	18	8	13
50		10	18	44	13	4	6
70		1	4	–	–	–	–
100		0	0	35	9	1	19

[a] *Salmonella typhimurium* TA92, 94, 100 and 1535 (base-pair change), and TA98 and 1538 (frameshift) were incubated with the various amounts of ACM without S-9 mix on the agar plate at 37° C

Pharmacokinetics

The kinetics of absorption, distribution, metabolism, and excretion of ACM have been investigated using radiolabeled drug and by chromatographic separation of parent drug and metabolites. A bioassay is available for ACM and its metabolites of the glycoside type, but it is insensitive to those of the aglycone type.

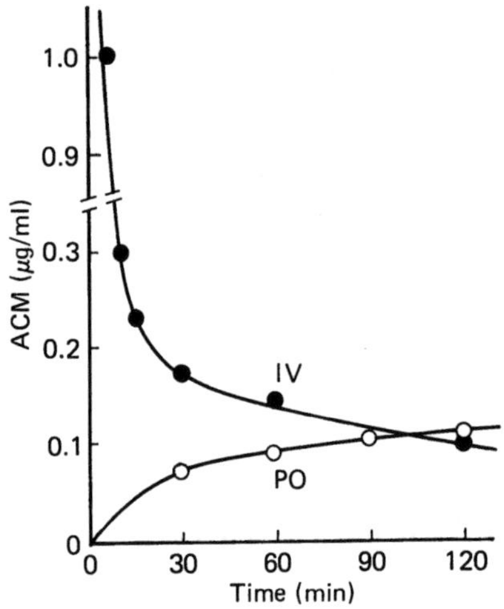

Fig. 3. Blood levels of aclacinomycin A in dogs after oral and IV administration of 15 mg/kg: IV, —●—, PO, —○—

After intravenous (IV) administration to dogs or rabbits, ACM concentrations rapidly declined with a half-life of about 2–5 min. Whole blood concentrations were greater than plasma concentrations, and this finding suggested an affinity of ACM to biologic components such as tissue and blood cells. A rebound in plasma levels was noted and was considered to be caused by enterohepatic circulation or by the release of ACM from tissues. The drug is absorbed orally, as shown by the concentration curve in Fig. 3.

Various metabolites have been found in the urine, feces, blood, bile, and tissues of mouse, rat, rabbit, dog, and man after ACM administration. The following metabolites were identified (their structures are presented in Fig. 4): glycoside type; M1, N1, S1, and 1-deoxypyrromycin, and aglycone type; aklavinone, Cl (7-deoxy-aklavinone), F (bisanhydroaklavinone), and E1.

Metabolic pathways of ACM were investigated with rat liver homogenates [5, 8, 9] and are shown in Fig. 4. Under anaerobic conditions, ACM was converted to Cl and F by reductive glycosidic cleavage in the presence of NADP or NADPH. The enzyme responsible for the reaction was identical to NADPH-cytochrome P450 reductase. This enzyme can utilize a wide variety of anthracycline glycosides and their aglycones as substrate and produce corresponding 7-deoxyaglycones by reduction at the C-7 position [9]. Aglycone-type compounds are biologically inactive.

Under aerobic conditions, ACM was converted to M1 and N1 by rat liver homogenates. The M1-forming enzyme was located in the soluble fraction of liver cells and required NADPH for the reduction. Two kinds of enzymes, one in the soluble fraction and the other in the microsomal fraction, were involved in the formation of N1. These enzymes were NADPH-dependent. Both N1 and M1 are glycosidic metabolites and have biologic activity comparable to that of ACM [4].

Figure 5 shows the changes in tissue levels of ACM, glycoside metabolites, and the aglycone metabolites in mice after IV injection of 50 mg/kg ACM. Initially, the concentration of ACM was greater than that of the metabolites in spleen and lung, but more M1 and N1 than ACM were in the spleen and lung after 4 h. In the spleen, the highest concentration of M1 and N1 metabolites was found at 5–8 h after dosing, with a high level retained for 24 h. In contrast, the aglycone metabolites were found chiefly in the liver and kidney.

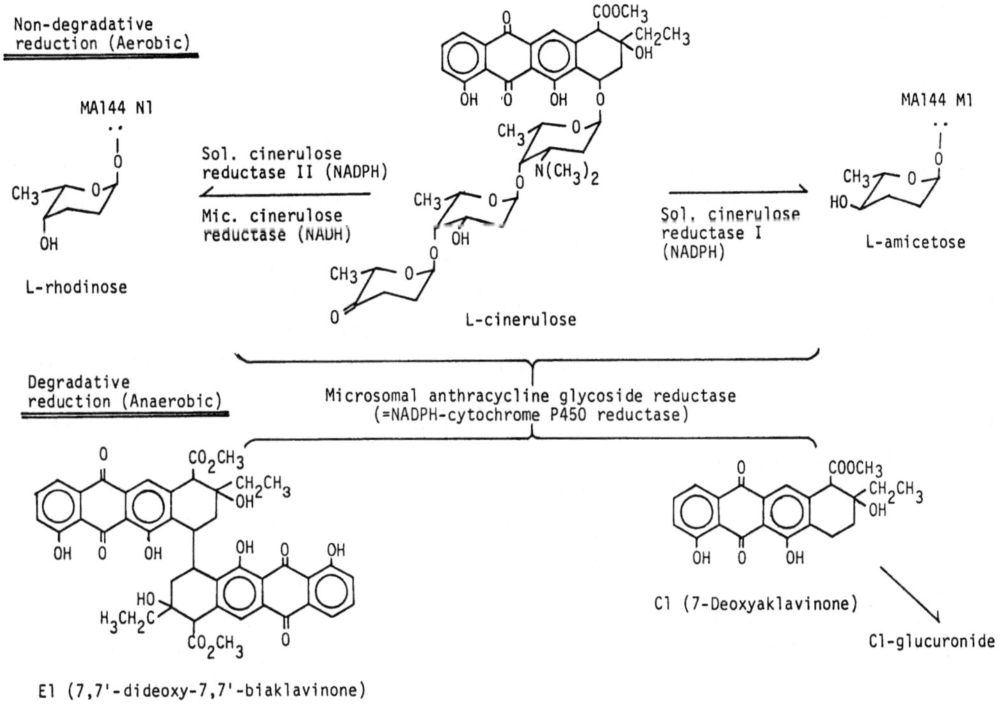

Fig. 4. Metabolism of aclacinomycin A

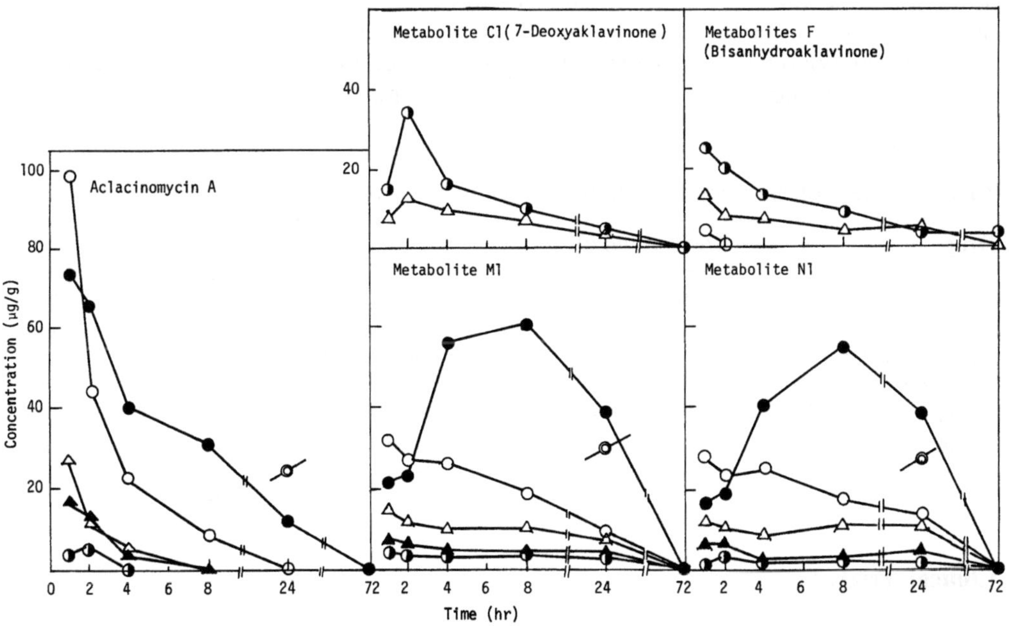

Fig. 5. Tissue levels of aclacinomycin A and its metabolites in mice after IV dose of 50 mg/kg (5 mice/group): liver, –◐–; kidney, –△–; heart, –▲–; lung, –○–; spleen, –●–; thymus, –◎–

Cardiotoxicity

Recently, Dantchev et al. [2] reported that electron microscopy detected almost no early lesions of myocardium in ACM-treated hamsters, but severe cardiac lesions, which are nonlethal and reversible, appeared after 4 weeks of treatment. We confirmed that ACM displayed transient and reversible effects on cardiac functions with both single and prolonged treatments at doses of more than 3–10 times those of ADM on the studies designed to assess the cardiotoxicity of ACM in hamsters, rats, rabbits, and dogs. Acute cardiotoxicity of ACM and ADM was examined in golden hamsters after a single IV administration [3]. Male golden hamsters, 4–8 per group, were anesthesized IP with sodium pentobarbital, and the test compound was injected into the femoral vein in a dose volume of 0.3 ml. Electrocardiograms were monitored by the standard Lead II. The incidence of ECG alterations is shown in Table 3. ADM had the highest incidence of acute ECG alteration, and adriamycinone aglycone still retained the acute effect on ECG at a dose of more than eight times that of ADM. In contrast, ACM caused similar ECG alterations at a dose of more than 15-fold that of ADM, but 7-deoxyaklavinone did not cause an ECG alteration, even at a dose of 100 mg/kg. Acute ECG alterations caused by ACM were reversible, but those by ADM were not.

Chronic cardiotoxicity was determined by studing the clinical and histopathologic alterations in rabbits treated IV with ACM at 1, 2, 4, and 8 mg/kg and with ADM at 2 mg/kg body weight once a week for 13 weeks. Electron-microscopic examination of the myocardium in rabbits treated with ADM revealed that muscle fibers were frequently fragmented and intracellular edema was quite remarkable. Intercalated disk was still preserved, but edema was so extensive that the muscle cells lost a normal shape and pinocytotic vesicles were scarcely seen. Mitochondria were swollen moderately, becoming round, but changes were not distinct compared with those of other organelles. On the contrary, in the heart muscle cells of rabbits treated with ACM at 8 mg/kg once a week for 13 weeks, every component of the muscle cells was well preserved and there was no perinuclear edema [13].

Table 3. Effect of anthracycline antibiotics on ECG of hamsters (single IV)

Drug	Dose (mg/kg)						
	1.56	3.13	6.25	12.5	25	50	100
Aclacinomycin A			(Abnormal/tested)		1/8	1/3	3/3
7-Deoxyaklavinone							0/3
Adriamycin · HCl	1/8	2/4	4/4	4/4	2/2		
Adriamycinone				0/3	2/3	2/2	1/1

Clinical Trials

A cooperative study group was organized and phase I trials were started in June 1976, and now 35 institutions throughout Japan are performing phase II trials employing various dose schedules (Table 4).

Table 4. Schedule model for the aclacinomycin phase II study[a]

Single dose (mg/kg)	Schedule	Average weekly dose (mg)
0.4	Daily	140
	Daily, q2w	70
0.6–0.8	×3/week, days 1, 2, 3	90–120
	×3/week, q2d	
0.8–1.2	×2/week, days 1, 2	80–120
	×2/week, q3d	
1.6–2.0	×1/week	80–120

[a] MTD = 4 mg/kg; safety dose index for weekly administration = 2 mg/kg

A phase I study revealed that Gl (gastrointestinal) toxicity was not related to the dose and well tolerated, but thrombocytopenia and leukopenia, and transient and reversible hepatic dysfunction, were dose-dependent and limited the treatment. Concerning hematologic toxicity, the maximum tolerated dose of ACM in man is considered to be 4 mg/kg/injection.

In the phase II trial from April 1978 to March 1979, 221 evaluable cases received ACM as a single agent, and the principal side effects related to cumulative dose of the drug are listed in Table 5. As described in the previous report by Oka [7], loss of hair to complete alopecia, stomatitis, and ECG changes were extremely rare. Various degrees of nausea, vomiting, and anorexia occurred in the large majority of patients, but were not related to the dose schedule. The major dose-limiting toxicity was hematologic with moderate and severe leukopenia, thrombocytopenia, and anemia increasing in frequency with a total dose greater than 6 mg/kg. Generally, thrombocytopenia reached a nadir a few days preceding leukopenia, and both returned to prior levels within a week with prompt recovery. The median WBC and platelet nadirs were related to the total dose and to the dose schedule. The toxic effects of ACM in the phase II study were predictable, usually reversible, and similar to those in the phase I study.

There were no clinical signs of congestive heart failure which were considered to be due to the treatment, but acute and reversible ECG changes; flattening or inversion or T wave, ST depression, and sinus tachycardia increased in the patients who received a large dose of ACM (more than 1000 mg in total or more than 2 mg/kg/dose).

Of the total number of patients with different types of solid tumor, 207 patients received the drug IV through rapid infusion with several dose schedules as described above; 19 patients with gastric cancer were administered IA (intraabdominal) daily or intermittently with a dose of 0.4–0.8 mg/kg through the abdominal aorta, 10 patients with metastatic peritonitis were given injections directly into the peritoneal cavity, and 11 patients having urinary bladder cancer were instilled with 20–30 ml of the ACM solution at a concentration of 200–1000 µg/ml into the bladder.

Table 5. Side effects related to cumulative dose in the phase II study (IV)

Total dosage/ patient (mg)	% of side effects					
	< 100	101–300	301–500	501–1000	> 1001	Total
	No. of cases					
	37	116	83	39	11	286
Fever	3	4	5	3	0	4
Anorexia	43	41	53	51	36	46
Nausea and vomiting	57	50	40	56	64	49
Diarrhea	5	3	6	10	9	5
Lassitude	11	13	13	23	0	14
Phlebitis and vascular pain	3	3	1	8	0	3
Loss of hair	0	1	1	0	0	1
Stomatitis	5	3	7	13	0	6
Leukopenia	8	30	41	51	45	34
Thrombocytopenia	8	25	33	41	9	27
Anemia	3	14	20	28	27	17
Hemorrhage	3	3	0	3	0	2
Liver impairment	3	5	7	10	9	6
Kidney impairment	0	0	0	0	0	0
ECG changes	5	5	0	8	18	5
Others	8	3	1	3	0	3

Table 6. Therapeutic effect of ACM alone on various recurrent and advanced cancers (IV + IP + IA)

Diagnosis	No. of cases	Karnofsky criteria			Response rate (%)
		< 0–C	I–A	> I–B	> IA
Breast cancer	39	31	7	1	21
Uterine cancer	6	6			
Ovarian cancer	11	8	3		27
Lung cancer	45	40	5		11
Esophageal cancer	3	2		1	
Gastric cancer	58	52	5	1	10
Intestinal cancer	14	13	1		7
Hepatoma	3	3			
Pancreatic cancer	6	6			
Urinary bladder cancer	11[a]	4	4	3	64
Sarcoma	7	5	1	1	
Head and neck cancer	5	4	1		
Miscellaneous	13	12		1	
Total	221	186	27	8	16

[a] Ten cases by instillation into the urinary bladder

Table 7. Response to malignant lymphoma by ACM treatment[a]

	No. of cases	NR	PR	CR
Lymphosarcoma	9	2	6	1
Reticulum cell sarcoma	9	4	3	2
Hodgkin's disease	7	4	2	1
Total	25	10	11	4

[a] Response rate ⩾ PR: 60%

Objective responses to IV and IP infusions or to bladder instillation were observed in patients with malignant lymphoma, breast cancer, ovarian cancer, lung cancer, gastric cancer, intestinal cancer, and urinary bladder cancer, as shown in Tables 6 and 7. As previously reported by MATHÉ et al. [6], SUZUKI et al. [11] recently observed a complete remission by using ACM in a case of acute myeloblastic leukemia which had not responded to five courses of conventional combination chemotherapy which had included DM.

Acknowledgments. The clinical study of ACM has been performed by members of the ACM Cooperative Study Group in collaboration with the following institutions: National Sapporo Hospital; Research Institute for Tuberculosis, Leprosy and Cancer, Tohoku University; National Cancer Center Hospital; National Medical Center Hospital; Cancer Institute Hospital; Cancer Chemotherapy Center; Keio University Hospital Group; Teikyo University Hospital; Tokyo University Hospital; Chiba Cancer Center Hospital; National Tachikawa Hospital; Shizuoka Red Cross Hospital; National Nagoya Hospital; Aichi Cancer Center Hospital; Nagoya University Hospital; Kyoto University Hospital; Research Institute for Microbial Diseases, Osaka University; The Center for Adult Diseases, Osaka; Okayama University Hospital; Research Institute for Nuclear Medicine and Biology, Hiroshima University, Kyushu University Hospital, National Kyushu Cancer Center Hospital. We express our sincere thanks to all participants in this study for their generosity to permit this publication.

References

1 Crooke ST, Duvernay VH, Galvan L, Prestayko AW (1978) Structure-activity relationships of anthracyclines relative to effects on macromolecular syntheses. Mol Pharmacol 14: 290–298
2 Dantchev D, Slioussartchouk V, Paintrand M, Bourut C, Mathé G, Macieira-Coelho A (1979) Comparative cardiac and skin toxicity of 8 anthracyclines: Adriamycin, daunorubicin, detrorubicin, 4-epi-adriamycin, adriamycin hydrochloride, rubidazone, aclacinomycin and AD32. Proc Am Assoc Cancer Res and Am Soc Clin Oncol 48
3 Hori S, Shirai M, Hirano S, Oki T, Inui T, Tsukagoshi S, Ishizuka M, Takeuchi T, Umezawa H (1977) Antitumor activity of new anthracycline antibiotics, aclacinomycin-A and its analogs, and their toxicity. GANN 68: 685–690
4 Komiyama T, Oki T, Inui T, Takeuchi T, Umezawa H (1978) NADH-dependent cinerulose reductase in rat liver microsomes. Biochem Biophys Res Commun 82: 188–195

5 Komiyama T, Oki T, Inui T, Takeuchi T, Umezawa H (1979) Reduction of anthracycline glycoside by NADPH-cytochrome P-450 reductase. GANN 70: 403–410
6 Mathé G, Bayssas M, Gouveia J, Dantchev D, Ribaud P, Machover D, Misset JL, Shearzenberg L, Jasmin C, Hayat M (1978) Preliminary results of a phase II trial of aclacinomycin in acute leukemia and lymphosarcoma. Can Chemother Pharmacol 1: 259–262
7 Oka S (1978) A review of clinical studies on aclacinomycin A – Phase I and preliminary phase II evaluation of ACM. Sci Rep Res Inst Tohoku Univ [C] 25: 37–49
8 Oki T (1977) New anthracycline antibiotics. Jpn J Antibiot 30: S-70–84
9 Oki T, Komiyama T, Tone H, Inui T, Takeuchi T, Umezawa H (1977) Reductive cleavage of anthracycline glycosides by microsomal NADPH-cytochrome C reductase. J Antibiot (Tokyo) 30: 613–615
10 Oki T, Matsuzawa Y, Yoshimoto A, Numata K, Kitamura I, Hori S, Takamatsu A, Umezawa H, Ishizuka M, Naganawa H, Suda H, Hamada M, Takeuchi T (1975) New antitumor antibiotics, aclacinomycins A and B. J Antibiot (Tokyo) 28: 830–834
11 Suzuki H, Kawashima K, Yamada K (1979) Aclacinomycin A, a new anti-leukemic agent. Lancet 8/2: 870–871
12 Tsuruo T, Yomori T, Naganuma K, Iida H, Tsukagoshi S, Sakurai Y (1979) Antitumor activity of aclacinomycin A against colon adenocarcinomas and lewis lung carcinoma by oral administration. Proc Jpn Cancer Assoc, p 188
13 Waka bayashi T, Oki T, Tone H, Hirano S, Omori K (1980) A comparative electron microscopic study of aclacinomycin and adriamycin cardiotoxicities in rabbits and hamsters. J Electron Microsc (Tokyo) 29: 106–118

Phase II Trial of Aclacinomycin in Acute Leukemia and Lymphosarcoma

G. Mathé, M.-A. Gil, M. Delgado, M. Bayssas, J. Gouvéia, P. Ribaud, D. Machover, J.-L. Misset, F. de Vassal, L. Schwarzenberg, C. Jasmin, and M. Hayat

Summary

A phase II trial of which preliminary results are available for 37 patients indicates that aclacinomycin applied in a continuous modality can induce complete or partial remissions in acute lymphoid leukemia resistant to all previously available drugs, and in lymphosarcoma. Bone marrow toxicity was the major side effect.

Daunorubicin (DRB) [1, 9] and adriamycin (ADM) [4] have been widely used, alone or in combinations [5], with remarkable oncostatic efficiency. In all conditions, however, their use has been limited because of two major side effects: (a) alopecia – some patients refuse to be exposed to a drug that suppresses hair growth; and (b) cardiotoxicity – although a given total dose has been calculated below which the myocardial risk is low [6], this risk is not nil and, in any case, the agent is generally not used beyond this total dose, which reduces its potential action.

Hence there is the considerable interest in other anthracyclines that have been considered to be less cardiotoxic and to cause less hair loss than ADM. We have systematically submitted all of them to a double test: electron-microscopic study of the myocardium and light-microscopic study of the skin of golden (cardiopathic) hamsters receiving three administrations per week of the dose corresponding (for mouse-hamster equivalence) to the optimally efficient dose, as far as survival is concerned, for murine L1210 leukemia [7]. The French detorubicin (DTR) [8, 12, 13] appears to be as cardiotoxic and to cause as much hair loss as ADM; the Italian 4′-epiadriamycin [3] is slightly less cardiotoxic, but causes the same hair loss as ADM; the American AD-32 [2] (*N*-trifluoroacetyl adriamycin-14-*O*-valerate) appears to be significantly less cardiotoxic and to induce no alopecia; the Japanese aclacinomycin (ACM) [11, 18] appears to be the least cardiotoxic and this preparation also induces no alopecia [7].

Hence, after the Japanese phase I trial in man [17], we started a phase II trial of aclacinomycin in man, the very preliminary results of which were reported in a short communication [16]. The results collected for the present meeting confirm the preliminary results.

Materials and Methods

Aclacinomycin, or 2-ethyl-1,2,3,4,6,11-hexahydro-2,5,7-trihydroxy-6,11-dioxo-4-(*O*-2,3,6-trideoxy-α-L-glycerohexopyranos-4-urosyl-(1–4)-*O*-2,6-dideoxy-α-L-lyxo-hexopyranosyl-(1–4)-2,3,6-trideoxy-3-(dimethylamino)-α-L-lyxohexopyranosyl)oxy

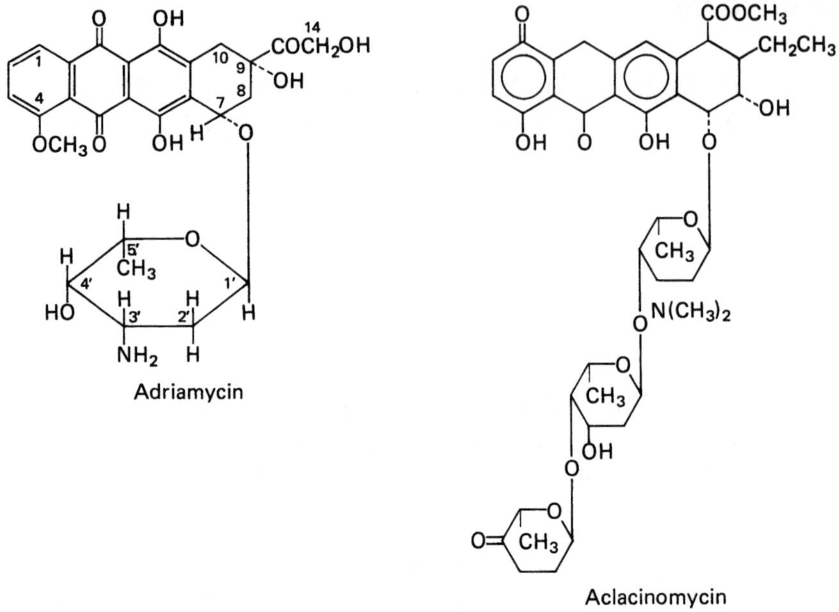

Fig. 1. Formula of aclacinomycin compared with that of adriamycin

Table 1. Phase II trial of aclacinomycin: Leukemias and hematosarcomas (continuous administration); eligibility

Diagnosis	Number of patients	Number of perceptible phases	Ages (years)	Sex	
				M	F
Acute lymphoid leukemia	16	2nd PP 5	11, 3, 3, 5, 22		
		3rd PP 7	5, 10, 12, 12, 12, 19, 47		
		4th PP 2	13, 10	11	5
		5th PP 1	17		
		8th PP 1	12		
Acute myeloid leukemia	6	1st PP 4	33, 32, 51, 9	4	2
		2nd PP 2	30, 12		
Blastic crisis of chronic myeloid leukemia	1	3rd PP 1	29		1
Hodgkin's disease	1	3rd PP 1	27	1	
Leukemic lymphosarcoma	9	1st PP 4	56, 16, 45, 29		
		2nd PP 2	7, 12	6	3
		3rd PP 3	12, 22, 31		
Lymphosarcoma	4	1st PP 4	38, 73, 73, 40	1	3
Total	37			23	14

-1-naphthacenecarboxilic acid methyl ester (Fig. 1), was discovered and produced by UMEZAWA [18], who showed its murine oncostatic activity and found it less cardiotoxic in mice than ADM.

The protocol chosen for leukemia and hematosarcomas involved continuous daily administration of the agent at the dose of 10–20 mg/m^2/day, the duration depending on the result and/or the toxicity. The total dose varied from 42–600 mg/m^2.

The criteria of eligibility for the trial were the same as for the EORTC phase II trials [10] and for our own methodologic and ethical concept of phase II trials [14]. The 37 subjects who were entered in the present trial and in whom the effect is evaluable are mentioned in Table 1, which indicates their age, sex, and disease and its phase of evolution (all were in a perceptible phase and all had been treated previously without success; none were in remission).

Results

Table 2 shows the present results: two complete (Fig. 2) and four incomplete remissions ($2 \geqslant 50\%$) were obtained in acute lymphoid leukemia (ALL) patients resistant to all previously available drugs active in this disease; two complete and six incomplete remissions ($3 \geqslant 50\%$) were obtained in patients with lymphosarcoma. One partial remission $> 50\%$ and one $< 50\%$ were obtained in acute myeloid leukemia. This makes about 40% responses in this preliminary trial on hematopoietic malignancies and almost 50% in the group composed of ALL and lymphosarcomas.

The four complete regressions were obtained with a total dose of 40–225 mg/m^2; the 12 partial regressions were obtained with doses varying between 200 and 285 mg/m^2;

Table 2. Phase II trial of aclacinomycin: Leukemias and hematosarcomas (continuous administration); results

Diagnosis	Number of patients evaluated	Complete regression	Partial regression		Failure
			≥ 50%	< 50%	
Acute lymphoid leukemia	16	2	2	2	10
Acute myeloid leukemia	6	–	1	1	4
Blastic crisis of chronic myeloid leukemia	1	–	–	–	1
Hodgkin's disease	1	–	–	–	1
Leukemic lymphosarcoma	9	2	1	2	4
Lymphosarcoma (stage IV)	3	–	2	–	1
Lymphosarcoma (stage III)	1	–	–	1	–
Total	37	4	6	6	21
Percentage		0.11	0.16		
		0.27 (complete + partial ≥ 50%)			
		0.43 (complete + partial ≥ 50% + partial < 50%)			

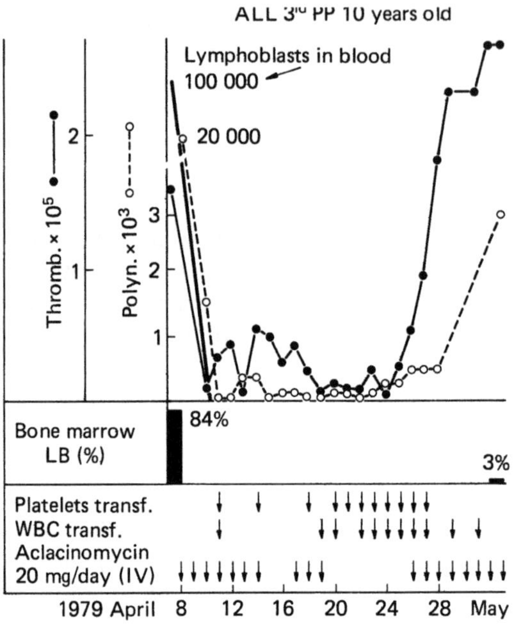

Fig. 2. Example of a complete remission induced with aclacinomycin in a patient suffering from a second relapse (third perceptible phase, 3rd PP) of acute lymphoid leukemia resistant to all conventional chemotherapies

thus in this small series, the response to the drug could not be related to the dose used. However, all the patients but one were submitted to a total dose of over 200 mg/m^2; toxicity precluded such a high dose in one case.

Toxicity

Table 3 shows the toxic manifestations recorded during and after the trial. ACM was myelotoxic in 27 of 35 patients in whom the hemopoietic effect was evaluable; two patients were not evaluable because of previously hypoplastic bone marrow. Of the 16 patients who had leukopenia, 11 had infections and seven of the 21 who had thrombocytopenia had hemorrhage. The details concerning the hematologic tolerance are presented in Table 4. It should be noted that all the patients who experienced a regression of their neoplasia had major toxicity with severe peripheral aplasia.
The digestive side effects were rare vomiting (6%); diarrhea was common at the end of the treatment (days 15–20), but could not be attributed to the drug alone, because of the patients' aplastic status.
It should be emphasized that only three patients of the 35 in whom the effect of ACM on the heart was evaluable presented a cardiac intolerance or had negative T waves in V_3–V_4 derivations after a total dose of 42 mg; the drug was discontinued and the ECG normalized after 20 days. One patient was a 3-year-old boy with ALL, and he entered complete remission under this very low dose of ACM. A 19-year-old patient suffering from ALL had elevated LDH, and 29-year-old patient with LSL had negative T waves V_1–V_4. None of the 12 patients in whom alopoecia was not present before ACM application suffered from this side effect.

Table 3. Phase II trial of aclacinomycin: Leukemias and hematosarcomas (continuous administration); toxicities

Types	Rate	
Hematologic	27/35	0.77
Anemia	10/35	0.29
Leukoneutropenia	16/35	0.46
Thrombocytopenia	21/35	0.70
Digestives		
Vomiting	2/35	0.06
Diarrhea[a]		
Cardiac[b]	3/35	0.09
Alopoecia[c]	0/12	

[a] Diarrhea was common but not only attributable to ACM in this kind of patient

[b] Cardiac: ALL 3 years old total dose 42 mg, complete remission – negative waves in V_3 and V_4, treatment discontinued, regression after 20 days, 1 ALL patient's LDH elevated

[c] Other patients were hairless before treatment

Table 4. Phase II trial of aclacinomycin: Leukemias and hematosarcomas (continuous administration); details of hematologic toxicity

Hemoglobin (% Fall)		Platelets ($10^3/mm^3$)		Neutrophils (mm^3)	
15	1	100	5	500–1000	1
15–30	5	50–100	4	100– 500	5
>30	4	50– 20	4	< 100	9
	10/35	< 20	8		16/35
	(0.28)		21/35		(0.46)
			(0.60)		

Discussion

The present results confirm the oncostatic efficiency of ACM in ALL and in lymphosarcoma, two very similar if not identical lymphoid neoplasias; and agree with that of our experimental study of myocardium and hair side effects, which were exceptional or absent in our trial as they were in our experiment in golden hamsters [7].

This correlation of the experimental tests of these toxicities is confirmed by our experience with adriamycin [15] and with detorubicin [8], which are toxic to heart and hair in both studies. Bone marrow toxicity appears to be the most important side effect of aclacinomycin in this trial and might be related to the continuous modality of administration.

References

1 Bernard J, Jacquillat C, Weil M, Boiron M, Tanzer J (1970) Present results in daunorubicin (rubidomycin, daunomycin). Recent Results Cancer Res 30:3–8
2 Blum RH, Garnick MB, Israel M, Canellos GP, Henderson IC, Frei E III (1979) Initial clinical evaluation of N-trifluoroacetyladriamycin-14-valerate (AD-32) an adriamycin analog. Cancer Treat Rep 63:919–923
3 Bonfante V, Bonadonna G, Villani F, Di Fronzo G, Martini A, Casazza AM (1979) Preliminary phase I study of 4′-epi-adriamycin. Cancer Treat Rep 63:915–918
4 Carter SK, Di Marco A, Ghione M, Krakoff IH, Mathé G (eds) (1972) Adriamycin. Springer, Heidelberg New York
5 Clarysse A, Kenis Y, Mathé G (1976) Cancer chemotherapy. Its role in the treatment strategy of hematologic malignancies and solid tumors. Springer, Berlin Heidelberg New York
6 Cortes EP, Lutman G, Wanka J, Wang JW, Pickren J, Wallace J, Holland JF (1975) Adriamycin (NSC-123127). Cardiotoxicity: A clinicopathologic correlation. Cancer Chemother Rep 6:215–225
7 Dantchev V, Slioussartchouk V, Paintrand M, Hayat M, Bourut C, Mathé G (1979) Electron microscopy of the heart and light microscopy of the skin after treatment of golden hamsters with adriamycin detorubicin, AD 32, and aclacinomycin. Cancer Treat Rep 63:875–888
8 EORTC Clinical Screening Group (1978) Detorubicin: Preliminary results of a phase II trial in solid tumors (abstr 37). Med Oncol 4:10
9 EORTC Leukemia and Hematosarcoma Cooperative Group (1970) Rubidomycin (or daunorubicin): A clinical evaluation. Recent Results Cancer Res 30:9–13
10 EORTC Screening Group (1972) Handbook of materials and methods. Eur J Cancer 8:185–196
11 Hori S, Shirai M, Hirano S, Oki T (1977) Antitumor activity of new anthracycline antibiotics, aclacinomycin A (NSC 208734) and its analogues, and their toxicity. Gann 68:685–690
12 Jacquillat Cl, Auclerc MF, Weil M, Maral J, Degos L, Auclerc G, Tobelem G, Schaison G, Bernard J (1979) Clinical activity of detorubicin: a new anthracycline derivative. Cancer Treat Rep 63:889–893
13 Maral R, Cucep JB, Farge D, Ponsinet G, Reisdorf D (1978) Préparation et activité antitumorale, expérimentale d'un nouvel antibiotique semi synthétique: la (diétoxyacétoxy)-14-daunorubicine (33921 RP) CR Acad Sci [D] (Paris) 286:443–446
14 Mathé G (1973) Clinical examination of a drug, a scientific and ethical challenge. Biomedicine 18:169–172
15 Mathé G, Amiel JL, Hayat M, De Vassal F, Schwarzenberg L, Schneider M, Jasmin C, Rosenfeld C (1972) Adriamycin in the treatment of acute leukemias. In: Carter SK, Di Marco A, Ghione M, Krakoff IH, Mathé G (eds) Adriamycin. Springer, Heidelberg New York, pp 168–172
16 Mathé G, Bayssas M, Gouveia J, Dantchev D, Ribaud P, Machover D, Misset JL, Schwarzenberg L, Jasmin C, Hayat M (1978) Preliminary results of a phase II trial of aclacinomycin in acute leukaemia and lymphosarcoma. An oncostatic anthracycline that is rarely cardiotoxic and induces no alopecia. Cancer Chemother Pharmacol 1:259–262
17 Ogawa M, Inagaki J, Horikoshi N, Inoue K, Chinen T, Ueoka H, Nagura E (1979) Clinical study of Aclacinomycin A. Cancer Treat Rep 63:931–934
18 Oki T, Matsukura Y, Yoshimoto A, Numata K, Kimatura I, Ori S, Takamatsu A, Umezawa H, Ishizuka M, Naganawa H, Suda H, Hamada M, Takeuchi T (1975) New antitumor antibiotics, aclacinomycins A and B. J Antibiot (Tokyo) 28:830–834

Ultrastructural Study of the Cardiotoxicity and Light-Microscopic Findings of the Skin After Treatment of Golden Hamsters with Seven Different Anthracyclines

D. Dantchev, V. Slioussartchouk, M. Paintrand, C. Bourut, M. Hayat, and G. Mathé*

Summary

Golden hamsters were administered seven anthracyclines: adriamycin (ADM), detorubicin (DTR), daunorubicin (DNR), 4′-epi-adriamycin (eADM), rubidazone (RBZ), aclacinomycin (ACM), and N-trifluoroacetyladriamycin-14-valerate (AD-32), three times a week during 4 weeks, at doses equivalent to $^{3}/_{4}$ of those which are optimally oncostatic on murine L1210 leukemia. We examined their myocardia by electron microscopy (EM) and their skin by light microscopy (LM), and report here the findings of these two examinations.

The mortality was very high for the groups of hamsters treated with ADM, DTR, DRB, eADM, and RBZ (all treated hamsters died before the end of the fourth week) and very low for those treated with ACM and AD-32 (for each drug, only one of the 21 treated animals died after 4 weeks of treatment). After the first week of treatment and chiefly after the second week, all treated hamsters, except those treated with ACM, showed very severe EM alterations of their myocardia. EM detected almost no early myocardial lesions in ACM-treated hamsters but, after 4 weeks of treatment, severe cardiac lesions also appeared which, like those after AD-32, were nonlethal and reversible.

LM of the skin detected degenerative lesions with atrophy of all epidermic layers and a loss of the hair (alopecia) in all treated hamsters except those treated with ACM and AD-32; the skin in these two groups preserved its normal histologic structure. These observations agree with phase I–II clinical ACM studies in which the rate of ECG abnormalities was 4.5% and the rate of alopecia 0%, and with an early AD-32 clinical study conducted by Blum [3].

Introduction

Anthracycline antibiotics possess significant antitumor activity against a wide range of murine and human malignancies. Some of these antibiotics, such as adriamycin (ADM), are the most promising agents, with useful clinical anticancer activity in hematologic malignancies and in solid tumors. Unfortunately, their therapeutic usefulness has been limited by their cardiotoxicity and alopecia, which are the two

* NCI-INSERM Franco-American Cooperation. This research was carried out with the technical assistance of I. Pignot, M. Bennoun, and G. Martin

important factors limiting their use [5]. Many anthracycline derivatives of adriamycin have been prepared in the hope that some would show reduced toxicities. In the phase II trials with detorubicin (DTR) [7] and aclacinomycin (ACM) [11], we observed that DTR produced cardiotoxicity (30%) and alopecia (90%) as frequently as adriamycin, whereas ECG changes were rare (4.5%) and alopecia was not induced by ACM. A lower incidence of cardiotoxicity and alopecia has also been reported with N-trifluoroacetyladriamycin-14-valerate (AD-32) [3].

Following an electron-microscopic study of the myocardia of golden hamsters submitted to optimal oncostatic doses of four anthracyclines [6], we report here our work on seven different anthracyclines, which was undertaken with the aim of determining whether the EM alterations would be predictive of myocardial toxicity in man, as has been shown by EM in the myocardia of subjects submitted to daunorubicin (DNR) [4] or ADM [2]. Simultaneously, we have examined the skin of these animals by light microscopy (LM) in an attempt to define a correlation between histologic changes in these experiments and the development of alopecia in man. Therefore, we compared the EM myocardial effects and the LM skin effects of ADM, DTR, DNR, 4′-epi-ADM (eADM), rubidazone (RBZ), ACM, and AD-32 in golden hamsters.

Materials and Methods

Twenty-one golden hamsters were used for each compound and 21 were kept as controls. Three times a week, the treated animals were injected intraperitoneally (IP) with a dose which, for each drug, was $^{3}/_{4}$ of the dose which, when given three times (days 1, 5, and 9), was optimally oncostatic on murine L1210 leukemia [9]. These doses are shown in Table 1.

Survival and weight were routinely followed. Three hamsters per treatment group and in the control group were killed each week. All tissues of interest were quickly removed and the ventricular cross (apices) was immediately fixed for transmission EM study in 5% cacodylate buffered glutaraldehyde adjusted to pH 7.25; the apex of the myocardium was minced under fixative into 1- to 2-mm^3 blocks. The remainder of the heart and other tissues (including lymph nodes, thymus, spleen, liver, lungs, kidneys,

Table 1. Doses (mg/kg for a single injection) and schedules of administration

Drug	Optimally oncostatic doses on murine L 1210 leukemia when injected 3 times at days 1, 5, and 9 after tumor cells inoculation	Doses repeated 3 times a week in golden hamsters for 1–4 weeks
ADM	4	3
DTR	4	3
DNR	4	3
eADM	8	6
RBZ	12	9
ACM	8	6
AD-32	40	30

intestine, bones, ovaries, muscles, and skin) were collected for LM examination and fixed in 10% neutral buffered formalin.

The blocks for transmission electron microscopy were post-fixed in 2% osmium tetroxide, dehydrated in graded ethanols, transferred to propylene oxide, and embedded in Epon. Thin sections cut at 300–500 Å with a Porter-Bloom ultramicrotome were mounted on Formvar-coated 300-mesh copper grids, stained with uranyl acetate and lead citrate, and examined with a Jeol 100 C ASSID electron microscope at 100 kV.

For histopathologic study, the tissues were embedded in paraffin, sectioned at 6 μm, and stained with hematoxylin-eosin. At the present time, only the heart and the skin have been examined by light microscopy.

Our grading system of EM alterations was derived from that proposed by BILLINGHAM et al. [2]. We used the grade 0 for a normal cardiac morphology on EM, and the grade 1 for the cases which contained some cardiac cells with mild alterations, i.e., swelling of mitochondriae with clearing of their matrices and lysis of their crests, lesions of myofilaments in some cells presenting a separation, a loss of their parallel orientation, and a lysis with disruption of Z-band registry. A grade 2 was given when some cardiac cells demonstrated the previous alterations, but more markedly: these included vacuolization of mitochondriae, appearance of myelinic figures, dilatation of sarcoplasmic reticulum, more intense loss of myofilaments, nuclear modifications with irregularity of the nuclear membrane and condensation or clumping of the chromatin into electron-dense masses adjacent to the nuclear membranes; and separation of the fascia adherens of the intercalated disks creating empty spaces between myocytes. In grade 3, changes of myocardium were diffusely affected by these very severe alterations, with a complete cell disorganization, vacuolization, loss of contractile elements, and, finally, the near cell death.

Using the grading system, in order to establish a possible comparative appreciation of the myocardial alterations, we have employed also the intermediate grades of 0–1, 1–2, and 2–3, which indicate that about half of myocardial cells showed the morphologic structure or changes of each of two grades, e.g., grade 0–1 signified that half of observed cells were normal (grade 0) and that grade 1 lesions were present in the others.

Results

Mortality

Table 2 summarizes the number of dead and surviving hamsters at the end of each week. Mortality was very high for the groups of hamsters treated with ADM, DTR, DNR, eADM, and RBZ, and very low for those treated with ACM and AD-32. Indeed, at the end of the second or third week of treatment, all treated animals were dead, except those treated with ACM and AD-32; in these last groups, only one of the 21 treated hamsters died due to toxicity after 4 weeks of treatment. Before death we observed a 30%–40% loss of initial weight in the first groups, i.e., hamsters treated with ADM, DTR, DNR, eADM, and RBZ, which suggested that death was probably not due, or not entirely only due, to cardiac failure. There was no weight loss in the second groups, e.g., ACM- and AD-32 treated hamsters. Moreover, hair loss was also evident in the first groups, but did not occur in the second groups or in the control group.

Table 2. Mortality by toxicity of drug-treated hamsters (21 hamsters were used for each drug)

Drug		End of			
		week 1	week 2	week 3	week 4
ADM	Dead	0	5	9	0
	Surviving	21	13	1	0
	Sacrificed	3	3	1	0
DTR	Dead	0	4	6	2
	Surviving	21	14	5	0
	Sacrificed	3	3	3	0
DNR	Dead	0	5	10	0
	Surviving	21	13	0	0
	Sacrificed	3	3	0	0
eADM	Dead	0	0	5	7
	Surviving	21	18	10	0
	Sacrificed	3	3	3	0
RBZ	Dead	0	9	6	0
	Surviving	21	9	0	0
	Sacrificed	3	3	0	0
ACM	Dead	0	0	1	0
	Surviving	21	18	14	11
	Sacrificed	3	3	3	3
AD-32	Dead	0	0	0	1
	Surviving	21	18	15	11
	Sacrificed	3	3	3	3
Controls	Dead	0	0	0	0
	Surviving	21	18	15	12
	Sacrificed	3	3	3	3

Cardiac Lesions Seen on Electron Microscopy

At the End of the First Week (i.e., After Three Drug Injections). The myocardia of all sacrificed hamsters in the groups treated with ADM, DTR, DNR, eADM, and RBZ already showed very important ultrastructural alterations in the mitochondria (clearing of their matrices, lysis of the crests, and formation of vacuoles and myelinic figures), the myofibrils (rents and loss of myofilaments with disappearance of Z bands), the sarcoplasmic reticulum and the transverse tubular system (vacuolization due to their swelling and dilatation), the nucleous (irregular membrane, separation of external membrane from internal membrane, condensation of the chromatin into electron-dense masses, most of which were adjacent to the nuclear membrane and to the nucleoli), and the intercalated disks (separations of their fasciae adherens, creating empty spaces between myocytes). Figures 1 and 2 show typical examples of these severe alterations. According to our semiquantitative grading system, these alterations were classified as grade 1–2; the lesions of DTR-treated animals were generally less severe (Fig. 2) and classified as grade 1.

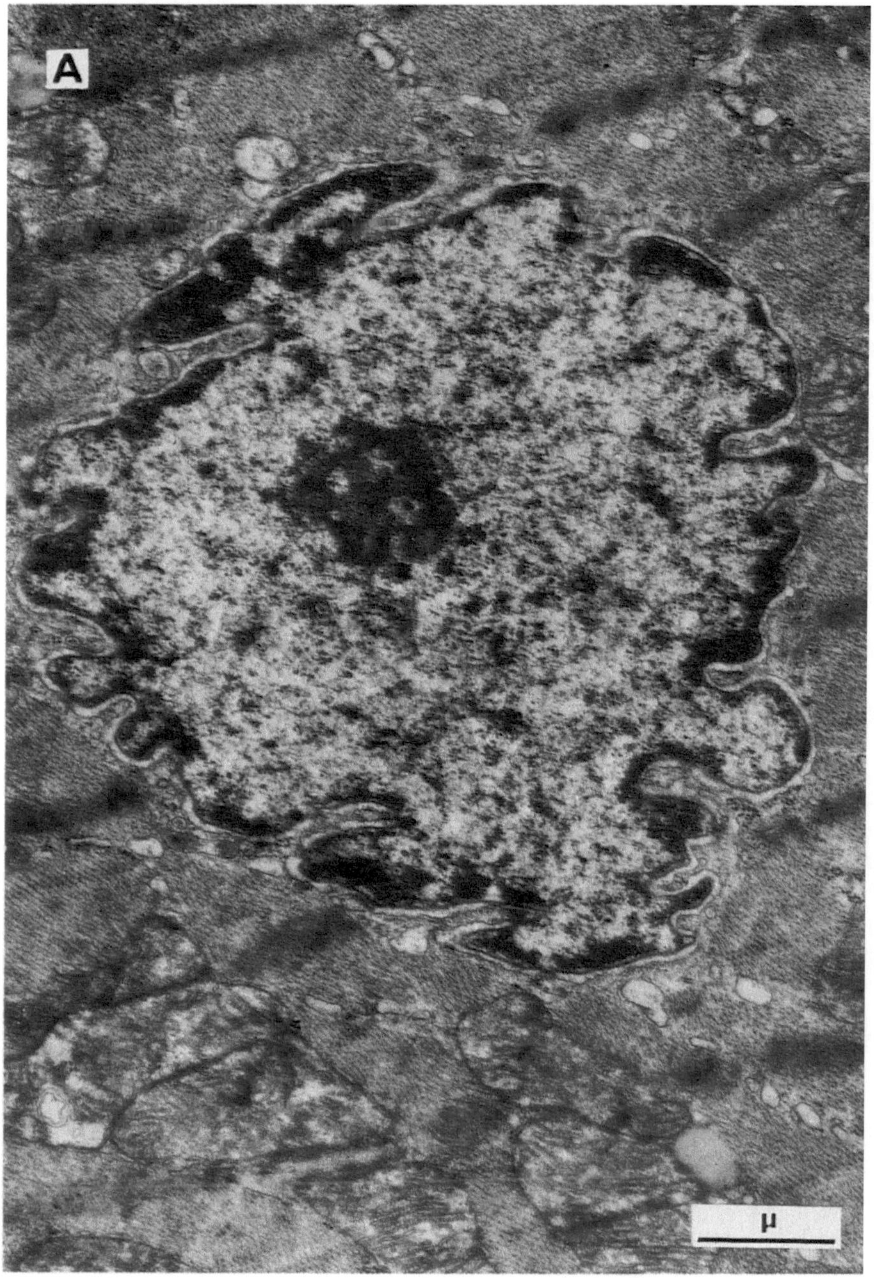

Fig. 1A–C. Myocardium from a golden hamster 7 days after treatment with adriamycin (ADM) (3 mg/kg/injection IP 3 times a week). Swelling of mitochondriae with clearing of their matrices, disappearance of their crests (**A**) and formation of vacuole and myelinic figures (**B**); rents and loss of myofilaments and widening of sarcoplasmic reticulum (**B**); irregular nuclear membrane, condensation of the chromatin into electron-dense masses adjacent to the nuclear membrane, and separation of external membrane from internal membrane of the nucleus (**A**): separation of fasciae adherens of the intercalated disks (**c**). Original magnification (6/9): **A** × 8,300; **B** × 8,300; **C** × 8,300

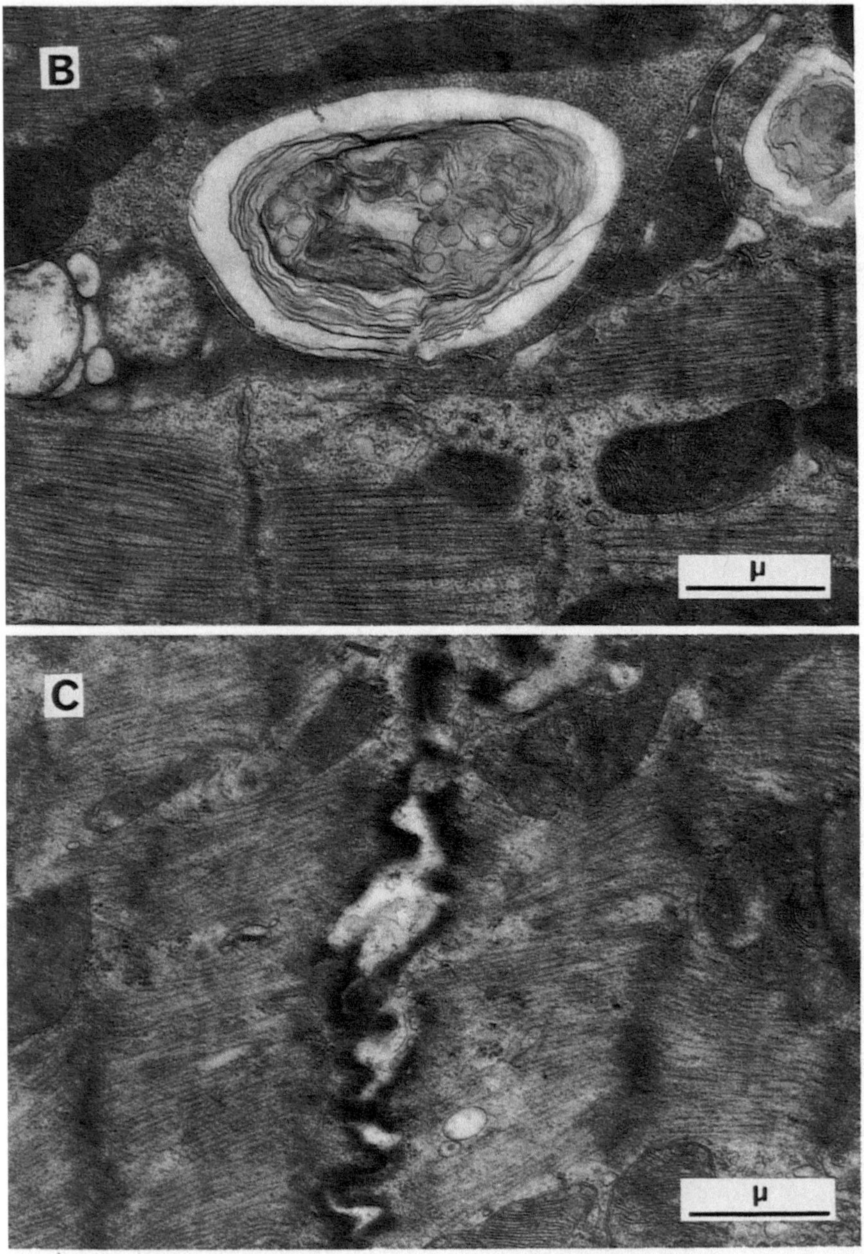

In the groups of ACM- and AD-32-treated hamsters, the myocardial lesions at the end of the first week of treatment were less frequent and much less severe. Generally, mitochondriae, myofilaments, and intercalated disks were well preserved, particularly in the group of ACM-treated animals; Fig. 3 shows an example of this, which is almost similar to that of controls and classified as grade 0 or 0–1. In the group of AD-32-treated animals, the lesions were therefore also less marked than those seen in the first groups of treated animals, but noticeable, consisting of moderate swelling of

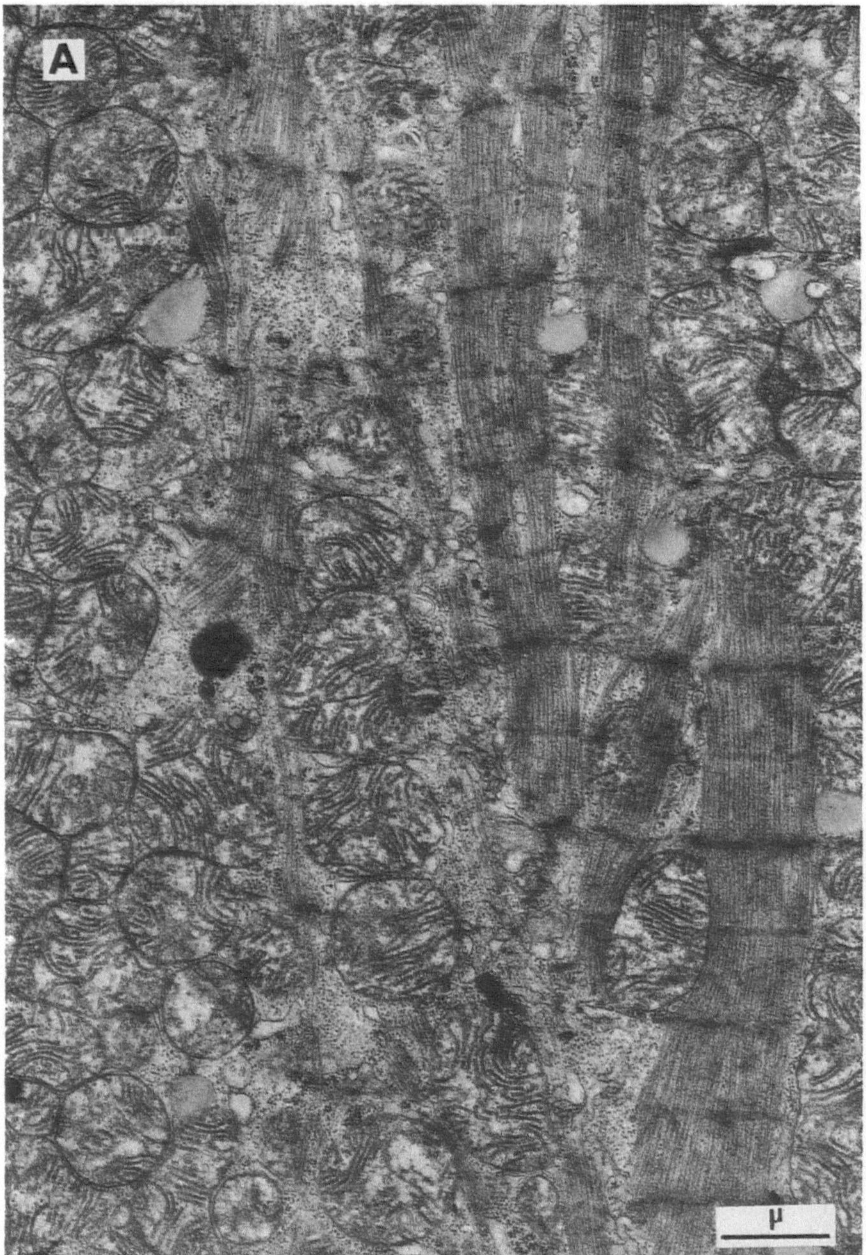

Fig. 2A, B. Myocardium from a golden hamster 7 days after treatment with detorubicin (DTR) (3 mg/kg/injection IP 3 times a week). Swelling of mitochondriae with clearing of their matrices and lysis of the crests (**A**); dilatation of sarcoplasmic reticulum (**B**); separation and lysis of myofilaments with disruption of Z-band registry and contraction of sarcomers (**B**). Original magnification (6/9): **A** × 8,300; **B** × 8,300

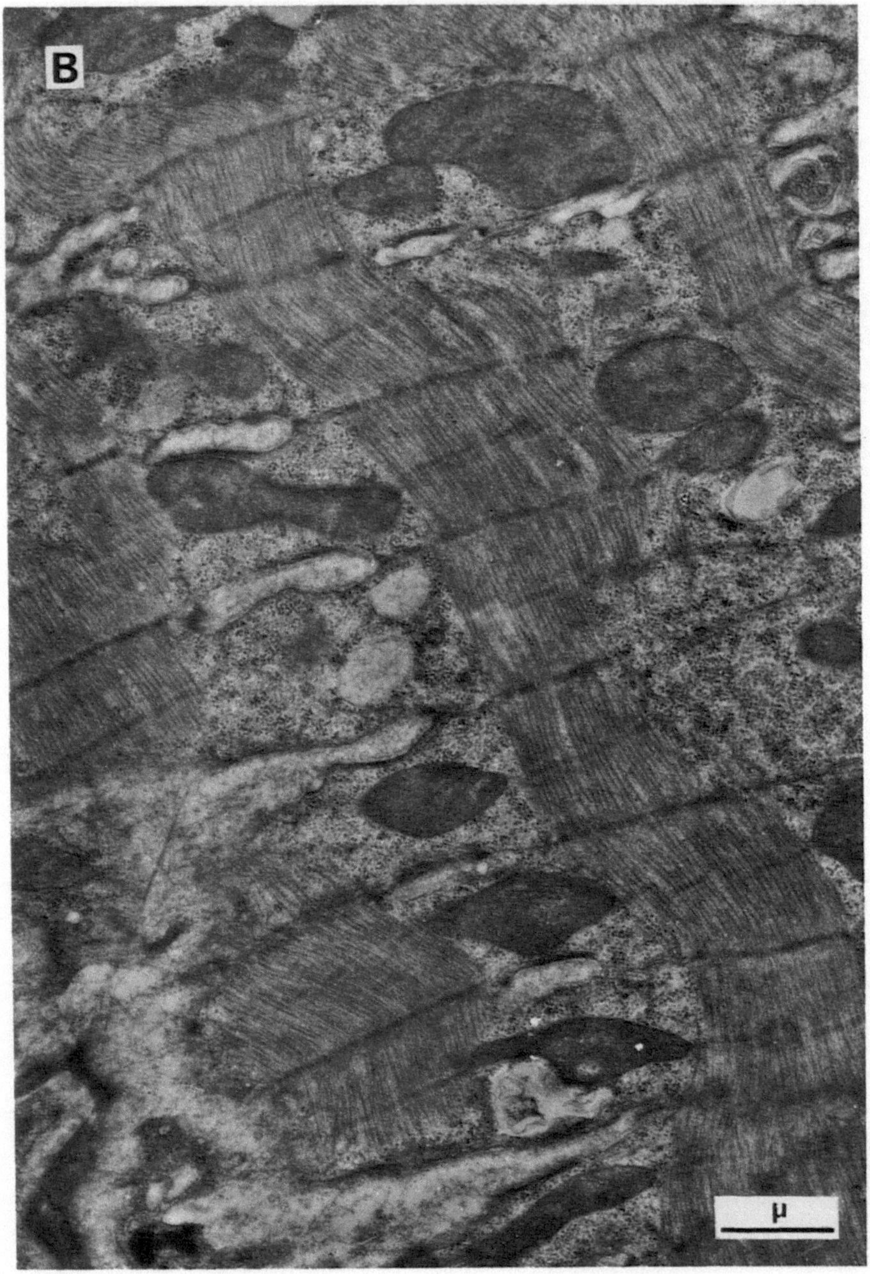

mitochondriae, clearing of their matrices, dilatation of sarcoplasmic reticulum, and lysis of myofilaments with disruption of Z bands. Figure 4 shows a typical example of these lesions classified as grade 1.

At the End of the Second Week (i.e., After Six Drug Injections). After 2 weeks of treatment, the myocardia of all hamsters treated with ADM, DTR, DNR, eADM, and

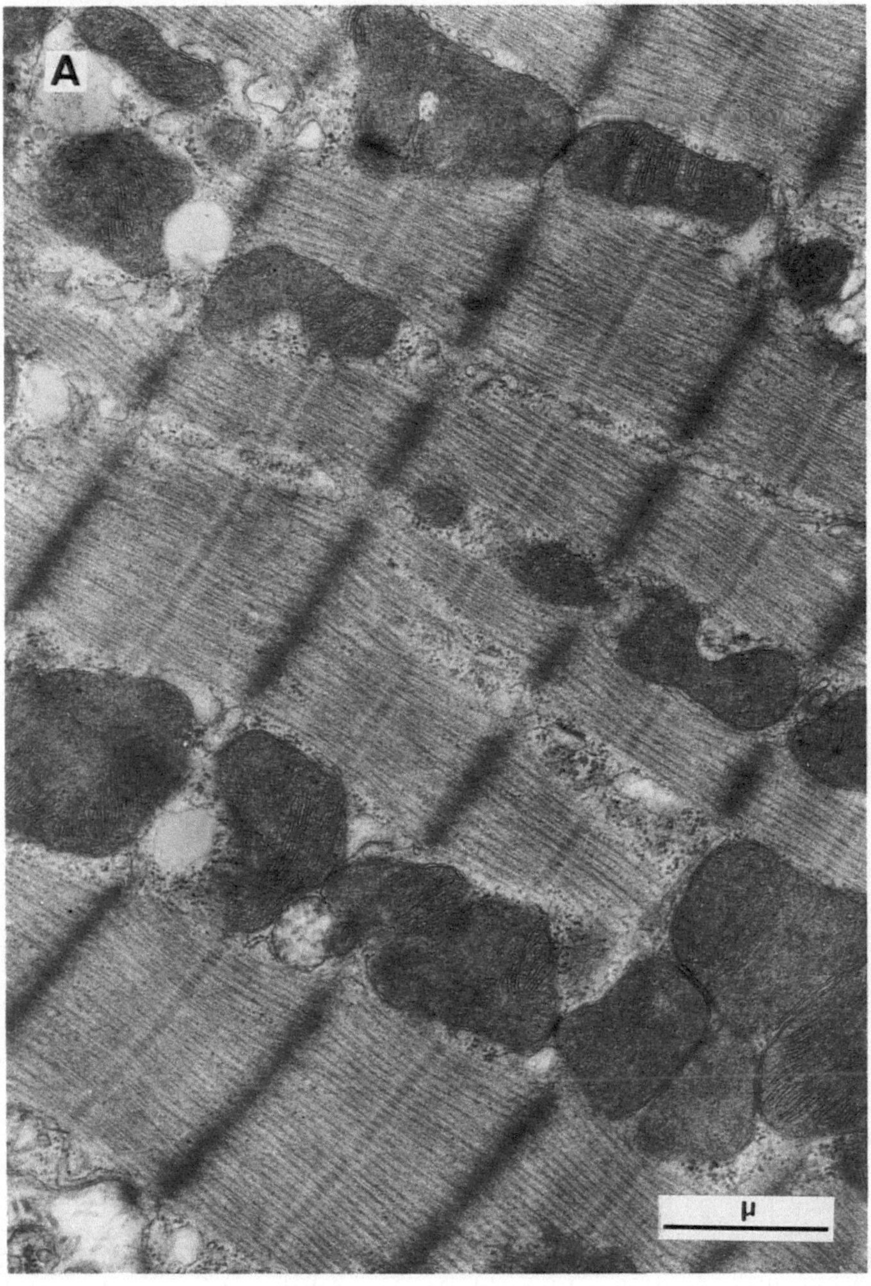

Fig. 3A–C. Myocardium from a golden hamster 7 days after treatment with ACM (6 mg/kg/injection IP 3 times a week). Generally, mitochondriae, myofilaments, and intercalated disks are well preserved (**A, B**), but it is possible to find clearing of the matrices of some mitochondriae and moderate dilatation of the sarcoplasmic reticulum (**C**). Original magnification (6/9): **A** × 10,000; **B** × 10,000; **C** × 8,300

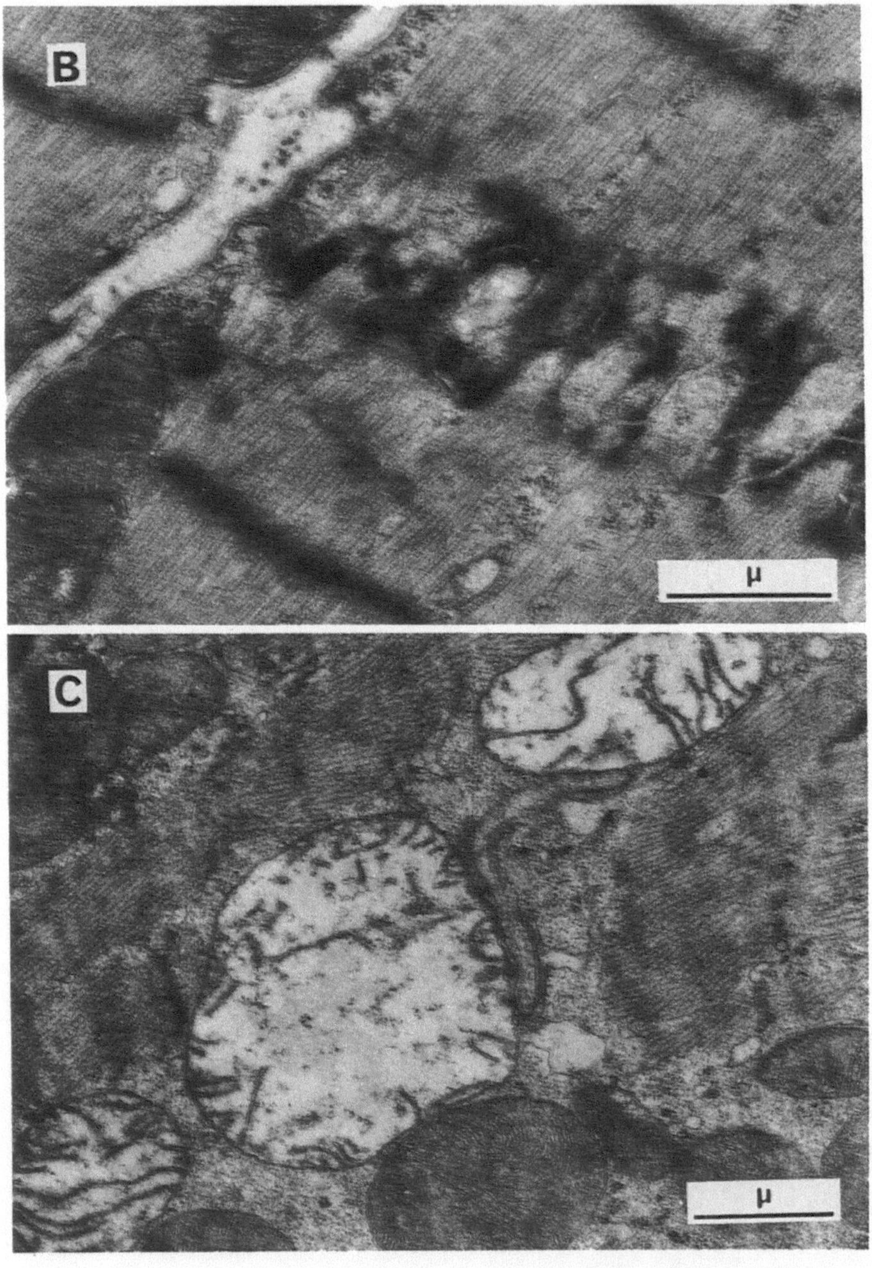

RBZ showed an increase in all alterations already found at the end of the first week. The swelling of mitochondriae with clearing of their matrices and lysis of their crests, the separation and lysis of myofilaments with disruption of Z-band registry, the formation of myelinic figures, the separation of fasciae adherens of the intercalated disks, the vacuolization of sarcoplasm, the condensation of nuclear chromatin, and the total disorganization of the myocytes were very severe alterations, which were classified as grade 2–3. Figures 5 and 6 show examples of these alterations.

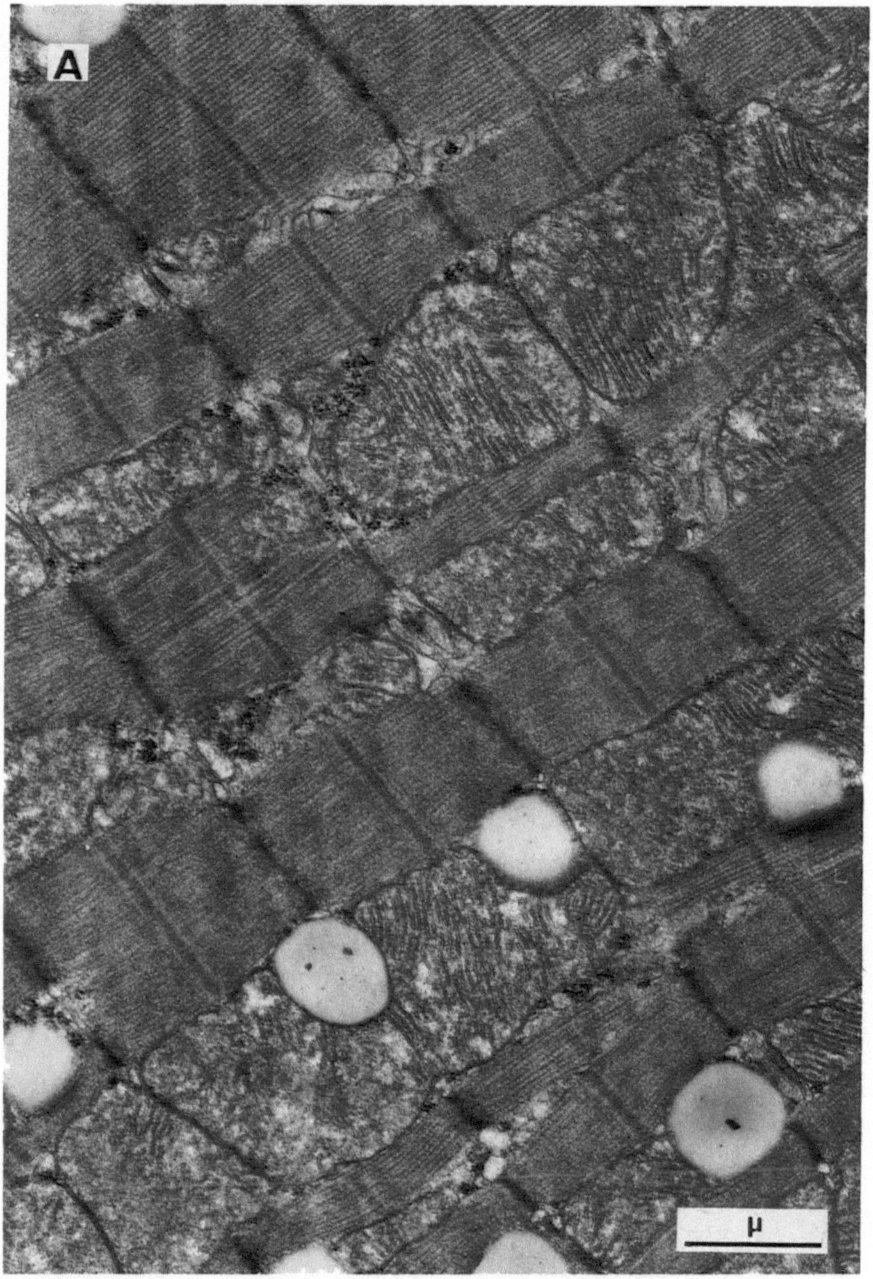

Fig. 4A, B. Myocardium from a golden hamster 7 days after treatment with AD-32 (30 mg/kg/injection IP 3 times a week). Swelling of mitochondriae with clearing of their matrices and lysis of the crests (**A**); dilatation of sarcoplasmic reticulum (**A, B**); separation and lysis of myofilaments with disruption of Z-band registry and contraction of sarcomers (**B**). Original magnification (6/9): **A** × 8,300; **B** × 8,300

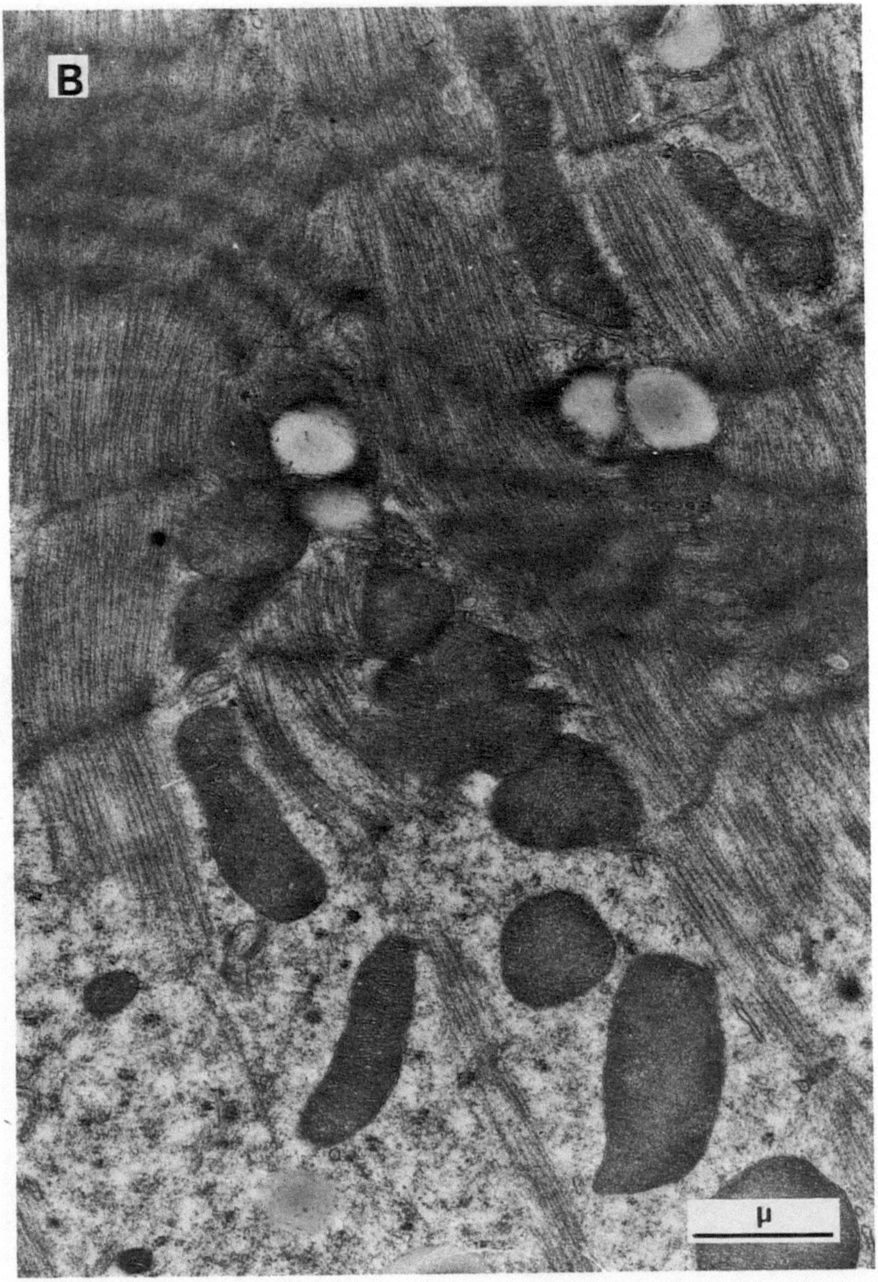

The lesions after AD-32 treatment were also very marked, but less intense than those after the preceding drugs, and were classified as grades 1–2 and 2 (Fig. 7). In ACM-treated animals, the lesions began to appear, but were still very mild. Most frequently, the myofilaments, mitochondriae, and intercalated disks were well preserved. Some myocytes showed swelling of mitochondriae with clearing of their matrices and lysis of crests. Contractions of sarcomers were also often seen (Fig. 8). These cases were classified as grades 0–1 and 1.

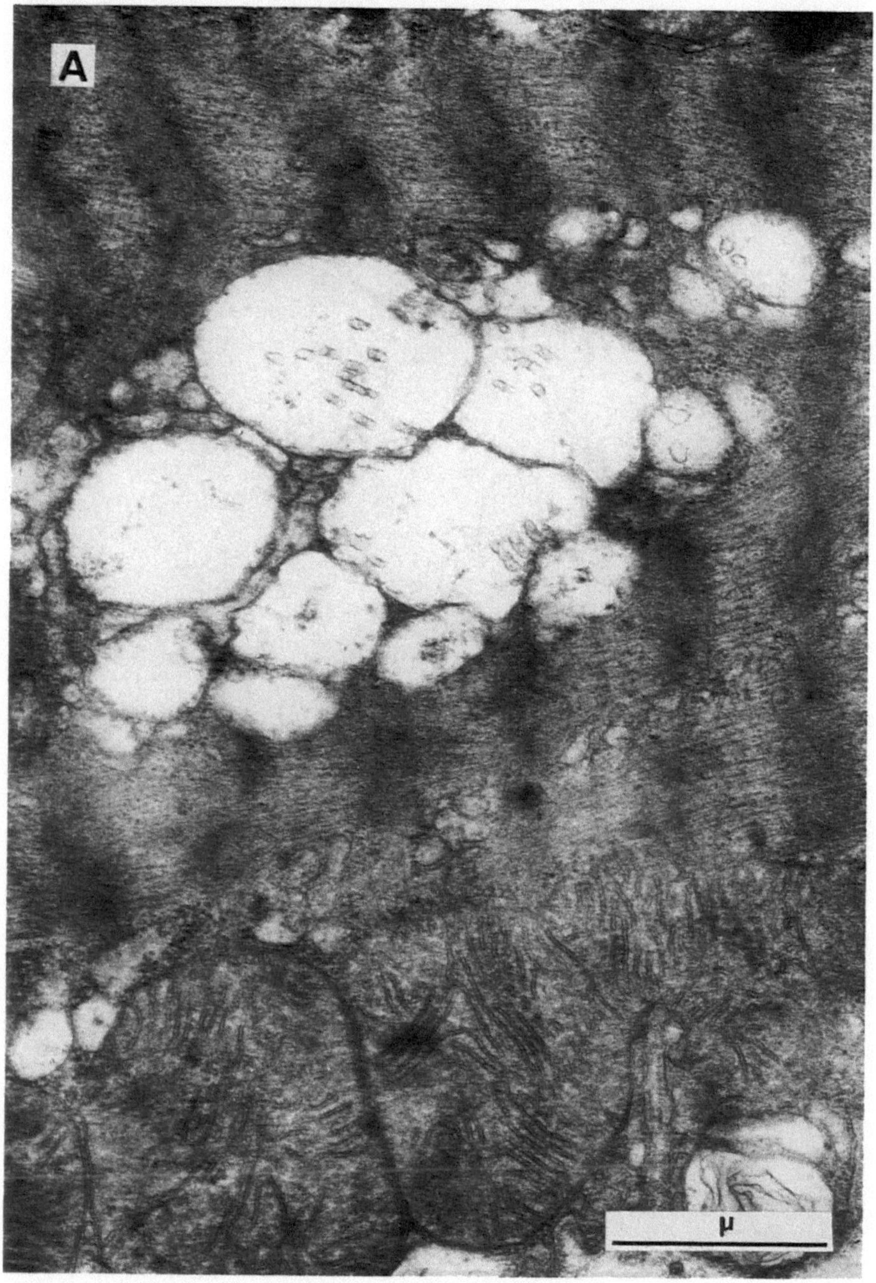

Fig. 5A, B. Myocardium from a golden hamster 14 days after treatment with ADM (3 mg/kg/injection IP 3 times a week). Swelling of mitochondriae with clearing of their matrices, lysis of their crests, vacuolization and formation of myelinic figures (**A**); separation, loss of parallel orientation and lysis of myofilaments with disruption of Z-band registry (**B**); contraction of sarcomers (**A**). Original magnification (6/9): **A** × 1,300; **B** × 1,300

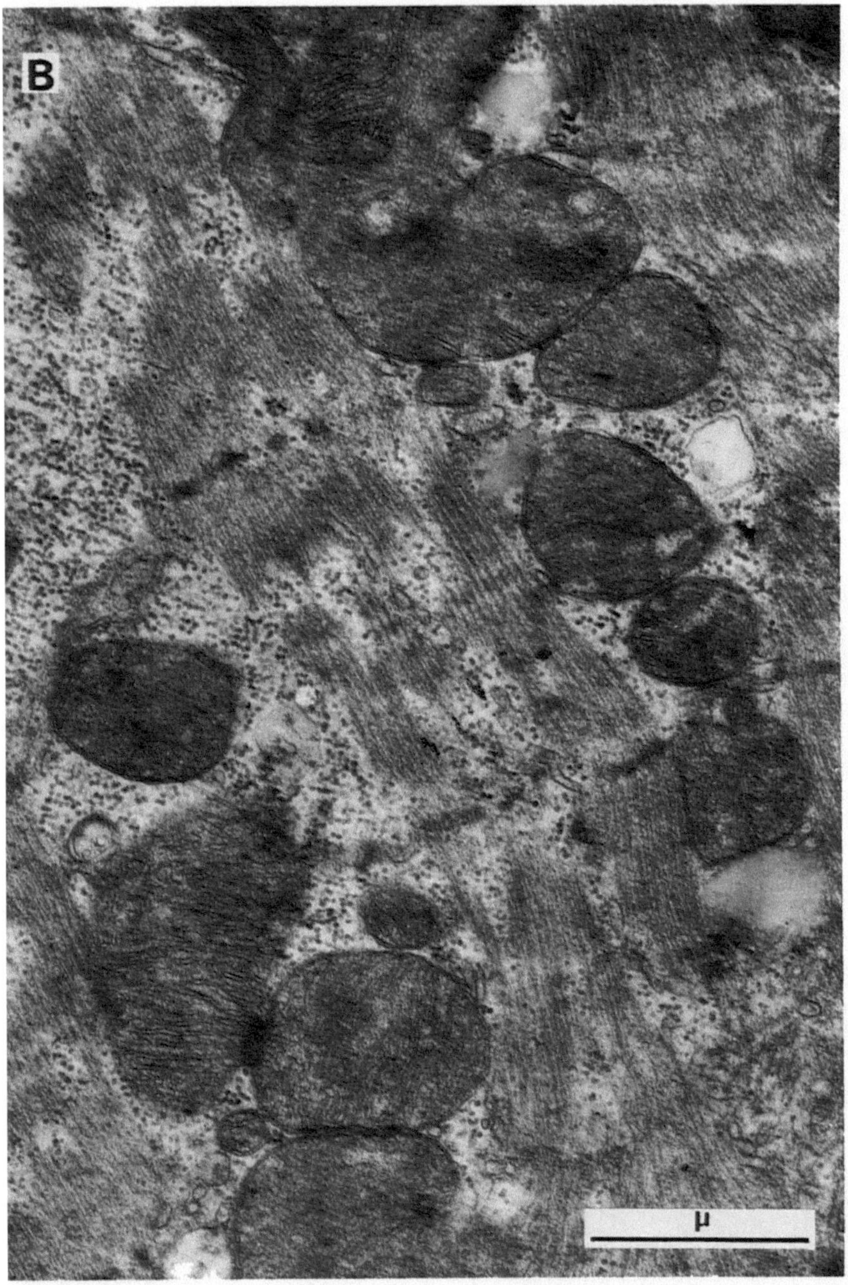

At the End of the Third Week (i.e., After Nine Drug Injections). Only one hamsters survived in the groups of ADM-treated animals, five in the DTR group, seven in the eADM group, 15 in the ACM group, none survived in the RBZ and DNR groups, and none died in the AD-32 group. The sacrificed hamsters in the groups treated with ADM, DTR, and eADM showed the same severe myocardial signs of degeneration as those seen at the end of the second week. However, some myocytes were only

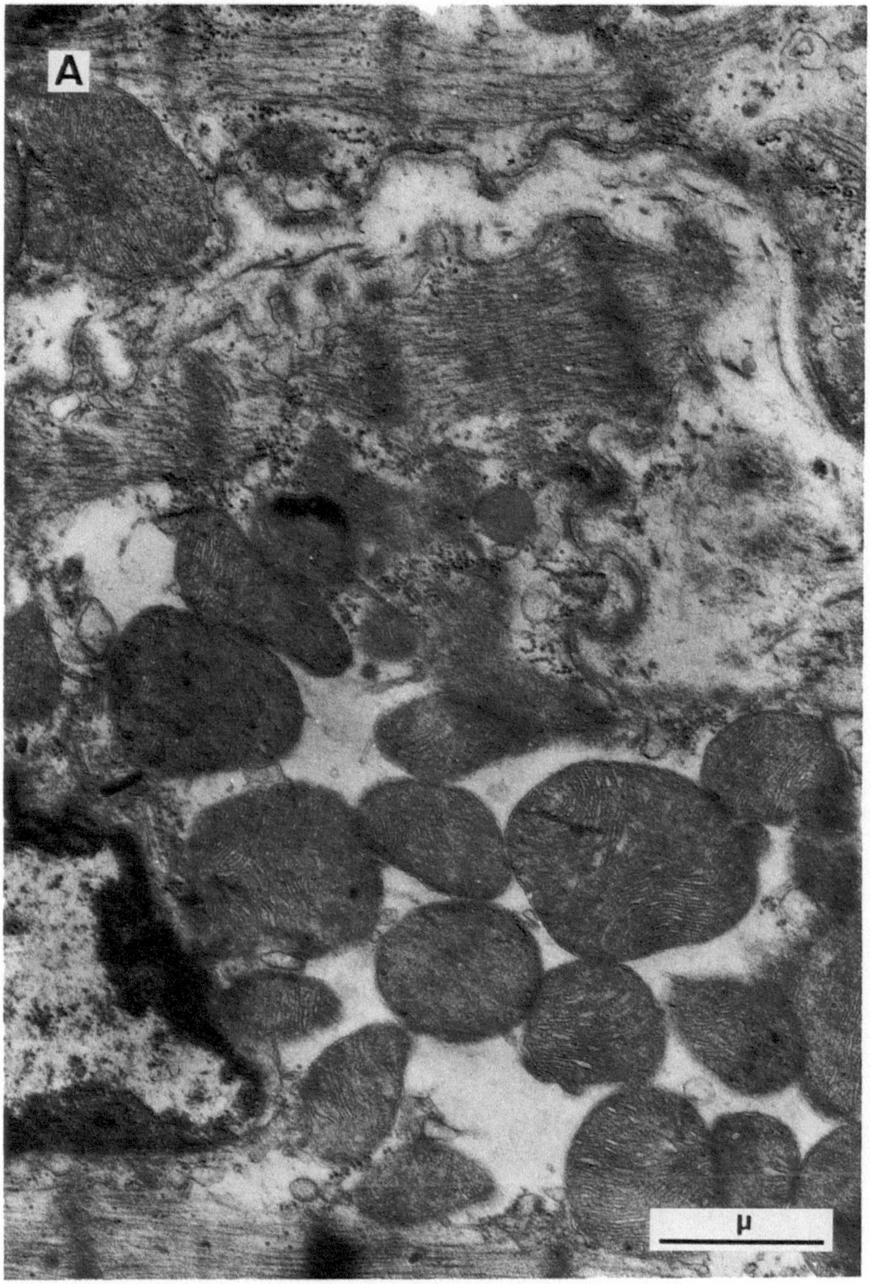

Fig. 6A, B. Myocardium from a golden hamster 14 days after treatment with daunorubicin (DNR) (3 mg/kg/injection IP 3 times a week). Homogenization and disappearance of crests of mitochondriae (**A, B**); dilatation of sarcoplasmic reticulum (**A, B**); separation of lysis of myofilaments (**A**); clumping of the chromatin into electron-dense masses which are adjacent to the nuclear membrane (**A**); separation of fasciae adherens with complete disorganization of intercalated disks and formation of extensive empty space between myocytes (**B**). Original magnification (6/9): **A** × 10,000; **B** × 8,300

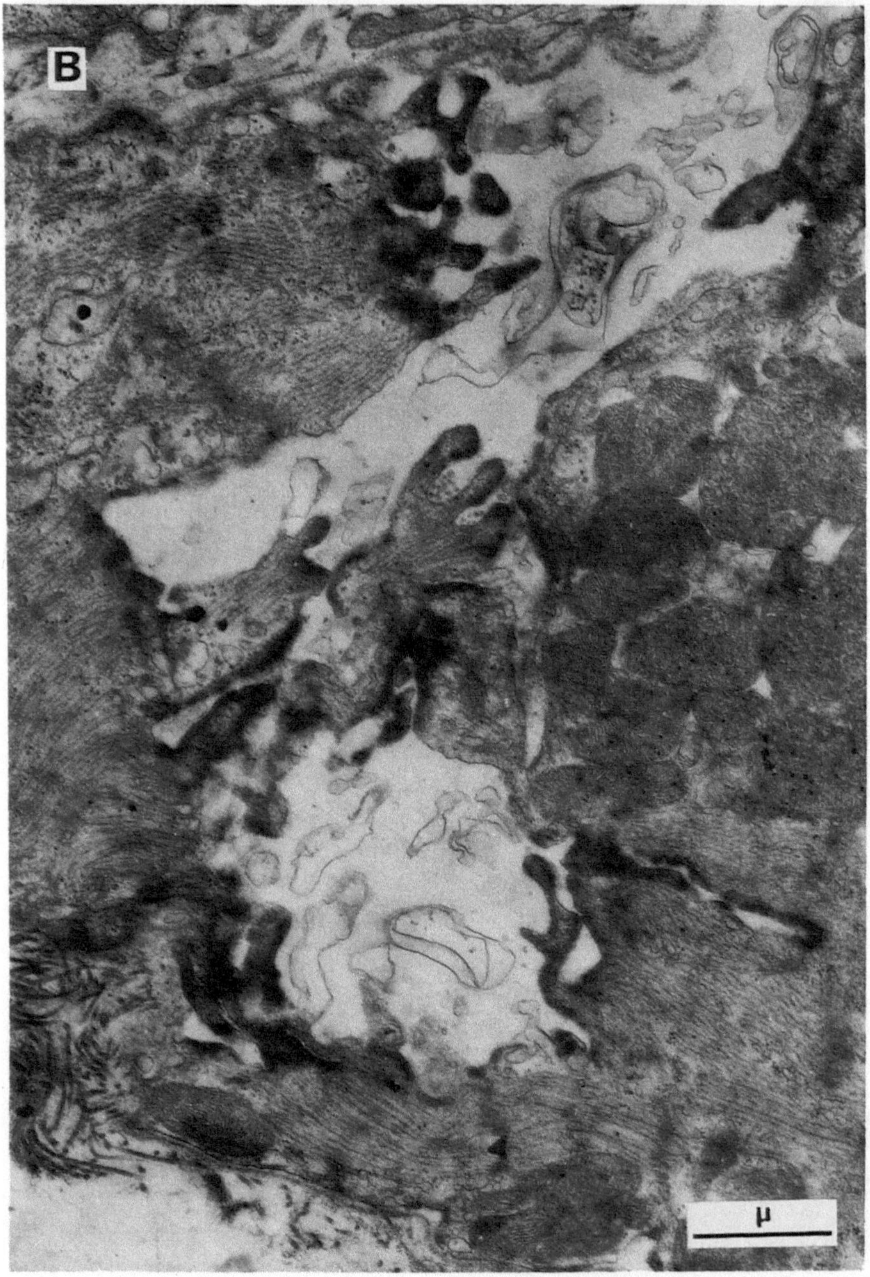

moderately altered and, moreover, some were relatively well preserved. These cases were classified as grade 2–3. The myocardia of AD-32-treated animals, even if no hamster was dead at that time, showed also severe alterations of the mitochondriae, myofilaments, and intercalated disks. These lesions were classified as grade 2. At the same time, the myocardia of ACM-treated animals still showed only changes moderate enough to be classified as grade 1–2.

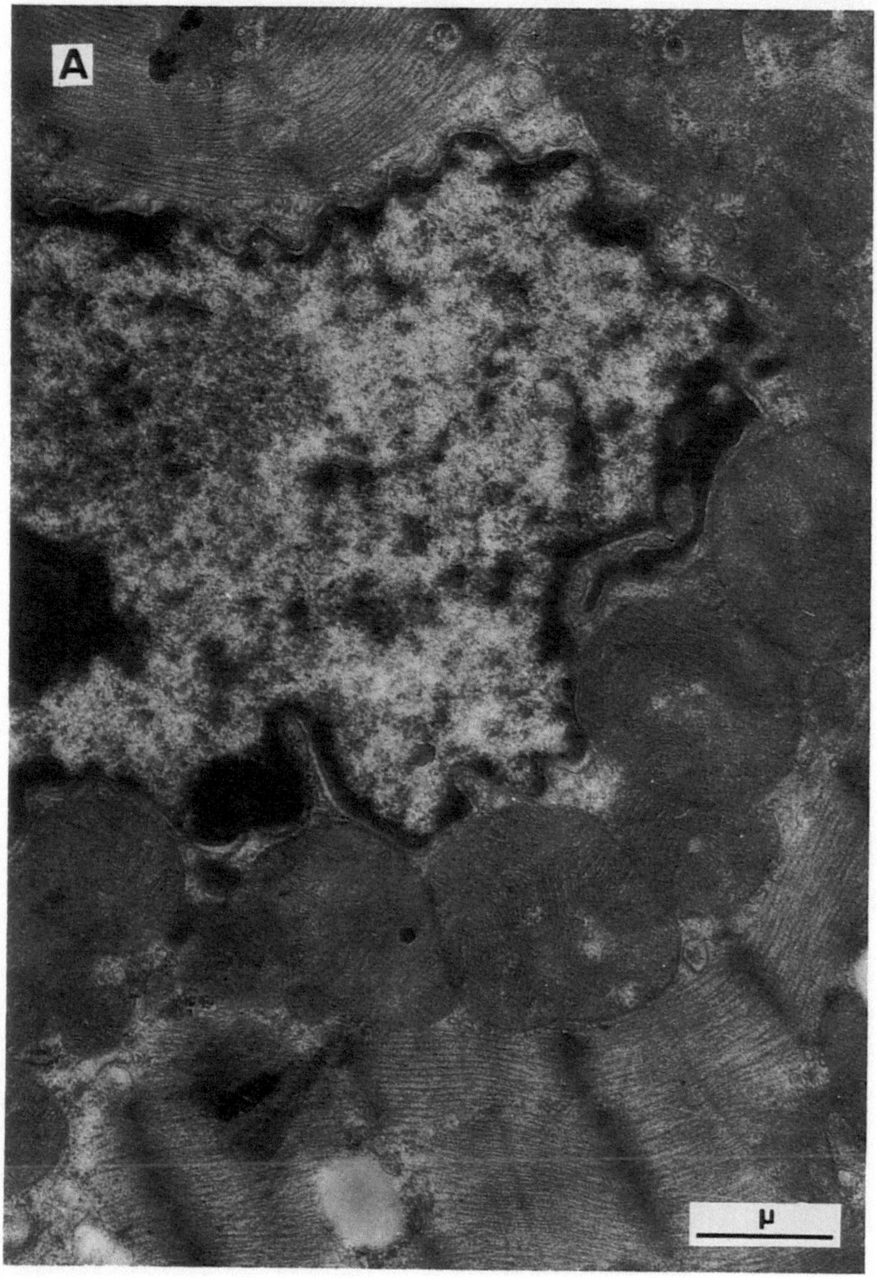

Fig. 7A–C. Myocardium from a golden hamster 14 days after treatment with AD-32 (30 mg/kg/injection IP 3 times a week). Irregular nuclear membranes and condensation of the chromatin into electron-dense masses which are adjacent to nuclear membranes (**A**); dilatation of sarcoplasmic reticulum and formation of myelinic figures (**B**); separation and lysis of myofilaments with disruption of Z-band registry (**C**). Original magnification (6/9); **A** × 8,300; **B** × 10,000; **C** × 8,300

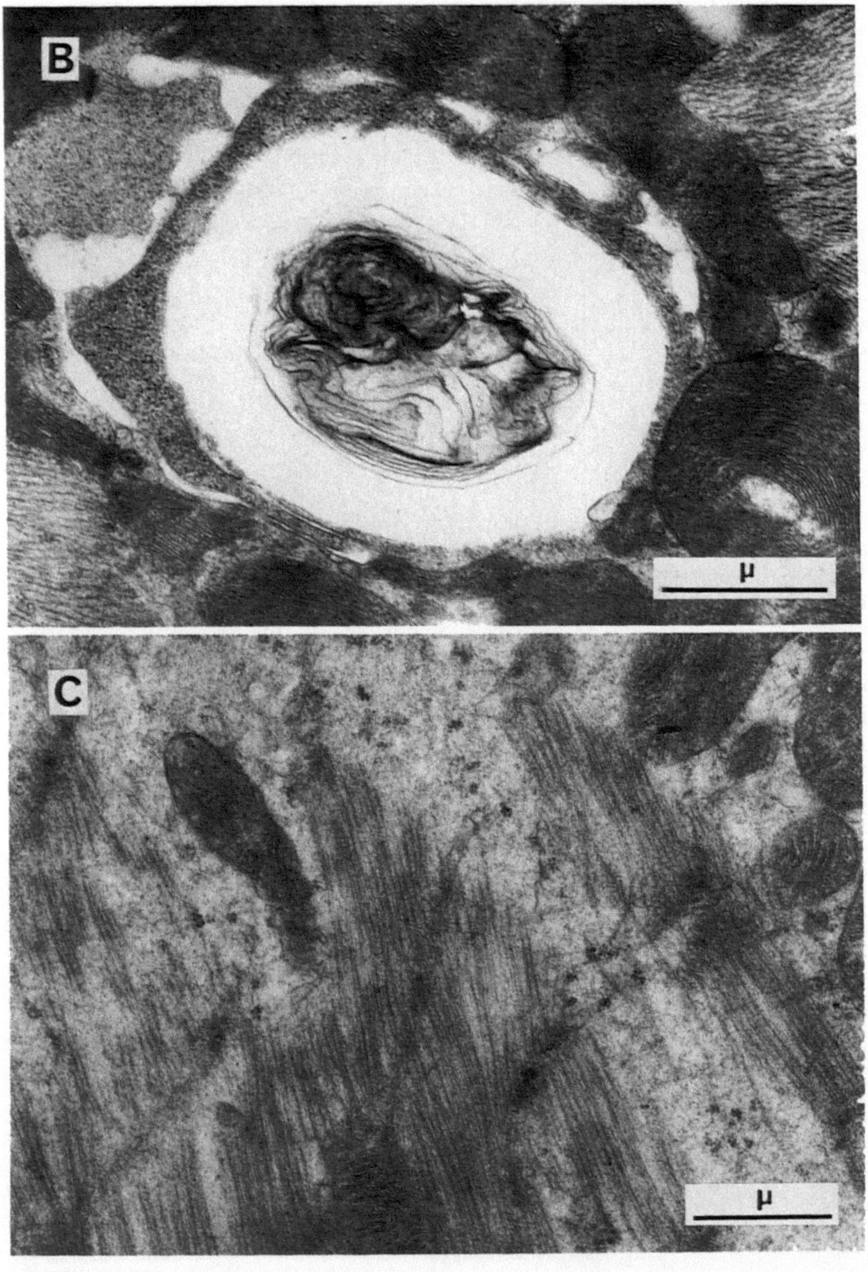

At the End of the Fourth Week (i.e., After 12 Drug Injections). Hamsters in only the ACM- and AD-32-treated groups survived (11 in each group). The myocardia of the sacrificed animals in these two groups contained almost all the types of previously described alterations, and some cells showed the same degree of cell degeneration as those of hamsters treated with the ADM, DTR, DNR, eADM, and RBZ, at the end of the second and third weeks (see Figs. 5–7). There was a clear difference, however, between the well-preserved general status of these ACM- and AD-32-treated hamsters

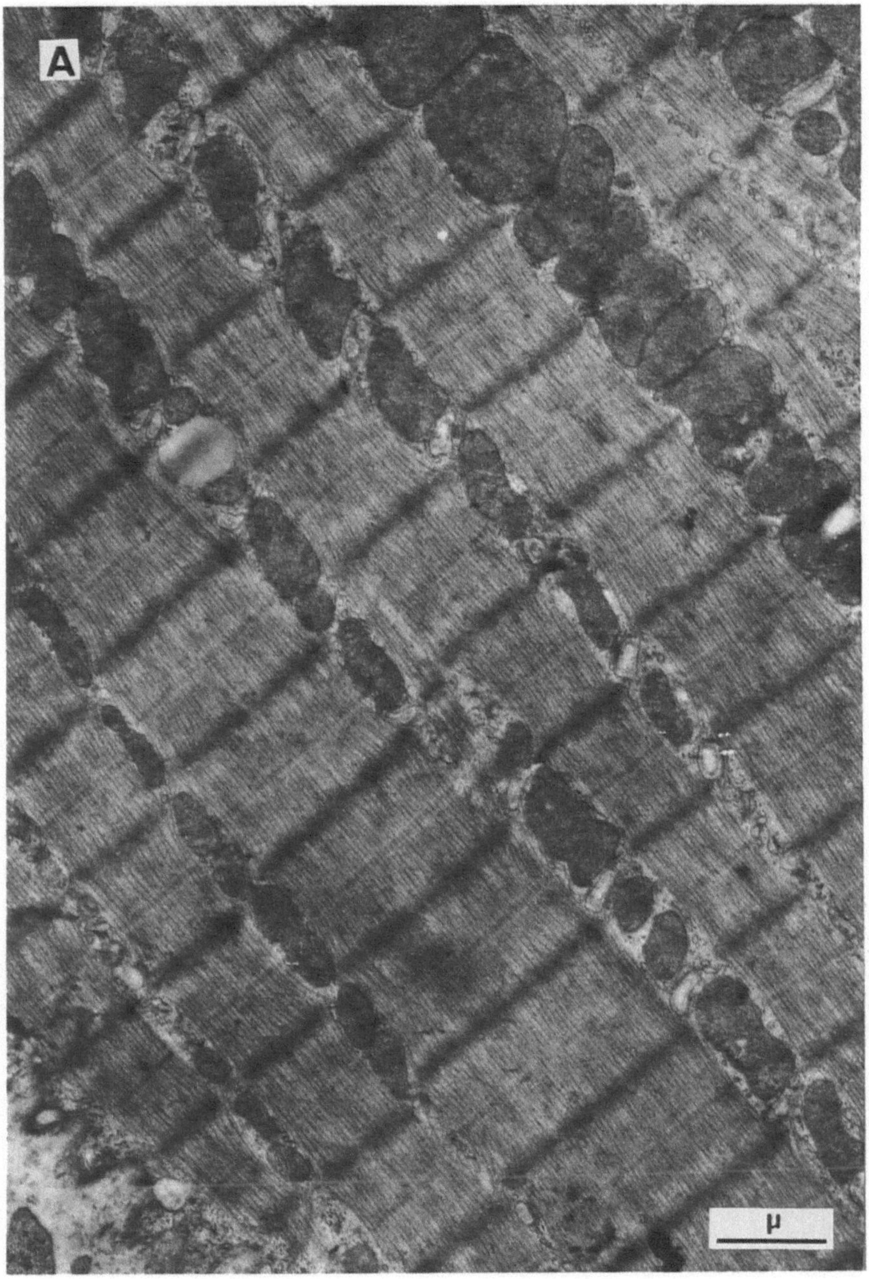

Fig. 8A–C. Myocardium from a golden hamster 14 days after treatment with ACM (6 mg/kg/injection IP 3 times a week). Most frequently myofilaments and mitochondriae are well preserved (**A**), but some myocytes show swelling of mitochondriae with clearing of their matrices and lysis of their crests, dilatation of sarcoplasmic reticulum (**B**), and contraction of sarcomers (**C**). Original magnification (6/9): **A** × 6,600; **B** × 10,000; **C** × 8,300

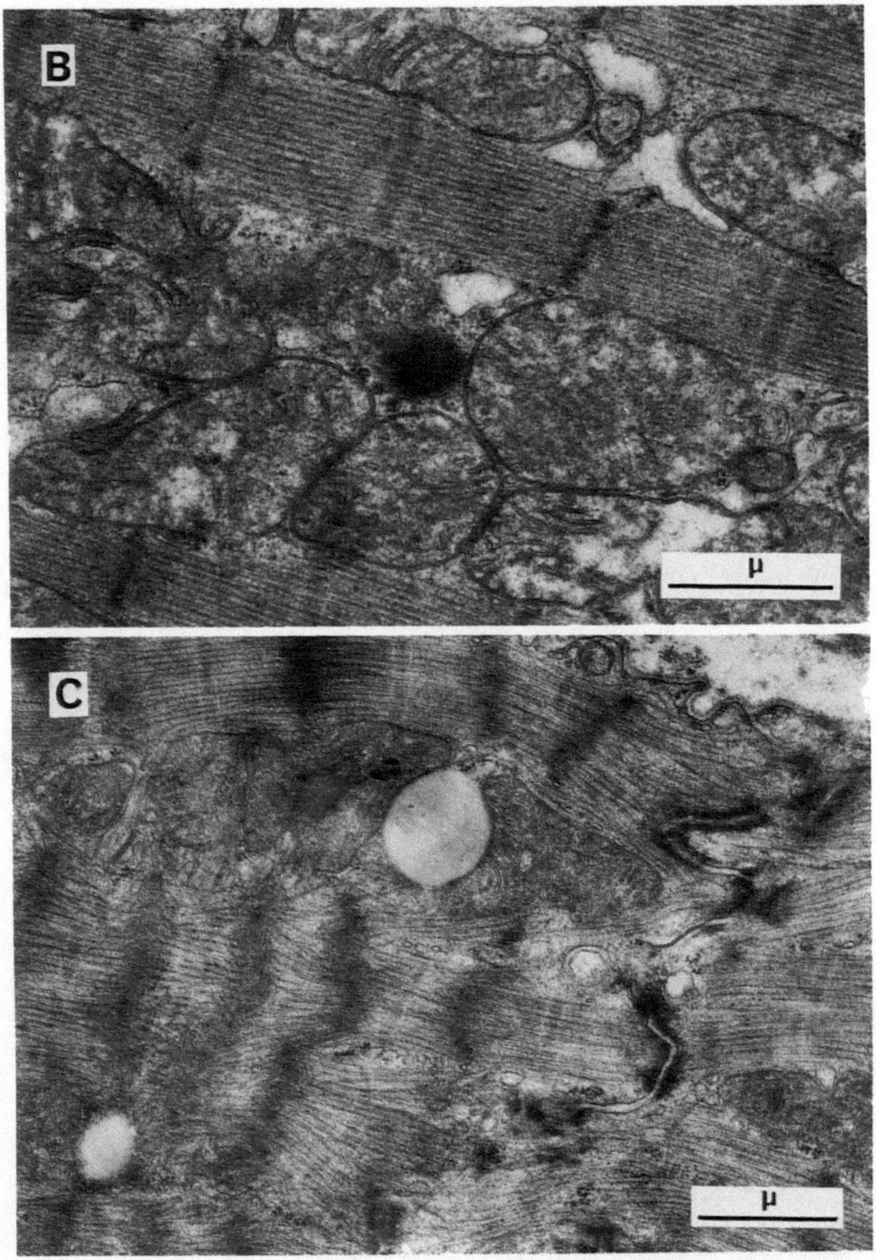

at the end of the fourth week, without weight loss and the very sick appearance of all other treated animals which lost 30%–40% of their weight at the time of their death. The ACM- and AD-32 myocardial lesions at the end of the fourth week were classified as grades 2 and 2–3, like those observed after all other drugs at the end of the second and third weeks. Table 3 summarizes the degree of myocardial EM alterations at the end of each week according to the semiquantitative grading system.

Table 3. Degree of myocardial EM alterations at the end of each week according to the semiquantitative grading system

At the end of	Drug							
	ADM	DTR	DNR	eADM	RBZ	ACM	AD-32	Controls
Week 1	1–2	1	1–2	1–2	1–2	0–1	1	0
Week 2	2–3	1–2 and 2	2–3	2–3	2–3	0–1 and 1	1–2 and 2	0
Week 3	2–3	2–3	–	2–3	–	1–2	2	0
Week 4	–	–	–	–	–	2 and 2–3	2 and 2–3	0

0 No cell pathologic alterations
1 Moderate cell alterations
2 Severe cell alterations
3 Very severe alterations just before cell death
For description of precise microscopic findings, see text

Recovery of Myocardial Alterations in Surviving ACM- and AD-32-Treated Hamsters, Two Months After Interruption of the Treatment

Two months after ACM and AD-32 treatment had been discontinued (i.e., after administration of 12 drug injections of each anthracycline during 4 weeks), three animals from each group were killed and their myocardia submitted to an EM study which revealed that their myofibrils and their mitochondriae were generally well preserved, particularly in ACM-treated animals, like those of controls. The rare EM abnormalities consisted of mild vacuolization of the cytoplasm and of some separations of the intercalated disks (Fig. 9). The morphologic aspects of the large number of myocytes were identical to those of controls.

Skin on Light Microscopy

In the groups of hamsters treated with ADM, DTR, DNR, eADM, and RBZ, the histopathologic study of the skin showed degenerative lesions which progressed every week. It was difficult to distinguish typical lesions at the end of the first week of treatment, but after the second week the skin showed a very marked atrophy of all epidermic layers and a loss of the hair (alopecia), as shown on Fig. 10. The skin of ACM- and AD-32-treated hamsters preserved its normal histologic structure, even after 4 weeks of treatment (Fig. 11).

Discussion

The experimental ultrastructural and histopathologic study of cardiotoxic alterations induced by some anthracyclines, and especially by ADM, DNM, and ADM-DNA, has been demonstrated by some authors [1, 2, 4, 8], who found numerous alterations of the

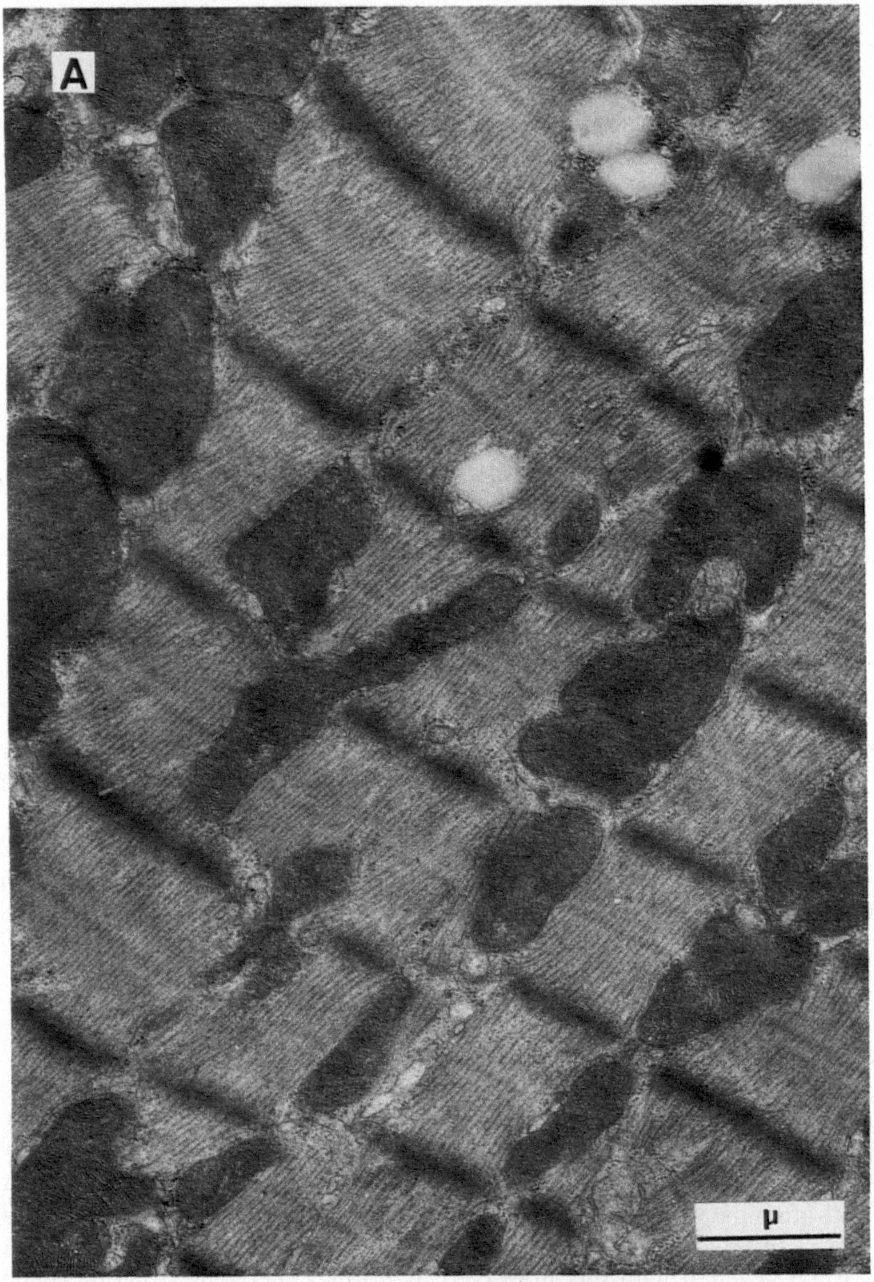

Fig. 9A–C. Myocardium from a golden hamster 8 weeks after administration of 12 ACM or AD-32 injections during 4 weeks. Generally, myofilaments and mitochondriae are in good condition (**A, B**), but some alterations persist, such as moderate vacuolization of the cytoplasm (**B**) and some separation of the intercalated disks (**C**). Original magnification (6/9): **A** × 8,300; **B** × 3,300; **C** × 8,300

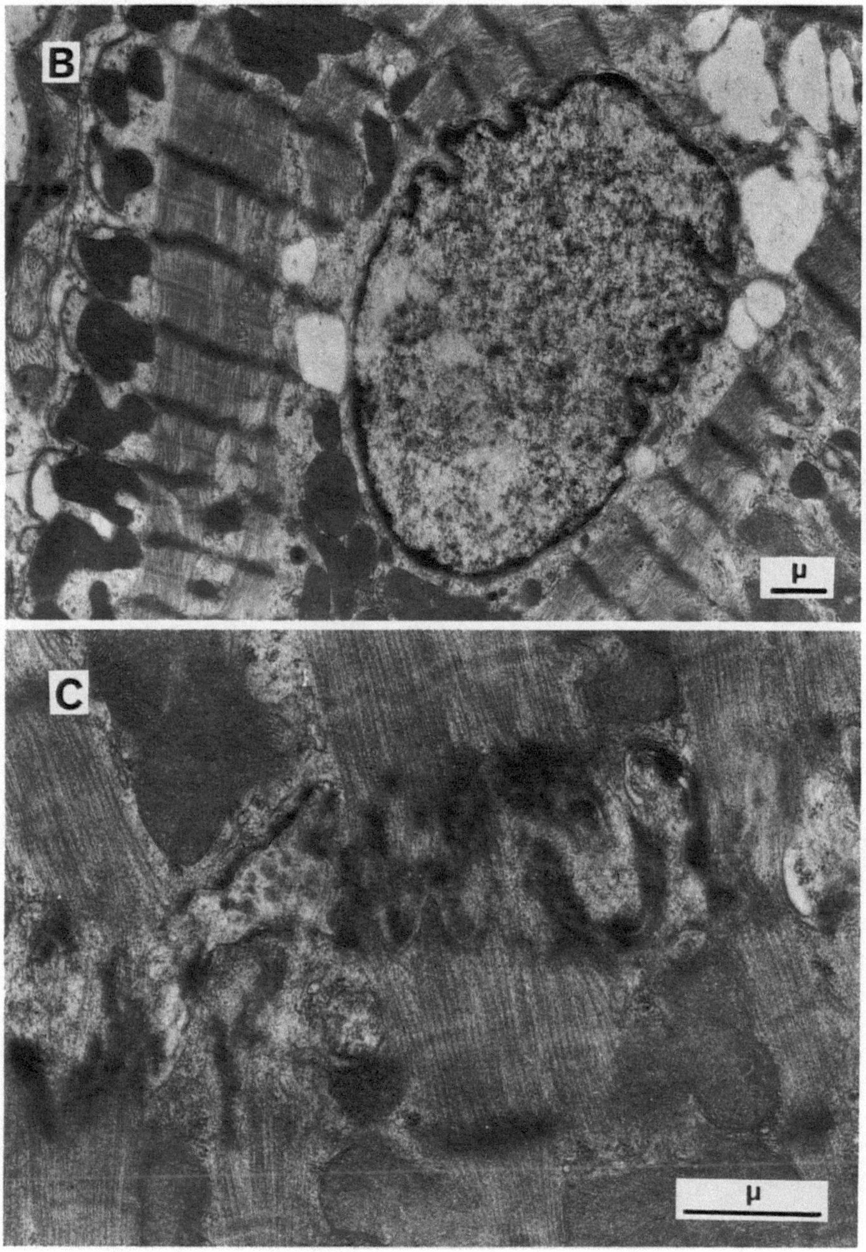

myocardium, which were similar to those in our experiments, after treatment with adriamycin and its derivatives. The findings of our comparative study of the cardiotoxicity and skin toxicity of seven anthracyclines allow us to draw several conclusions concerning their toxicity, animal survival after administration of equivalent doses, and consequently the advantages and/or disadvantages of each drug.

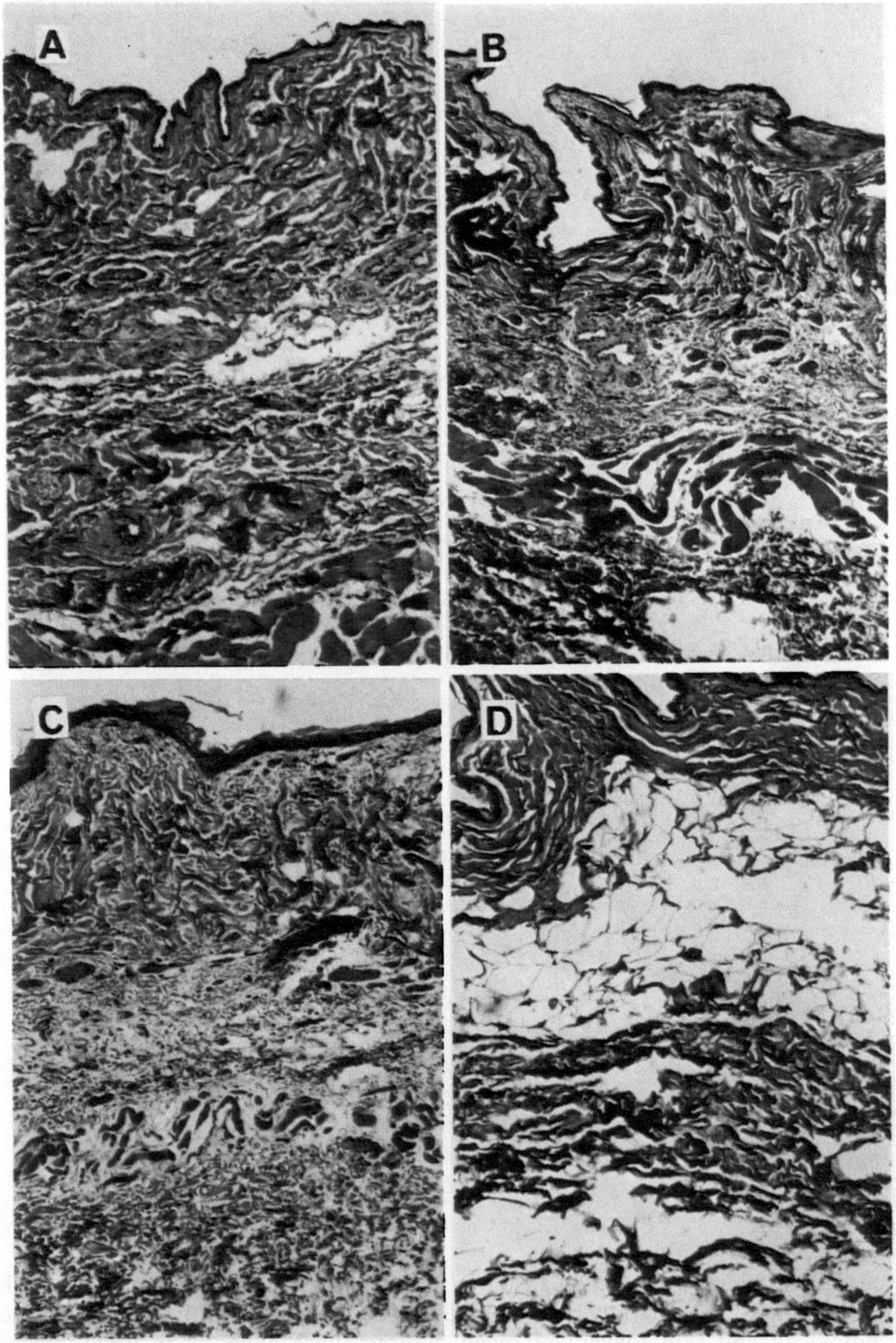

Fig. 10A–F. Histopathologic alterations of the skin of golden hamster after 3-week treatment with ADM (**A**), DTR (**B**), DNR (**C**), eADM (**D**), ADM (**E**), and RBZ (F). Atrophy of all layers of the epidermis and loss of the hair (alopecia). Original magnification (24/36): **A–F** × 140

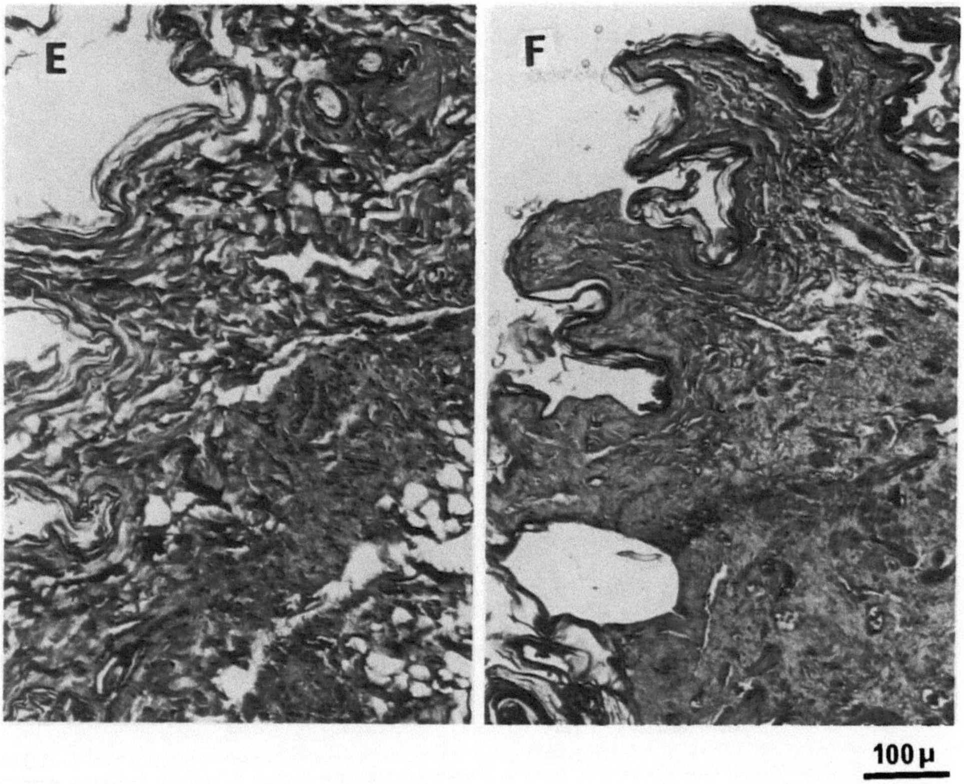

Comparing the results of the mortality of eight groups of hamsters (Table 1), with or without loss of weight and hair, and digestive disorders, it is obvious that ACM and AD-32, under our experimental conditions, are much less toxic than ADM, DTR, DNR, eADM, and RBZ. On the other hand, EM study of the myocardium indicates also a lower degree of cardiotoxicity with the first two drugs, especially during the first 2 weeks in ACM-treated hamsters, as compared with the five other drugs. These results are very consistent with clinical data presently available with these compounds: in early clinical trials, ACM and AD-32 were rarely cardiotoxic and induced little or no alopecia [3, 11, 12], while the other anthracyclines, i.e., ADM and DTR, were highly cardiotoxic and caused alopecia [5, 7, 10].

Nevertheless, at the end of the fourth week of treatment, ACM- and AD-32-treated hamsters showed almost the same degree of myocardial degeneration (grade 2–3) as the hamsters treated with the other anthracyclines at the end of the second or third week just before their death. Besides the conservation of their hair, however, all surviving ACM- and AD-32-treated hamsters preserved their weight and a good general state without diarrhea, while all the hamsters treated with the other anthracyclines lost their hair and 30%–40% of their weight, and presented very serious digestive symptoms, particularly abundant diarrhea. These findings seem to indicate that cardiotoxicity is probably not the main cause of animal death under our experimental conditions. As it has been shown by certain authors [8], the toxic effects of anthracyclines cause severe problems in many organs and metabolites. We also hope to study completely and to answer this question to a certain extent after a careful LM analysis of all organ samples collected in sacrificed animals.

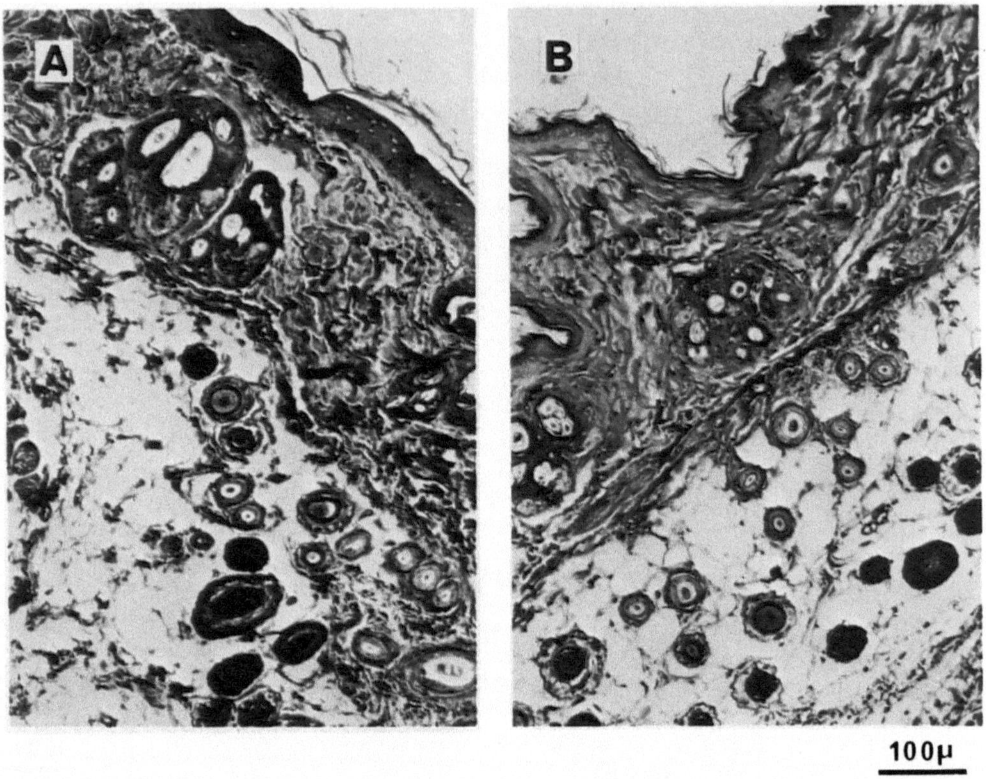

Fig. 11A, B. Histopathologic alterations of the skin of a golden hamster after 4-week treatment with ACM (**C**) and AD-32 (**D**). Normal histologic structure of epidermal cell layers and of the hair (no alopecia). Original magnification (24/36): **A** × 140; **B** × 140

Myocardial lesions were observed with all seven anthracyclines in our study, and most interesting was the observation of a possible recovery of these lesions. This occurred quite rapidly and was demonstrated after ACM and AD-32 treatment, but might also occur with other cardiotoxic anthracyclines; the practical impact of these findings remains to be established in man.

Except for these hamsters treated with ACM and AD-32, shortly after treatment all the others receiving one of the five remaining drugs began to lose their hair. Histopathologic study of the skin confirmed this fact and showed an impressive atrophy of epidermal cell layers (Fig. 10). In the group of ACM- and AD-32-treated hamsters, however, the skin and the hair were preserved and showed a histologic structure similar to that of controls (Fig. 11); this is another advantage of these two new drugs which are already very much appreciated in their clinical application.

In conclusion, after seven different anthracyclines were administered IP at equivalent doses and under the same experimental conditions in golden hamsters, the comparative study of mortality, EM alterations of the myocardium, and the LM histopathologic alterations of the skin showed that ACM was the least toxic drug, followed by AD-32; if with this lower toxicity the further clinical observations confirm a good antitumor activity of these two drugs, they will offer an important contribution to the chemotherapy of neoplasias.

References

1 Benjamin RS, Mason YW, Billingham ME (1978) Cardiac toxicity of adriamycin-DNA complex and rubidazone: Evaluation by electrocardiogram and endomyocardial biopsy. Cancer Treat Rep 62: 935–939

2 Billingham MA, Mason JW, Briston MR, Daniels JR (1978) Anthracycline cardiomyopathy monitored by morphologic changes. Cancer Treat Rep 62: 865–872

3 Blum RH, Garnick MB, Israel M, Canellos GP, Henderson IC, Frei III E (1979) Initial clinical evaluation of N-trifluoroacetyladriamycin-14-valerate (AD-32), an adriamycin analog. Cancer Treat Rep 63: 919–925

4 Buja LM, Ferrans VJ, Mayer RJ, Roberts WC, Henderson ES (1973) Cardiac ultrastructural changes induced by daunorubicin therapy. Cancer 32: 771–788

5 Clarysse A, Kenis Y, Mathé G (1976) Cancer chemotherapy. Its role in the treatment strategy of hematologic malignancies and solid tumors. Springer, Berlin Heidelberg New York

6 Dantchev D, Slioussartchouk V, Paintrand M, Bourut C, Hayat M, Mathé G (1979) Electron microscopy of the heart and light microscopy of the skin after treatment of golden hamsters with adriamycin, detorubicin, AD32 and aclacinomycin. Cancer Treat Rep 63: 875–889

7 E.O.R.T.C. Clinical Screening Group (1980) Clinical study of detorubicin. Recent Results Cancer Res 74: 194–201

8 Ferrans VJ (1978) Overview of cardiac pathology in relation to anthracycline cardiotoxicity. Cancer Treat Rep 62: 955–961

9 Freireich EJ, Gehan EA, Rall DP, Schmidt LM, Skipper HE (1966) Quantitative comparison of toxicity of anticancer agents in mouse, rat, hamster, dog, monkey and man. Cancer Chemother Rep 50: 219–245

10 Jacquillat CL, Auclerc MF, Weil M, Maral J, Degas L, Auclerc G, Tobelem G, Schaison G, Bernard J (1979) Clinical activity of detorubicin: a new anthracycline derivative. Cancer Treat Rep 63: 889–895

11 Mathé G, Bayssas M, Gouveia J, Dantchev D, Ribaud P, Machover D, Misset JL, Schwarzenberg L, Jasmin C, Hayat M (1978) Preliminary results of a phase II trial of aclacinomycin in acute leukemia and lymphosarcoma. Cancer Chemother Pharmacol 1: 259–262

12 Ogawa M, Inagaki J, Horikoshi N, Inoue K, Chinen T, Ueoka H, Nagura E (1979) Clinical study of aclacinomycin A. Cancer Treat Rep 63: 931–935

m-AMSA: A New Anticancer Agent

M. Rozencweig, D. D. Von Hoff, S. S. Legha, R. L. Cysyk,
and F. M. Muggia*

Summary

4′-(9-Acridinylamino)methanesulfon-*m*-anisidide (*m*-AMSA; NSC-249992) is a new anticancer agent that has undergone extensive experimental investigation. Clinical trials have recently been initiated and current data suggest a wide spectrum of antitumor activity in human cancer.

Introduction

The antitumor activity of acriflavine, an acridine dye, was first reported by MELLANBY in 1933 [17]. Since then, numerous acridine derivatives have been produced in a search for compounds with enhanced therapeutic index. 4′-(9-Acridinylamino)methanesulfon-*m*-anisidide (*m*-AMSA; NSC-249992) is one of the many acridine derivatives synthesized by CAIN and ATWELL [1] (Fig. 1). This review summarizes the preclinical information that has accumulated on this compound as well as the preliminary data obtained in early clinical studies.

Preclinical Information

Animal Tumor Data

m-AMSA is active against a wide spectrum of murine tumors [1, 2, 18]. These include the ascitic form of the L1210 and the P388 leukemia, Lewis lung carcinoma, spontaneous C3H mammary adenocarcinoma, and mammary tumor in $CD8F_1$ mice. There is no clear evidence of schedule dependency of this antitumor activity. Of particular interest, the drug is curative in the commonly resistant B16 melanoma. This has been related to an enhanced localization of *m*-AMSA in melanoma cells, followed by a binding to melanin granules [21]. The drug is considered inactive against intracerebrally inoculated L1210, transplantable colon tumors 36 and 38, colon xenografts, and MX1 breast xenograft in nude mice.

* This work was supported by grant 3.4535.79 from the "Fonds de la Recherche Scientifique Médicale" (FNRS, Belgium), and by contract NIH NO1/CM53840 from the National Cancer Institute, Bethesda, Maryland, USA

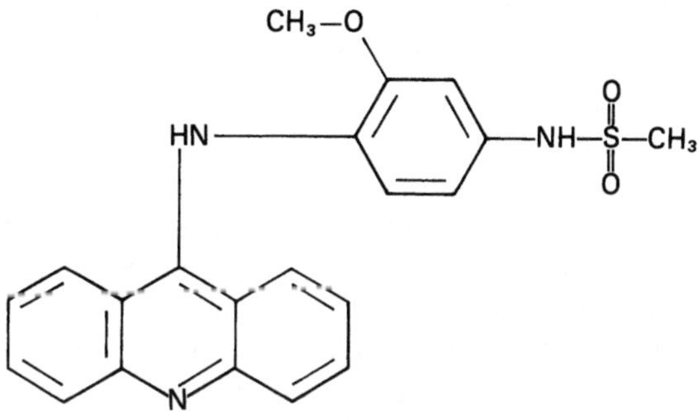

Fig. 1. Chemical structure of *m*-AMSA

Mechanism of Action

Since the acridines, as a class, interact with DNA, attempts to define the mechanism of cytotoxicity of *m*-AMSA have so far been directed at studying DNA effects [27]. However, *m*-AMSA is structurally dissimilar to simple acridines in that the 9-methanesulfonanilide moiety is orthogonal to the acridine ring system [1] and thus might be expected to interfere with intercalation [26]. GORMLEY et al. [9] studied the interaction of *m*-AMSA with calf thymus DNA and various chemically defined synthetic copolymers. They found that *m*-AMSA does intercalate into DNA base pairs, that it interacts with both AT and GC base pairs, and that the drug alters the template properties of DNA as determined by inhibition of nucleic acid polymerizing enzymes. A study by FURLONG et al. [7] on the effects of *m*-AMSA on macromolecular synthesis in L1210 cells in vivo and in vitro demonstrated that DNA synthesis is substantially inhibited at *m*-AMSA concentrations that do not interfere with RNA synthesis. In addition, *m*-AMSA was found to produce DNA fragmentation in L1210 cells (exposed in vivo or in vitro) as shown by centrifugation of cell lysates on alkaline sucrose gradients. In vivo experiments have revealed cross-resistance to *m*-AMSA of a subline of P388 leukemic cells resistant to a variety of DNA intercalating agents [12].

The kinetic response to *m*-AMSA was investigated in cycling and noncycling cells [23]. In these experiments, CHO cells were exposed to the drug for 2 h and the cell-cycle distributions were determined 30 h later. Cycling cells were shown to accumulate in G2, and this phenomenon was dose-dependent. CHO cells arrested in G1 were also treated prior to return to cycle. At moderate concentrations, these noncycling cells were 2–4 times more resistant to the drug than were cycling cells. At higher doses, the cell kill effects were similar in cycling and noncycling cells, but the progression through the cell cycle was not markedly affected in noncycling cells. Overall, the kinetic response to *m*-AMSA resembled that observed with adriamycin.

m-AMSA was also found to induce cell-cycle-specific chromosome damages in CHO cells [5]. In these experiments, synchronized cells were exposed to *m*-AMSA at various phases of the cell cycle. Severe damages were seen especially after treatment during the early G2 phase with more than 20 breaks/cell. This is in contrast to adriamycin, which induces more chromosome damage in the S phase than in G2.

Experimental Pharmacology

A preclinical pharmacologic study [3] using ^{14}C-*m*-AMSA labeled in the acridine nucleus in rodents showed that radioactivity was well distributed to all tissues except the brain. The pharmacologic disposition of *m*-AMSA appeared to be related to the susceptibility of the 9-carbon atom of the acridine ring to nucleophilic attack by endogenous thiols. This results in the release of the 9-methanesulfanilide moiety and the formation of the corresponding 9-alkylthioether of acridine. Biliary excretion was the primary route of elimination, with more than 50% of the administered dose eliminated in the bile within 2 h after intravenous (IV) administration. Less than 2% of the biliary radioactivity was unchanged *m*-AMSA. The glutathione-9-thioether of acridine was detected in the bile by field desorption mass spectroscopy. The major metabolite of *m*-AMSA is actively excreted into the bile by a transport mechanism that is saturable with therapeutic doses in rats.

Multiphasic plasma decay curves were observed with an early rapid component followed by a more gradual decline. This pattern of disappearance is believed to be due to an interaction of *m*-AMSA with thiol groups of protein, forming stable protein-acridine complexes and thus causing prolonged retention of the acridine moiety in plasma and certain tissues. By 24 h, 11% of the administered radioactivity had been recovered in the urine, with approximately 22% of it being unchanged *m*-AMSA. Although thiolysis can occur nonenzymatically, *m*-AMSA is an excellent substrate for glutathione-S-transferase purified from rat liver. Plasma levels and biliary excretion of *m*-AMSA and its metabolite can be influenced by the in vivo manipulation of glutathione-S-transferase activity and glutathione levels. Enhancement of in vivo transferase activity by phenobarbital pretreatment produced a decrease in the plasma half-life of unchanged *m*-AMSA and a corresponding increase in biliary excretion. Diethyl-maleate-induced depletion of glutathione levels resulted in a prolonged plasma half-life of unchanged *m*-AMSA and a corresponding decrease in biliary excretion [20].

Preliminary experiments with oral administration of ^{14}C-*m*-AMSA to rats (100 mg/kg) indicated that 60%–90% of the radioactivity was recovered in the bile (M. Rozencweig and R. L. Cysyk, unpublished data). At doses achieving similar levels of radioactivity in the liver, considerably lower concentrations of *m*-AMSA, particularly in its unchanged form, were seen in most other organs as compared with IV administration [4].

m-AMSA is only modestly effective against L1210 implanted intraperitoneally (IP) when given orally. This is probably a consequence of its rapid uptake by the liver. The following experiment was carried out by Cysyk and co-workers [4] to determine whether the high levels of drug in the liver might result in an antitumor effect in liver disease. *m*-AMSA was given orally at various dose levels 5 days after IV L1210 inoculation to groups of ten mice. The liver was removed 24 h thereafter and bioassayed for content of tumor cells. At the highest doses, no L1210 cells were detected in the liver in most animals. These findings point to the potential of *m*-AMSA for the treatment of liver metastases, particularly with the oral route.

Animal Toxicology

Toxicologic studies of *m*-AMSA in beagles and rhesus monkeys showed that the dog was the more sensitive of the two animal species (M. C. Henry et al., Report II TRI-TOX 2499992-76-2, NCI, Oct. 20, 1976). The toxic dose low and the toxic dose high for the beagle were 31.2 and 62.5 mg/m^2, respectively, on a single-dose IV schedule. After oral (PO) administration, the corresponding figures were 125 and 500

mg/m^2. In dogs and monkeys, the most frequently observed toxic effects were related to the liver, gastrointestinal, lymphatic, and hematopoietic systems. The liver abnormalities seen at higher doses included elevated alkaline phosphatase, SGOT, SGPT, and bilirubin levels. Histologic alterations included cytoplasmic vacuolization, congestion, hemosideroris, and hemorrhage. Gastrointestinal toxicity was manifested by anorexia, emesis, and bloody diarrhea. There was congestion, hemorrhage, degeneration, and necrosis of intestinal mucous membranes. Lymphatic tissues showed hemorrhage, congestion, and necrosis.
Anemia and leukopenia were noted in peripheral blood and were dose-related. Thrombocytopenia, however, was not a prominent manifestation of toxicity in the dogs and monkeys. Dose-related, but reversible, hypoplastic effect was noted in the animals' bone marrow. Other side effects included local tissue reactions at injection sites. In the dog, reversible congestion and hemorrhage in the kidneys were noted with transient increases in BUN and serum creatinine levels accompanied by hematuria and proteinuria.

Clinical Studies

Method of Drug Administration

For clinical IV use, *m*-AMSA is formulated as two sterile liquids that are aseptically combined prior to use. Each 2-ml flint ampule contains 1.5 ml of a 50-mg/ml solution of *m*-AMSA in anhydrous *N,N*-dimethylacetamide. Each 20-ml amber vial contains 13.5 ml for 0.0353 *M* L-lactic acid. The flint ampule (1.5 ml) containing 75 mg of *m*-AMSA is added to the vial of L-lactic acid solution and the contents are mixed. The

Table 1. Phase I clinical trials with IV *m*-AMSA

Schedule	Dose (mg/m^2)			Reference
	Starting	Highest escalation	Maximum tolerated	
Solid tumors				
Weekly × 4	20	90	90	[19]
q 2 Weeks × 3	10	175	70[a]	[24]
q 3 Weeks	10	120	90[a]	[8]
q 4 Weeks	10	160	120[a]	[25]
Daily × 3 q 3 weeks	4	50	40	[15]
Acute leukemia				
Daily × 5	40	90	90	[8]
Daily × 5 q 2–3 weeks	–	150	150	[19]
Daily × 3–10 q 10–28 days	120	750[b]	–	[14]

[a] Dose for good-risk patients. Dosage reductions recommended if extensive prior chemotherapy or radiotherapy and/or hepatic dysfunction
[b] Total dose over 10 days

resulting orange-red solution contains 5 mg/ml of *m*-AMSA. Because of phlebitis occurring at a dose of ≥ 70 mg/m², it has been recommended that the drug be diluted in 200–500 ml of 5% dextrose in water and infused IV for 30–60 min [8, 25]. Of note, the drug precipitates in chloride-containing solutions.

A variety of schedules have been explored in phase I clinical trials (Table 1). The drug has been given IV on a weekly basis or as a single dose repeated every 2, 3, or 4 weeks. Divided daily administration for 3, 5, and 7–10 days has also been investigated especially for the treatment of acute leukemia [14, 22]. A maximally tolerated dosage has been defined in most of these studies (Table 1). Clinical investigations are also being actively pursued with oral *m*-AMSA [6].

Toxic Effects

Leukopenia has been the major dose-limiting toxicity in all phase I clinical trials with *m*-AMSA. Leukopenia has been dose-related, reproducible, and reversible with IV administration of the drug. Thrombocytopenia has generally been mild in patients treated for solid tumors, but may become significant in patients with bone marrow impairment [13].

Severe phlebitis can develop when doses of 70 mg/m² or more are infused without adequate dilution. The effect of drug extravasation has not yet been ascertained.

Nausea and vomiting have been infrequent with *m*-AMSA, even with the high doses used in acute leukemia. Drug-induced mucositis and alopecia have been occasionally encountered. Mild elevations in liver function tests have also been noted, but have always been reversible [8, 25]. Grand mal seizures have occurred in three acute leukemia patients and in one patient with breast cancer [13, 14]. It is not clear whether these seizures were drug-related. Headache and dizziness have also been experienced by some patients [13]. Finally, drug-related cardiac toxicity cannot be ruled out at this point.

Antitumor Activity

m-AMSA exhibited a broad range of antitumor activity in phase I studies, including responses in patients with ovarian cancer [25], Hodgkin's disease [8], chronic lymphocytic leukemia [8], desmoid fibrosarcoma [19], liposarcoma [24], adenocarcinoma, and squamous cell carcinoma of unknown primary [24].

Phase II trials with *m*-AMSA have recently been initiated. In one series of 26 evaluable patients with far-advanced breast cancer, four patients achieved partial remission for 3–11+ months [13]. Two of these remissions occurred in patients whose disease did not respond to first-line combination chemotherapy regimen that included adriamycin. Two partial responses were achieved in 30 evaluable patients with malignant melanoma previously treated with DTIC-containing regimens [10]. Finally, in a phase I–II study, three complete and one partial remission were reported in 22 evaluable leukemia patients [14]. Further studies are under way in all of the signal tumors.

Clinical Pharmacology

Limited clinical pharmacology studies have been reported for m-AMSA [6, 11, 18, 24, 25]. Utilizing ^{14}C-radiolabeled m-AMSA, Von Hoff and colleagues [25] reported pharmacokinetics in one patient who received 160 mg/m^2 of m-AMSA. Plasma radioactivity displayed an apparent biphasic decline with an early-phase half-life of 11 min and a second-phase half-life of 4.5 h.

Following the extraction of free m-AMSA [3], the plasma levels of parent drug were shown to decline biphasically with an early-phase half-life of 12 min and a second-phase half-life of 2.5 h. Plasma samples obtained at 22 h showed no detectable parent compound. Of the administered dose, 20% appeared in the urine within the first 8 h after the start of the infusion. By the end of the third day after the infusion, urinary radioactivity accounted for 42% of the administered dose.

Hall and co-workers [11] studied the pharmacokinetics in 19 patients. In five patients with normal hepatic and renal function, the mean terminal plasma half-life was 33.9 h for radiolabeled (^{14}C) and 7.4 h for unchanged m-AMSA. In patients with severe hepatic dysfunction, these figures increased to 68.7 h and 17.2 h, respectively. Using a high-pressure liquid-chromatographic assay, other investigators have also documented a prolonged terminal plasma half-life of m-AMSA with hepatic dysfunction [16]. The 72-h cumulative biliary excretion of ^{14}C was 8% and 36% in two patients with severe hepatic dysfunction [11]. The 72-h cumulative urinary excretion showed progressive increases with the severity of liver disease. In a patient with severe renal impairment, the terminal plasma half-life for m-AMSA was prolonged to 10.8 h [11]. Cerebrospinal fluid ^{14}C specific activities in three patients were below 2% of the concurrent plasma ^{14}C activities [11].

Overall, m-AMSA has a mean terminal half-life for the parent compound ranging from 2.5–7.4 h in patients with normal hepatic and renal function. Biliary excretion is an important route of elimination while urinary clearance is of lesser importance. In patients with liver disease, dosage reduction should be considered.

Discussion

m-AMSA is a new antitumor agent that is generating increasing interest. Drug-induced toxic manifestations are generally mild, predictable, and reversible. Much larger clinical experience is needed to assess properly the spectrum of its single-agent antitumor activity and its degree of cross-resistance with compounds commonly employed in current anticancer therapy. Numerous ongoing phase II studies should rapidly help elucidate the ultimate role of m-AMSA in the treatment of cancer.

References

1 Cain BF, Atwell GJ (1974) The experimental antitumour properties of three congeners of the acridylmethanesulphonanilide (AMSA) series. Eur J Cancer 10: 539–549
2 Corbett TH, Griswold DP Jr Roberts BJ, Peckham JC, Schabel FM Jr (1977) Evaluation of single agents and combinations of chemotherapeutic agents in mouse colon carcinomas. Cancer 40: 2660–2680

3 Cysyk RL, Shoemaker D, Adamson RH (1977) The pharmacologic disposition of 4′-(9-acridinylamino)methanesulfon-*m*-anisidide in mice and rats. Drug Metab Dispos 5: 579–590
4 Cysyk RL, Shoemaker D, Ayers OC, Adamson RH (1978) Oral absorption and selective tissue localization of 4′-(9-acridinylamino)-methanesulfon-*m*-anisidide. Pharmacology 16: 206–213
5 Deaven LL, Oka MS, Tobey RA (1978) Cell-cycle-specific chromosome damage following treatment of cultured Chinese hamster cells with 4′-[(9-acridinyl)-amino]methanesulphon-*m*-anisidide-HCl. J Natl Cancer Inst 60: 1155–1161
6 De Jager R, Body JJ, Dupont D, Klastersky J, Kenis Y (1979) Phase I study of oral 4′-(9-acridinylamino)methanesulfon-m-anisidide (*m*-AMSA, NSC 249992). Proc Am Assoc Cancer Res and Am Soc Clin Oncol 20: 429
7 Furlong NB, Sato J, Brown T, Chavez F, Hurlbert RB (1978) Induction of limited DNA damage by the antitumor agent Cain's acridine. Cancer Res 38: 1329–1335
8 Goldsmith MA, Bhardwaj S, Ohnuma T, Greenspan EM, Holland JF (1979) Phase I study of *m*-AMSA in patients with solid tumors and leukemias. Proc Am Assoc Cancer Res and Am Soc Clin Oncol 20: 344
9 Gormley PE, Sethi VS, Cysyk RL (1978) Interaction of 4′-(9-acridinylamino)methanesulfon-m-anisidide with DNA and inhibition of oncornavirus reverse transcriptase and cellular nucleic acid polymerases. Cancer Res 38: 1300–1306
10 Hall SW, Benjamin RS, Legha SS, Gutterman JU, Burgess MA, Bodey GP (1979) AMSA: A new acridine derivative with activity against metastatic melanoma. Proc Am Assoc Cancer Res and Am Soc Clin Oncol 20: 372
11 Hall SW, Benjamin RS, Legha SS, Gutterman JU, Loo TL (1979) Clinical pharmacokinetics of the new antitumor agent AMSA. Proc Am Assoc Cancer Res and Am Soc Clin Oncol 20: 175
12 Johnson RK, Chitnis MP, Goldin A (1976) Characteristics of resistance and cross-resistance in vivo of a subline of P388 leukemia resistant to adriamycin. Pharmacologist 18: 173
13 Legha SS, Blumenschein GR, Buzdar AU, Hortobagyi GN, Bodey GP (1979) Phase II study of 4′-(9-acridinylamino)methanesulfon-*m*-anisidide (AMSA) in metastatic breast cancer. Cancer Treat Rep 63: 1961–1964
14 Legha SS, Bodey GP, Keating MJ, Blumenschein GR, Hortobagyi GN, Buzdar AU, McCredie K, Freireich EJ (1979) Early clinical evaluation of acridinylamino-methanesulfon-*m*-anisidide (AMSA) in patients with advanced breast cancer and acute leukemia. Proc Am Assoc Cancer Res and Am Soc Clin Oncol 20: 416
15 Legha SS, Gutterman JU, Hall SW, Benjamin RS, Burgess MA, Valdivieso M, Bodey GP (1978) Phase I clinical investigation of 4′-(9-acridinylamino)methanesulfon-*m*-anisidide (NSC-249992), a new acridine derivative. Cancer Res 38: 3712–3716
16 Malspeis L, Khan MN, Blat HB (1979) HPLC determination of 4′-(9acridinyl-amino-methanesulfon)m-anisidide (m-AMSA; NSC 249992) in the plasma of a patient with hepatic dysfunction. Proc Am Assoc Cancer Res and Am Soc Clin Oncol 20: 384
17 Mellanby E (1933) Report on work carried out in the pharmacological laboratory, Sheffield University. British Empire Cancer Campaign 10th Annual Report, pp 102–103
18 Osieka, R, Houchens DP, Goldin A, Johnson RK (1977) Chemotherapy of human colon cancer xenografts in athymic nude mice. Cancer 40: 2640–2650
19 Schneider R, Sklaroff R, Ochoa M Jr, Young C (1979) Phase I trial of AMSA [4′-(9-acridinylamino)-methanesulfon-m-anisidide]. Proc Am Assoc Cancer Res and Am Soc Clin Oncol 20: 114
20 Shoemaker D, Ayer O, D'Anna M, Cysyk R (1979) Effect of diethyl maleate and phenobarbital on the metabolism and biliary excretion of 4′-(9-acridinylamino)-methanesulfon-m-anisidide (m-AMSA; NSC-141549) in rats. Proc Am Assoc Cancer Res and Am Soc Clin Oncol 20: 280
21 Shoemaker DD, Legha SS, Cysyk RL (1978) Selective localization of 4′-(9-acridinylamino)methanesulfon-m-anisidide in B16 melanoma. Pharmacology 16: 221–225

22 Tan C, Haghbin M, Rosen G, Miller DR (1979) Acridinylamino anisidide (AMSA) in children with advanced cancer. Proc Am Assoc Cancer Res and Am Soc Clin Oncol 20: 154
23 Tobey RA, Deaven LL, Oka MS (1978) Kinetic response of cultured Chinese hamster cells to treatment with 4′-[(9-acridinyl)amino]methanesulphon-*m*-anisidide-HCl. J Natl Cancer Inst 60: 1147–1153
24 Van Echo DA, Gormley P, Lichtenfeld JL, Scoltock M, Wiernik PH (1979) A phase I study of m-AMSA. Proc Am Assoc Cancer Res and Am Soc Clin Oncol 20: 422
25 Von Hoff DD, Howser D, Gormley P, Bender RA, Glaubiger D, Levine AS, Young RC (1978) Phase I study of methanesulfonamide, *N*-[4-(9-acridinylamino)-3-methoxyphenyl]-(*m*-AMSA) using a single-dose schedule. Cancer Treat Rep 62: 1421–1426
26 Waring MJ (1976) DNA-binding characteristics of acridinylmethanesulphonanilide drugs: Comparison with antitumour properties. Eur J Cancer 12: 995–1001
27 Wilson WR (1973) Studies on mechanism of action of an experimental antitumor drug. Chem NZ 37: 148–152

The Rediscovery of DON (6-Diazo-5-oxo-L-norleucine)

D. L. Kisner, R. Catane, and F. M. Muggia

Summary

DON (6-diazo-5-oxo-L-norleucine) and azotomycin are glutamine antagonists that were tested in human malignancies in the 1950s. Azotomycin demonstrated significant activity in colorectal cancer. DON is probably the active form of azotomycin. Recent impressive results for both of these agents in human tumor xenografts (especially the CX-2 colon tumor) have stimulated renewed clinical interest in DON, the more readily available agent. DON mechanism of action, clinical pharmacology, previous clinical data, and current phase I studies are discussed.

Introduction

The compound 6-diazo-5-oxo-L-norleucine (DON) is an antibiotic that was isolated from a *Streptomyces* in 1953. It is a diazo analogue of L-glutamine and interferes in several reactions present in the synthesis of nucleic acids and proteins in which L-glutamine participates as a nitrogen source [5]. DON demonstrated antitumor activity against choriocarcinoma [4] in trials performed in the late 1950s. A second glutamine antagonist, azotomycin, showed considerable activity against human colorectal carcinoma [15]. Azotomycin, a polymer of two molecules of DON and one glutamic acid residue, is converted in vivo to its active form, which is DON [10]. Because of this fact and the recent demonstration of significant activity in tumor xenografts in nude mice [5, 9], there has been renewed interest in further clinical trials with DON. DON has been selected for further development because it is more readily available than azotomycin. This paper briefly reviews the biochemical actions of DON, its clinical pharmacology, past clinical studies of DON (and azotomycin where appropriate), the recent data dealing with human xenograft tumors, and currently ongoing phase I trials.

Biochemical Actions

L-Glutamine donates its amide nitrogen in at least 12 biologically significant pathways [11]. DON is chemically closely related to L-glutamine (Fig. 1) and interferes with a variety of transamidation reactions using L-glutamine as a substrate [5].

DON

6-diazo-5-oxo-L-norleucine

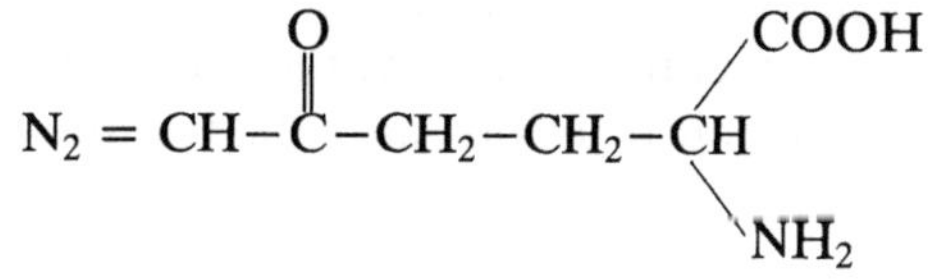

L-Glutamine

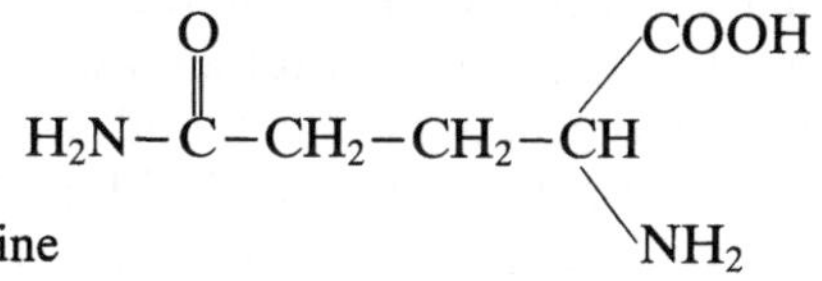

Fig. 1. Clinical structures of DON and L-glutamine

Purine Synthesis. DON inhibits all de novo purine synthesis early in the pathway chiefly by retarding synthesis of 2-*N*-formylglycinamidine ribotide (FGAM) from 2-*N*-formylglycinamide ribotide (FGAR) [8]. This is apparently accomplished by DON competition with L-glutamine for FGAR amidotransferase. The result is reduced synthesis of inosinic acid for incorporation into adenosine monophosphate (AMP) and guanosine monophosphate (GMP).

Pyrimidine Synthesis. DON has been demonstrated to inhibit the enzyme system responsible for conversion of uridine triphosphate (UTP) to cytosine triphosphate (CTP). However, this occurs only at concentrations of DON at least ten times those necessary to inhibit completely de novo synthesis of purine nucleotides [7]. This makes the inhibition of UTP $\rightarrow$ CTP less likely to be the principal cytotoxic lesion of DON.

Additionally, DON has been shown to inhibit glutamine-dependent carbamyl phosphate synthetase found in several malignant cell lines [5]. Carbamyl phosphate is an initial substrate in the orotic acid pathway in pyrimidine synthesis. The overall importance of this action of DON is unsettled.

Protein Synthesis. More recently, the importance of DON inhibition of L-asparagine synthetase has been emphasized [5, 12]. This enzyme catalyzes the reaction L-aspartic acid + L-glutamine (or NH_3) $\rightarrow$ L-asparagine + L-glutamic acid. Tumor cells deficient in this enzyme are sensitive to the effects of L-asparaginase. DON has been found in vitro competitively to inhibit glutamine utilization by asparaginase synthetase in Gardner lymphosarcoma cells [5], and from the L-asparaginase-resistant leukemia L5178/AR [12] as well as other cell lines. Potent inhibition of L-asparagine synthetase in vivo in L5178Y/AR cells in male BDF mice was also demonstrated [12]. In a subsequent publication, COONEY et al. [2] demonstrated that DON was not synergistic with L-asparaginase in leukemia L1210 in mice, despite the theoretical advantage in cellular deprivation of asparagine. They also demonstrated that DON shares a membrane transport system for cellular uptake with L-asparagine, L-glutamine, and two other glutamine antagonists in L5178Y/AR cells. Additionally, the increased

antitumor activity of DON over that of other glutamine antagonists tested appeared to be related to increased intracellular tumor concentrations of the drug in vivo.
In summary, the inhibition of de novo purine biosynthesis and the inhibition of L-asparagine synthetase are felt to be significant actions of DON. The inhibition of carbamyl phosphate synthetase is of unclear importance. The question of the critical biochemical lesion must be regarded as unsettled.

Clinical Pharmacology

MAGILL et al. reported the clinical pharmacology of DON in man [6]. DON is rapidly removed from plasma. After an intravenous (IV) dose of 0.2–0.3 mg/kg, peak serum levels are reached in the blood within 5–15 min. Levels rapidly decrease with complete disappearance in 8–24 h, depending on the dose given. Intramuscular absorption is delayed with peak levels $^1/_2$–1 h after injection. Oral administration of 0.4–2.5 mg/kg results in good absorption, but with delayed peak levels from 15 min to 2 h. Less than 1% of DON is excreted in the urine in the active form within 24 h of administration.
In this trial [6], most patients received the drug in an oral or IV daily schedule. Clinical toxicity included mucositis, diarrhea, nausea and vomiting, and bone marrow suppression.

Past Clinical Data

DON received limited clinical testing in the late 1950s, almost entirely in a daily dose schedule orally or parenterally at 0.2–1.1 mg/kg/day [4, 6, 13]. The single-agent activity of DON is demonstrated in Table 1. No significant activity was noted except in

Table 1. Single-agent activity of DON

Disease	Number of responders/ number of evaluable patients	Reference
Breast adenocarcinoma	2/14	[6]
Lung carcinoma	2/9	[6]
	0/18	[13]
Gastric and colon carcinoma	1/6	[6]
Melanoma	0/4	[6]
	0/5	[13]
Lymphoma	1/4	[6]
	0/7	[13]
Leukemia	0/1	[6]
Hodgkin's disease	2/11	[13]
Choriocarcinoma	3/4	[4]
Miscellaneous tumors	1/9	[6]

choriocarcinoma [4]. It is of interest that the one patient responding with gastric/colon was a patient with colorectal carcinoma [6].
Table 2 demonstrates clinical results with azotomycin as a single agent suggesting promising results in colon cancer, sarcomas, and melanoma. In 1970, WEISS and MASTRANGELO [14] reported reponses in 10 of 22 patients with advanced colorectal cancer receiving combination therapy with azotomycin + 5-fluorouracil. Subsequent to that trial, the reduced availability and expense of azotomycin essentially discontinued its development.

Table 2. Single-agent activity of azotomycin

Disease	Number of responders/ number of evaluable patients	Reference
Colorectal carcinoma	11/64	[15]
	0/2	[3]
Sarcoma	4/14	[15]
	0/1	[3]
Lung cancer	2/21	[15]
	0/2	[3]
Melanoma	3/21	[15]
	0/1	[3]
Lymphoma	2/7	[15]
Breast carcinoma	1/15	[15]
Head and neck squamous cell carcinoma	1/21	[15]
	0/1	[3]
Miscellaneous solid tumors	1/32	[4]
	0/2	[3]

Table 3. Drug activity against human tumor xenografts[a]

Drug	Activity[b]			
	Lung (LX-1)	Colon (CX-2)	Colon (CX-1)	Breast (MX-1)
DON	++	++	−	++
Azotomycin	++	+	−	++
Methotrexate		−		+
6-Mercaptopurine	−		−	−
5-Fluorouracil		+	−	+
Cyclophosphamide	−	+		++
Adriamycin	−			
BCNU		−		+

[a] Modified from OVEJERA et al. [9] and CATANE et al. [1]
[b] Activity: +, retards tumor growth; ++, elicits tumor regression; −, not active

Studies with Human Tumor Xenografts

Because azotomycin has shown significant activity against human colorectal cancer [14, 15], and DON may be the active form of azotomycin [10], the two drugs were compared in a panel of human tumor xenografts, along with several other standard chemotherapeutic agents [1, 9]. Human tumor lines used for testing included two colon adenocarcinomas (CX-1 and CX-2), a small cell lung cancer (LX-1), and a premenopausal breast cancer (MX-1). Table 3 displays the results of these studies. Both DON and azotomycin produced tumor regressions in the LX-1 lung tumor, but DON was more active than azotomycin in the CX-2 colon tumors. DON, azotomycin, and cyclophosphamide were active in the breast tumor.

Conclusion

The encouraging early clinical results in colorectal cancer with azotomycin coupled with the superior activity of DON in the CX-2 colon xenograft tumor strongly suggest the need for additional clinical trials with DON. This drug has not been sufficiently tested in virtually any of the tumors in the Division of Cancer Treatment Clinical panel.

Negative early results with DON might have been related to the daily dose schedule, since this drug has shown marked schedule dependency in animals [2]. With this in mind, two new phase I studies have been initiated to systematically determine toxicity and maximum tolerated dose for DON in intermittent schedules. Memorial Sloan-Kettering Cancer Center is performing a trial using a biweekly IV bolus regimen beginning at 100 mg/m^2. The Mayo Clinic is initiating a trial utilizing an every-three-week regimen by IV bolus starting at 150 mg/m^2. At present, no phase I study is exploring the use of a prolonged infusion with DON. In light of the drug's short serum half-life, a longer infusion time might alter efficacy and toxicity. It is anticipated that DON will be ready for phase II testing in an intermittent schedule before the end of 1979. Emphasis will be placed initially on colorectal cancer.

References

1 Catane R, Ovejera AA, Houchens DP, Von Hoff DD, Davis HL Jr, Wolpert MK, Rozencweig M, Muggia FM (1978) Rationale for further clinical trials with 6-diazo-5-oxo-L-norleucine (DON) (abstr). Proc Am Assoc Cancer Res and Am Soc Clin Oncol 19:317

2 Cooney DA, Jayaram HN, Milman HA, Homan ER, Pittillo R, Geran RI, Ryan J, Rosenbluth RJ (1976) DON, CONV and DONV-III, pharmacologic and toxicologic studies. Biochem Pharmacol 25:1859–1870

3 Hill GJ, Larsen RR, Sas EM (1973) Cancer chemotherapy II. Results of 603 courses of therapy in 400 consecutive patients followed for 18–52 months. Oncology 27:137–152

4 Li MC (1961) Management of chariocarcinoma and related tumors of the uterus and testis. Med Clin North Am 45:661–676

5 Livingston RB, Vendetti JM, Cooney DA, Carter SK (1970) Glutamine antagonists in chemotherapy, vol 8. Academic, New York, pp 62–83

6 Magill GB, Myers WPL, Reilly HC, Putnam RC, Magill JW, Sykes MP, Escher GC, Karnofsky GC, Burchenal JH (1957) Pharmacological and initial therapeutic observations on 6-diazo-5-oxo-L-norleucine (DON) in human neoplastic disease. Cancer 10: 1138–1150
7 Moore E, Hulbert R (1961) Biosynthesis of RNA cytosine and RNA purines; differential inhibition by 6-diazo-5-oxo-L-norleucine. Cancer Res 21: 257–261
8 Moore EC, LePage GA (1957) In vivo sensitivity of normal and neoplastic mouse tissues to azaserine. Cancer Res 17: 804–808
9 Ovejera AA, Houchens DP, Barker AD (1977) Chemotherapeutic sensitivity to anticancer agents of human tumor xenografts in athymic mice. Current Chemotherapy: Proc. 10th International Congress on Chemotherapy 2: 1144–1146
10 Pittillo RF, Wooley C, Brockman RW, Ho DH (1971) Azotomycin (NSC-1566454): Biologic fate in mice and man. Cancer Chemother Rep 55: 47–52
11 Prusiner S, Stadtman ER (eds) (1973) The enzymes of glutamine metabolism. Academic, New York
12 Rosenbluth RJ, Cooney DA, Jayaram HN, Milman HA, Homan ER (1976) DON, CONV, and DONV.-II, inhibition of L-asparaginase synthetase in vivo. Biochem Pharmacol 25: 1851–1858
13 Veterans Administration Cancer Chemotherapy Study Group (1959) A clinical study of the comparative effect of nitrogen mustard and DON in patients with bronchogenic carcinoma, Hodgkin's disease, lymphosarcoma and melanoma. J Natl Cancer Inst 22: 433–439
14 Weiss AJ, Mastrangelo MJ (1970) Phase I study of a combination of azotomycin + 5-FU in malignant disease. Cancer Chemother Rep 54: 109–111
15 Weiss AJ, Ramirez G, Grage T, Strawitz J, Goldman L, Downing V (1968) Phase II study of azotomycin. Cancer Chemother Rep 52: 611–614

The Use of Peritoneal Dialysis for Delivery of Chemotherapy to Intraperitoneal Malignancies

J. L. Speyer and C. E. Myers

Summary

We have utilized peritoneal dialysis via semipermanent Tenckhoff catheters to administer methotrexate and 5-fluorouracil to 16 patients with cancer whose tumor was confined to the intraabdominal space. The method of dialysis is described. The therapy was well tolerated by the patients. The major risks were bacterial peritonitis, local drug-induced peritonitis, and the systemic effects of the drugs. Theoretic modeling predicted that far greater concentrations of drug can be safely delivered by this route with less toxicity than when lower concentrations are administered by conventional routes. Furthermore, much higher concentrations should be achieved in the dialysate to which the tumor is exposed than in the systemic plasma. These predictions were confirmed.

A significant problem in the treatment of many tumors is assuring that an adequate amount of drug is delivered to the malignant tissue in question. Unfortunately, all too often one cannot simply alter the dosage or schedule of a drug to achieve higher concentrations in the tumor, because of limiting systemic toxicity that develops. This is particularly a problem when tumors are located in areas such as the central nervous system or peritoneum, where peak drug concentrations achieved with intravenous (IV) or oral (PO) administration are frequently much lower than that found in the systemic plasma. In the case of the central nervous system, clinicians have turned to local modalities such as radiotherapy or intrathecal drug administration. In the case of ovarian cancer, tumor even in advanced disease (stage III) is usually confined to the intraperitoneal (IP) space with diffuse studding of the peritoneum and omentum (Fig. 1). This intraabdominal extension is in fact the most frequent cause of death in these patients, through gastrointestinal involvement and inanition.

Ovarian cancer and similar tumors such as gastric, colon, and endometrial cancer, because of the tendency to stay localized within the abdominal cavity, would seem amenable to direct local instillation of drugs into the peritoneal cavity, thereby facilitating high drug concentrations at the actual tumor location. Moreover, theoretic arguments developed by Dedrick et al. [1] and data on the uptake of substances from peritoneal fluid in rats reported by Torres et al. [5] and Jones et al. [3] predict that if many cancer drugs are placed directly into the intraperitoneal space, they will be cleared less rapidly from the peritoneal space than from the systemic circulation. This differential clearance establishes a concentration difference between the intraperitoneal space and the systemic circulation, with intraperitoneal tumor being exposed to high drug concentrations and the target organs such as marrow and gastrointestinal

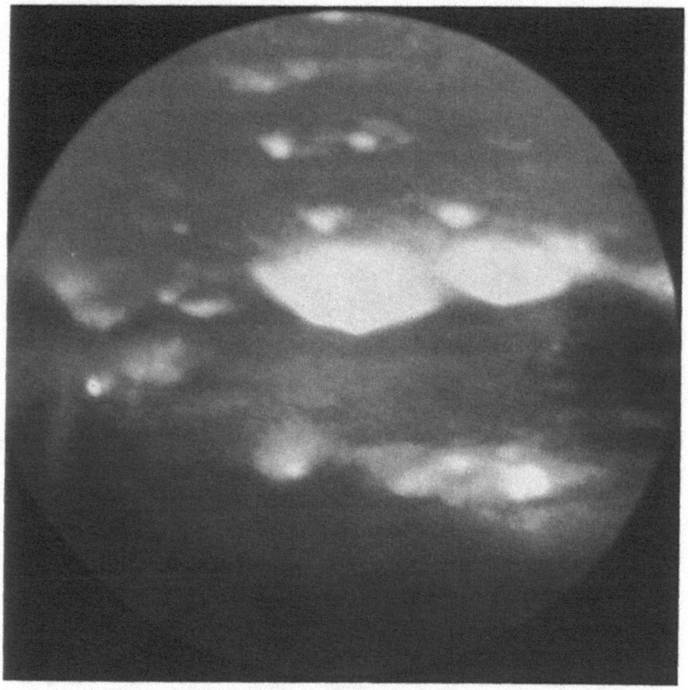

Fig. 1. Metastatic nodules of ovarian cancer on the inner surface of the peritoneum as viewed through the peritoneoscope. Nodules are 1–2 cm across

epithelium being exposed to lower drug concentrations. DEDRICK et al. did point out that such therapy could only be effective in sensitive tumors where there was a dose-response relationship and that its value could be maximized by (a) treating small tumor volumes in order to permit good drug penetration, (b) instilling the drugs in large volumes of fluid to facilitate good distribution and maximal exposure of intraabdominal tumor, and (c) administering drugs in the absence of other substances which might reduce their renal or hepatic clearance.

We have attempted to follow these guidelines in humans with ovarian and colon cancer. We administered drug in large volumes of fluid via peritoneal dialysis to patients with disease confined to the abdomen. To facilitate repeated dialysis, a semipermanent Tenckhoff catheter (a flexible silastic tube with fenestrations at one end) was placed through the abdominal wall via a subcutaneous tunnel with a single Dacron cuff around it to decrease the possibility of leakage or contamination (Fig. 2).

The patients were taught by the nursing staff to don mask and gloves and, with sterile technique, clean the catheter with Betadine and apply fresh sterile gauze pads once a day. After the initial healing of a small surgical scar, the catheter did not interfere with daily functions, including exercise, work, or bathing.

The dialysis fluid consisted of 2 l of a commercially prepared peritoneal dialysate of 1.5% dextrose in a balanced salt solution (Inpersol, Abbot Labs, North Chicago, Illinois) to which was added 1000 units of heparin and 8 meq of KCl as well as the chemotherapeutic agent. The pH of this dialysate is 4.5. At this pH some drugs may either be insoluble or unstable. We have found that sodium bicarbonate may be added

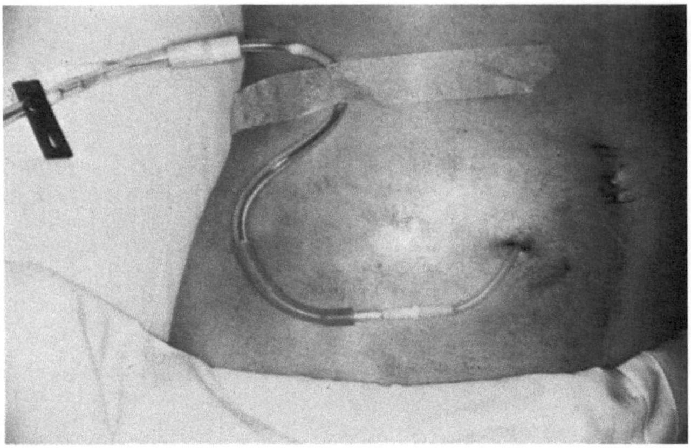

Fig. 2. Patient with ovarian cancer in whom the Tenckhoff catheter attached to a dialysis set is placed to the right of a midline abdominal incision

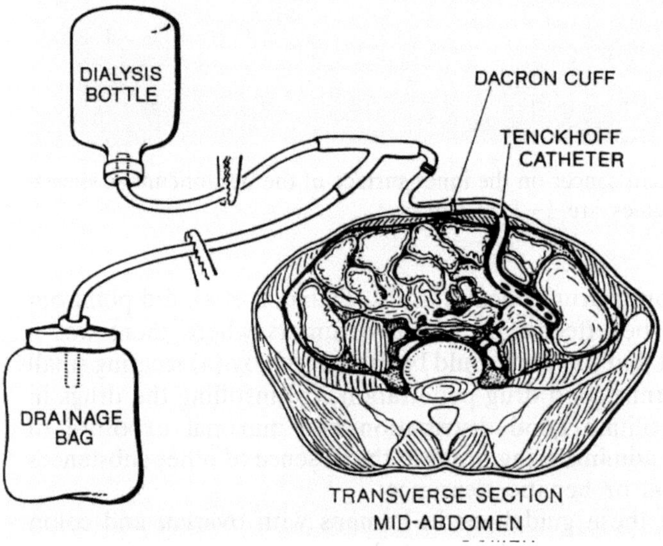

Fig. 3. The Tenckhoff catheter is placed into the peritoneal cavity through a subcutaneous skin tunnel. The external end of the catheter is connected to a Y tube, connecting both the dialysis bottle and drainage bag in a closed system. Dialysate bottles are changed at the distal end of the Y tube and fluid is removed from the drainage bag through a drain in the bottom. The Y-tube catheter connection is broken only at the beginning and end of the course of treatment

to raise the pH to as high as 8.0 without causing localized chemical irritation. When 5-fluorouracil (5-FU) was used, 50 meq of sodium bicarbonate was added to increase the drug solubility. Methotrexate in concentrations from 0.01–0.07 m*M* or 5-FU in concentrations from 0.005–5 m*M* was added to the dialysate. Even with 2 l of dialysis fluid in the abdomen, most patients are able to ambulate, although they all experience a feeling of fullness and sometimes generalized mild abdominal discomfort. Occasionally, the instillation of fluid can put painful temporary pressure on surgical adhesions.

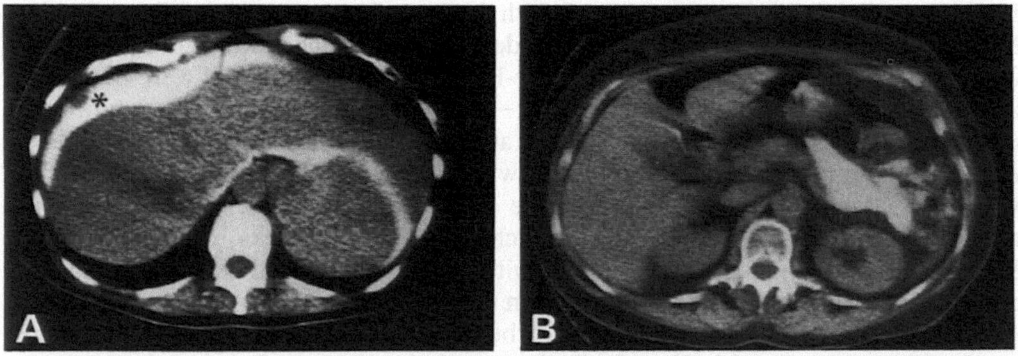

Fig. 4A, B. Contrast CAT scans of the abdomen. In *panel a*, contrast dialysate is seen flowing up and over the liver as well as in the left and mid-abdomen. Peritoneal metastases (*) are visualized as negative images. In *panel b*, contrast material is seen only in the mid and left abdomen. There is poor distribution of fluid over the liver in the *right upper quadrant*

To lessen the risk of infection, dialysate was administered with a closed system. The 2-l bottle and a plastic bag for collecting drainage were connected to the external end of the catheter via a Y tube with clamps on the inlet and outlet. In this way the system was only "broken" at the initial connection of the Y tube and for the connection of fresh bottles of dialysate (Fig. 3).

Dialysate may be administered either as a continuous series of exchanges, each with a dwell time from 1–6 h, or as a series of daily instillations of dialysate where the fluid is not drained. We have found that over 24 h most patients will absorb 2 l of fluid and not require drainage before the next instillation. The flexibility of this system is to allow the physician to tailor the dialysate procedure to the specific pharmacologic properties of a range of chemotherapeutic agents. The capacity for frequent dialysate exchanges facilitates the maintainance of high intraperitoneal drug levels.

Patients treated by this modality are likely to have adhesions secondary to previous abdominal surgery in addition to intraperitoneal tumor. This can lead to difficulty with proper catheter placement and/or fluid distribution. To evaluate this, we developed a modification of the conventional computerized axial tomography (CAT) scan technique. Proper distribution of dialysate within the abdomen is determined by adding Hypaque dye (Winthrop Labs, New York, New York) (150 cm^3 of a 25% solution to 2 l of dialysate not containing drug) and performing a CAT scan of the abdomen [2]. This has the added advantage of helping to noninvasively visualize peritoneal metastases which might otherwise be difficult to visualize or follow (Fig. 4).

The actual dialysis was well tolerated by the patients. As noted, there is often fullness and mild but tolerable discomfort. The major risk of the dialysis procedure alone is bacterial peritonitis. We have had three episodes of bacterial peritonitis in 19 patients treated. In two of these cases the catheter ceased functioning and required replacement. All three patients were treated successfully with IV and IP antibiotics. One additional patient developed a subcutaneous infection along the catheter track that did not seed the peritoneum but which did require replacement of the catheter. Although this complication of dialysis therapy is related to the number of times the catheter integrity is violated, its incidence can be reduced by careful attention to sterile technique when handling and dressing the catheter.

Phase I studies have been conducted with both methotrexate and 5-fluorouracil. Methotrexate testing was limited by the development of chemical peritonitis at a 0.07-m*M* dialysate concentration. The dose-limiting toxicities of 5-FU were the same as when the drug is given by other routes – nausea, vomiting, mucositis, and bone marrow suppression – which were reached at a dialysate concentration of 5 m*M*. The details of these trials will be presented elsewhere. In our current trials with IP 5-FU, we are treating patients with a dialysate concentration of 4 m*M* 5-FU. This is administered for eight consecutive 4-h exchanges every 2 weeks.

We have currently treated seven patients with ovarian cancer and eight patients with colon cancer with IP 5-FU. There have been two responses in the ovarian group. One was a partial response in a patient with bulky disease who had previously failed combination therapy with HexaCAF (hexamethylmelamine, Cytoxan (cyclophosphamide), methotrexate, and IV 5-FU) [6] and single-agent cis-diamminodichloroplatinum. She had a greater than 50% shrinkage of a pelvic mass for 2 months. The second patient had a complete remission. She had previously received L-phenylalanine mustard and abdominal radiation. At repeat laparotomy, after therapy, all previously noted tiny peritoneal nodules were completely gone. Four of the patients with colon cancer metastatic to liver are currently evaluable and all have progressed on IP 5-FU therapy. There were no responses in the five patients treated with methotrexate.

Our work in this form of cancer treatment has as its theoretic basis the pharmacokinetic analysis reported by Dedrick et al. [1]. We have now studied methotrexate and 5-FU levels in plasma and peritoneal fluid to determine the pharmacokinetics of the drug when given to patients by this route. We are now in a position to evaluate the validity of the earlier predicitions of a concentration difference between the peritoneal fluid and plasma. The measurements do confirm the suggestion of Dedrick et al. that peritoneal clearance will be substantially slower than total body clearance. This was adequately borne out for both drugs, as noted in Table 1. As predicted by the model, this difference in clearance rates was translated into a difference in drug concentration between peritoneal fluid and plasma (Table 1). Peritoneal clearance for humans was predicted from measurements of methotrexate and 5-FU absorption in rats [3], with the assumption that effective peritoneal surface area was proportional to body surface area.

Table 1. Differential clearances with intraperitoneal chemotherapy

	Peritoneal clearance[a] (ml/min)		Total body clearance[b] (ml/min)		Peritoneal fluid concentration/ plasma concentration
	Predicted	Measured	Predicted	Measured	
Methotrexate [4]	8	5	180	135	23
5-Flourouracil	14	14	3,000–6,000	2,000–6,000	298

[a] Peritoneal clearance is measured as the permeability-product; predictions are based upon clinical studies of similar-sized molecules in humans and confirmed by preliminary studies in the rat, where percent uptake data was scaled up to man [1]

[b] Total body clearance predictions are based upon literature values for human continuous infusion data

Additional preliminary studies indicate that portal vein concentrations achieved by this route of administration are several times systemic plasma levels, indicating that not only the peritoneal space but the liver parenchyma are exposed to higher than normal drug levels. Presumably due to hepatic metabolism, these higher levels are not observed in the hepatic vein or peripheral blood (J. L. Speyer et al., unpublished work).

At this time, the measurement of systemic levels of 5-FU does not clearly correlate with clinical toxicity. Further investigations in our laboratory are pursuing the relationship between 5-FU metabolites and clinical toxicity.

In summary, intraperitoneal administration via peritoneal dialysis is a feasible and interesting route for delivering chemotherapy to patients in whom tumor is confined to the intraabdominal space. Most patients tolerate the procedure well. Its major risks are chemical and bacterial peritonitis and the systemic effects of the drug. While we have seen responses in patients with ovarian cancer who have failed systemic chemotherapy, far too few patients have been treated for us to assess the clinical utility of this form of therapy. For this reason, it should be clearly stated that at this point, although preliminary results are interesting, it is too early to assign an improved therapeutic efficacy to this route of administering chemotherapy. The pharmacologic confirmation of a predicted improved concentration ratio between peritoneal fluid and systemic plasma does, however, make it attractive to pursue further clinical trials in patients with localized malignancies.

Acknowledgments. Other investigators without whom this work would not have been possible are Drs. Murray Brennan and Paul Sugarbaker of the Surgery Branch of the National Cancer Institute, Dr. Vincent DeVita, Director of the Division of Cancer Treatment of the National Cancer Institute, Drs. Jerry Collins and Robert Dedrick of the Division of Research Services of the National Institutes of Health, and Dr. N. Reed Dunnick of the Department of Diagnostic Radiology of the Clinical Center of the National Institutes of Health.

References

1 Dedrick RL, Myers CE, Bungay PM, DeVita VT (1978) Pharmacokinetic rationale for peritoneal drug administration. Cancer Treat Rep 62: 1–13
2 Dunnick NR, Jones RB, Doppman JL, Speyer JL, Myers CE (1979) Intraperitoneal contrast infusion for assessment of intraperitoneal metastases and fluid dynamics. Am J Roentgenol 133: 221–223
3 Jones RB, Myers CE, Guarino AM, Dedrick RL, Hubbard SM, DeVita VT (1978) High volume intraperitoneal chemotherapy ("belly bath") for ovarian cancer. Cancer Chemother Pharmacol 1: 161–166
4 Myers C, Jones E, Londer H, Hubbard S, Brennan M, Balow J, Dedrick R, Ozols R, DeVita VT Jr (1978) Pharmacology of high-dose methotrexate (MTX) administered via peritoneal dialysis. Proc Am Soc Clin Oncol 19: 390
5 Torres IJ, Litterst CL, Guarino AM (1978) Transport of model compounds across the peritoneal membrane in the rat. Pharmacology 17: 330–340
6 Young RC, Chabner BA, Hubbard SP (1978) Advanced ovarian adenocarcinoma. A prospective clinical trial of melphalan (L-PAM) versus combination chemotherapy. N Engl J Med 299: 1261–1266

The Development of Mesna for the Inhibition of Urotoxic Side Effects of Cyclophosphamide, Ifosfamide, and Other Oxazaphosphorine Cytostatics

N. Brock

Summary

Urotoxic side effects on the kidneys and urinary bladder are a limiting factor in chemotherapy with oxazaphosphorine cytostatics such as cyclophosphamide and ifosfamide. Acrolein was found to be the causative factor which is spontaneously formed in the urine from the primary metabolites eliminated via the kidneys. Sodium 2-mercaptoethanesulfonate (INN: mesna) enables regional detoxification of acrolein in the kidneys and deferent urinary tract. The author reports on the pharmacotherapeutic bases and the mechanism of action of this new combination therapy and its clinical results. The untoward urotoxic side effects can be avoided with mesna without interfering with the chemotherapeutic effect on the tumor.

Introduction

During the 12th International Cancer Congress held in Buenos Aires in 1978, the problem of side effects of cytostatics was the focus of interest. Numerous authors reported results obtained in studies aimed at decreasing the organotoxic effects of some important agents, such as the cardiotoxic effects of doxorubicin, induction of pulmonary fibrosis by bleomycin, and the urotoxic action of the oxazaphosphorines cyclophosphamide and ifosfamide.

The urotoxic side effects of oxazaphosphorines, especially hemorrhagic cystitis, are due to the renal elimination of aggressive metabolites, and their intensity depends on the concentration in the urine. For clinical prevention of these urotoxic effects, various measures have been recommended, e.g., extensive supply of fluids, diuretics, alkalinization of the urine, and, for topical treatment, the instillation of mercapto compounds into the bladder. However, the efficacy and practicability of this standard preventive method are not at all satisfactory. Even the systemic use of mercapto compounds such as *N*-acetylcysteine did not yield a clinical benefit, since not only the drug's urotoxicity, but also its antitumor potency, was reduced. Thus we aimed at developing a uroprotective agent which would enable regional detoxification and thus add to solving the problem of urotoxicity of the oxazaphosphorines [1–6].

Materials and Methods

For the analysis of the potency of an uroprotective drug, it was necessary to develop an experimental model for urotoxicity which enables rapid and safe assessment of the agents under test.

Table 1. Criteria for assessment

% Increase in weight of the moist bladder and/or extractable trypan blue	Macroscopic assessment	Score
Control animals	Normal	0
< 30	Slight swelling, slight blue staining	1
$> 30 - < 60$	Moderate swelling, moderate staining	2
> 60	Intense swelling, intense staining	3

Rats of strain BD II proved to be particularly suited for this purpose, since they show inflammatory signs in bladder and kidneys as early as within 24 h following intravenous (IV) injection of cyclophosphamide. Criteria for urotoxicity are the macroscopic signs of inflammation: swelling, hemorrhages, and increased capillary permeability.
For accurate assessment of urotoxicity, the individual parameters were quantitatively determined, the increase in weight of the moist bladder being the criterion for swelling, and the blue coloration of the bladder due to IV trypan blue injection that for capillary permeability. The extravasal amount of stain was determined semiquantitatively by photometry.
These two parameters of inflammation (weight of moist bladder and extractable trypan blue) are closely related to each other. They enable a graded macroscopic assessment in terms of scores and thus readily reproducible results in a large series of tests (Table 1).
In the systemic tests for urotoxicity, all compounds were tested in rising doses by the IV and intraperitoneal (IP) routes. The animals were killed 24 h after administration of the agents under test, 21.5 mg/kg of trypan blue being given by IV injection 0.5 h before the animals were killed. The dose-action regression line enables the evaluation of the lowest definitely urotoxic dose (ED_{95}), which was found to correspond to score 1.5 ($D_{1.5}$).
In the intravesical test, rising concentrations of the compounds were given to female rats by means of a PVC catheter under pentobarbital anesthesia. Subsequently, the urethra was compressed by means of a fine clamp, the test solution being left to act in the bladder for 1 h. Then the bladder was repeatedly washed with normal saline. After 24 h, the animals were killed, trypan blue being given 0.5 h before. The dose-action regression lines enable the assessment of the definitely urotoxic concentration which was found to correspond to score 1.5 ($C_{1.5}$).

Results

Experimental Induction of Hemorrhagic Cystitis in the Rat by Systemic Administration

Out of the great number of alkylating agents studied, only relatively few exerted a urotoxic effect on systemic administration. These compounds (including cyclophosphamide and ifosfamide), summarized in Table 2, have one characteristic feature in common – the oxazaphosphorine ring, which is hydroxylated at the 4-position and spontaneously converted into directly alkylating phosphoric acid diamides and

Table 2. Compounds exerting urotoxic effects by systemic administration (ILVL) in rats. $D_{1.5}$: definitely phlogogenic dose

Compound	Structural formula	$D_{1.5}$ (mg/kg)
Cyclophosphamide	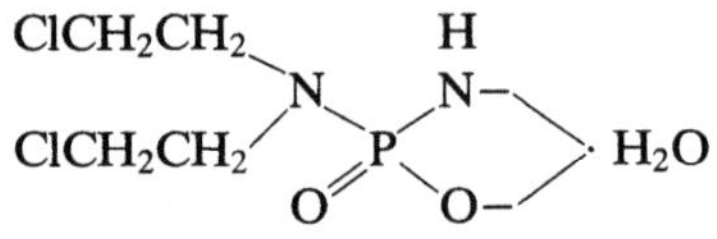	40.0
Ifosfamide	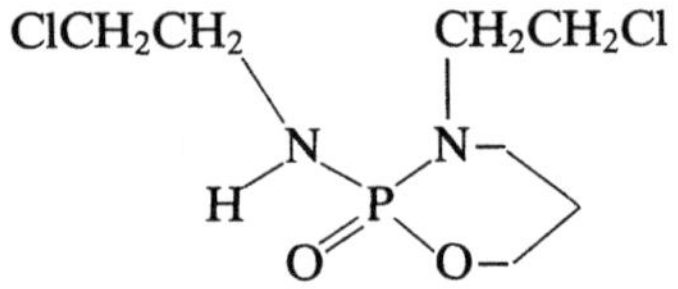	46.4
Trofosfamide	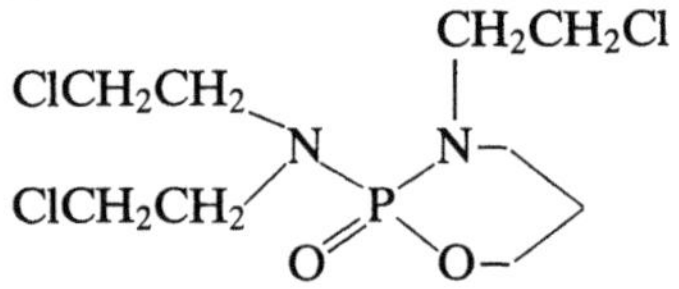	51.1
Sufosfamide	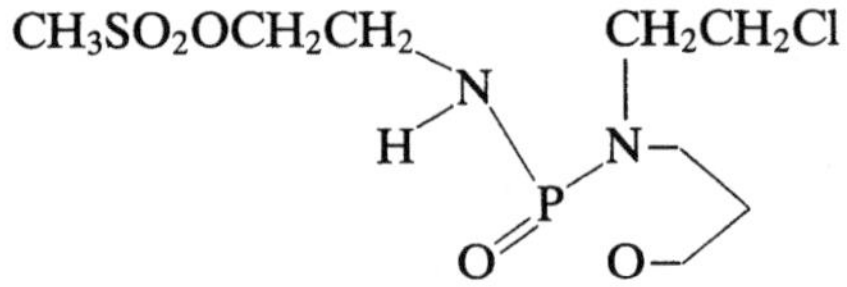	68.1
ASTA B-516	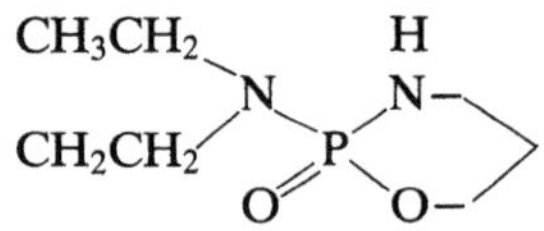	100
ASTA B-707	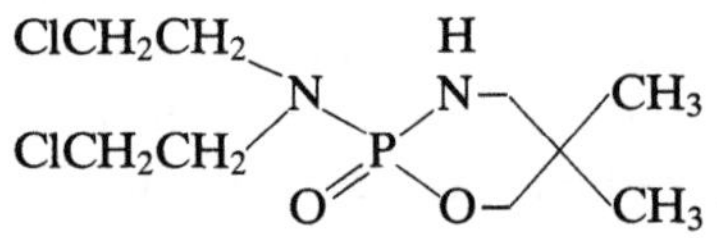	> 100 (no effect)

acrolein. The metabolites resulting from the oxazaphosphorine ring had preferably to be studied for their urotoxic effects. The presence of an alkylating group is not necessary for their urotoxic effect to occur: cf., ASTA B-516.

Even enzymatic hydroxylation at C-4 is per se not sufficient for the urotoxic action: like cyclophosphamide, ASTA B-707 is hydroxylated at the 4-position, but without producing any urotoxic effect. In contradistinction to cyclophosphamide, ASTA B-707 does not liberate acrolein. Since the directly alkylating phosphoric acid diamides are only slightly urotoxic on systemic administration, these results suggest acrolein to be the causative factor of urotoxic side effects.

Table 3. Concentrations of oxazaphosphorine compounds and metabolites inducing cystitis after 1 h instillation into the urinary bladder of rats. $C_{1.5}$: definitely phlogogenic concentration

Compound	Structural formula	$C_{1.5}$ (μmol/ml)
Cyclophosphamide	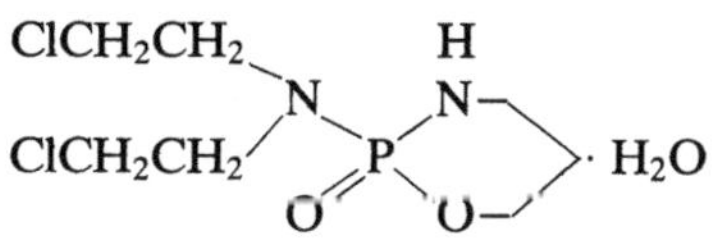	> 100
Ifosfamide	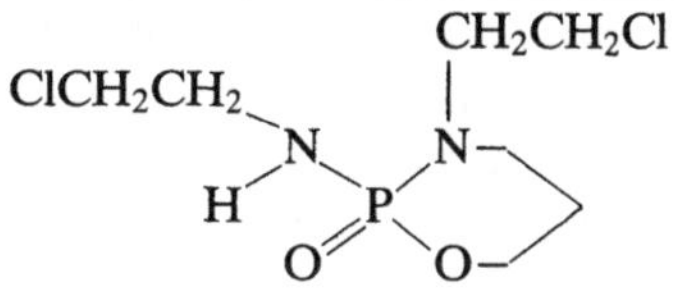	> 100
Trofosfamide	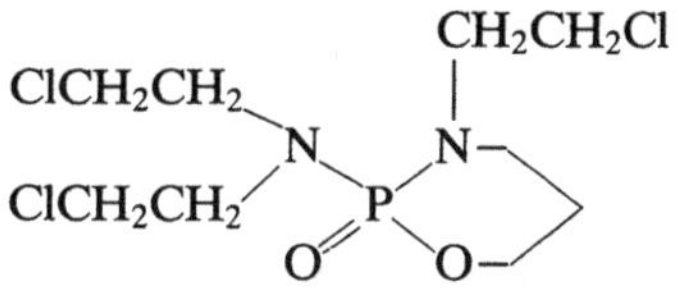	> 100
ASTA 6635	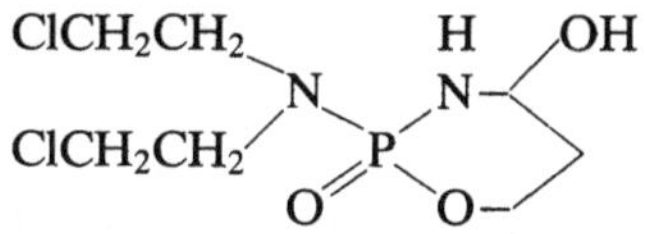	10[a]
ASTA 6569	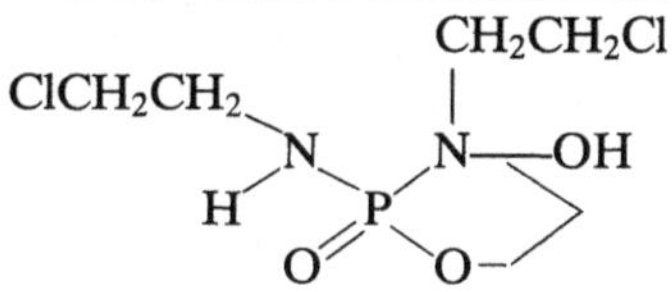	10[a]
ASTA 7169	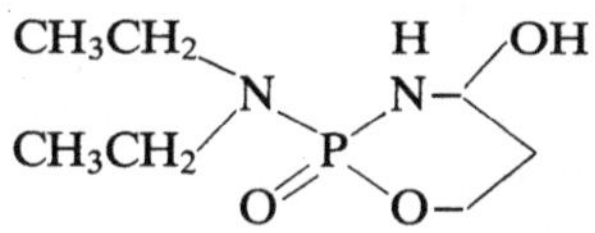	10[a]
Acrolein	$CH_2 = CH—CHO$	1
ASTA 5317	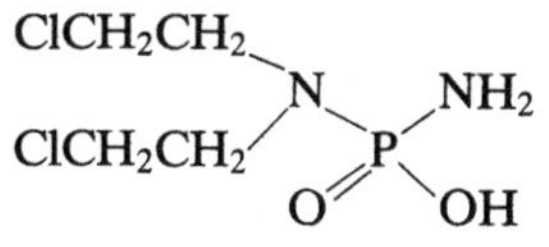	> 50
ASTA 5333	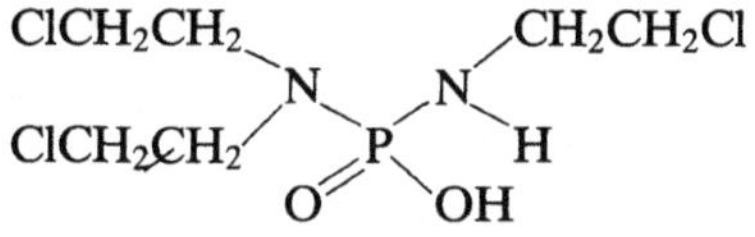	> 50

[a] The urotoxic action of buffered solutions of 4-hydroxymetabolites at different pH values is being studied at present

Experimental Induction of Hemorrhagic Cystitis in the Rat by Intravesical Administration

For further elucidation of the etiology of hemorrhagic cystitis, we studied the systemically urotoxic compounds and their renal metabolites by instilling them directly into the urinary bladder of rats. Table 3 shows that acrolein proved to be the most potent urotoxic agent of all compounds tested. Its urotoxicity is by one order of magnitude greater than that of the 4-hydroxy metabolites, which become biologically active only by their spontaneous breakdown. The resulting directly alkylating phosphoric acid diamides exert a relatively slight urotoxic effect, even on topical application, which again suggests that acrolein is the causative factor in urotoxicity. After glomerular filtration of the compounds hydroxylated at position 4 of the oxazaphosphorine ring, acrolein is liberated in the urine. In this protein-free medium, the highly reactive acrolein molecule exclusively attacks the renal and vesical epithelia, which explains its extremely high urotoxicity.

Studies on the Uroprotective Action of Sodium 2-Mercaptoethanesulfonate (INN: Mesna)

Subsequently, we studied the question of how the specific urotoxicity of the oxazaphosphorines could be avoided. The uroprotective agent should immediately react with acrolein and block the 4-hydroxy metabolites in the kidneys and deferent urinary tract, thus preventing the liberation of acrolein. From the viewpoint of chemical reactivity, mercapto compounds should preferably be used, since they largely comply with this twofold requirement. The desired compound should show a completely different pharmacokinetic behavior in comparison with the mercapto compounds known so far: it should not penetrate into the tissues, so as to avoid weakening the therapeutic effect of the cytostatics, but should be excreted rapidly and completely by the kidneys.

Out of the great number of mercapto compounds, only sodium 2-mercaptoethanesulfonate (INN: mesna) complies with these very strict chemical and pharmacokinetic requirements. It is rapidly and completely eliminated through the kidneys. In the rat, its half-life for elimination is 1.48 h on IV injection, its tissue distribution pattern being practically negligible, since it does not penetrate into the tissues.

Regional protection of kidneys and urinrary bladder can only be expected if the oxazaphosphorine metabolites and the mercapto compound are simultaneously excreted through the kidneys. In preliminary tests, we found the detoxifying action of mesna in the rat to be particularly favourable if its administration was synchronized as closely as possible with that of the oxazaphosphorines.

From among the great number of results obtained under varied conditions, we shall only discuss those of cyclophosphamide detoxification. Table 4 shows the urotoxic effect of 68.1 mg/kg of cyclophosphamide to be completely relieved if 31.6 mg/kg of mesna is given 15 min before. A dose of 21.5 mg/kg of mesna already reduces the urotoxicity to such an extent that slight swelling and small amounts of stain occur in a few isolated cases only. With other oxazaphosphorines, such as ifosfamide and trofosfamide, we observed the same protective effect. This combination therapy, for the first time enables the separation of specific organotoxic side effects from the desired cancerotoxic effect.

Table 4. Protective action of mesnum against urotoxic side-effects of cyclophosphamide (IV injection)

Cyclophosphamide (mg/kg)	Mesnum (mg/kg)	No. of rats	Assessment of urinary bladder	
			Inflammation (score)	Bleeding (%)
68.1	–	40	2.6	45
68.1	10.0	10	2.3	20
68.1	14.7	10	2.6	0
68.1	21.5	10	1.1	0
68.1	31.6	10	0	0
68.1	68.1	5	0	0

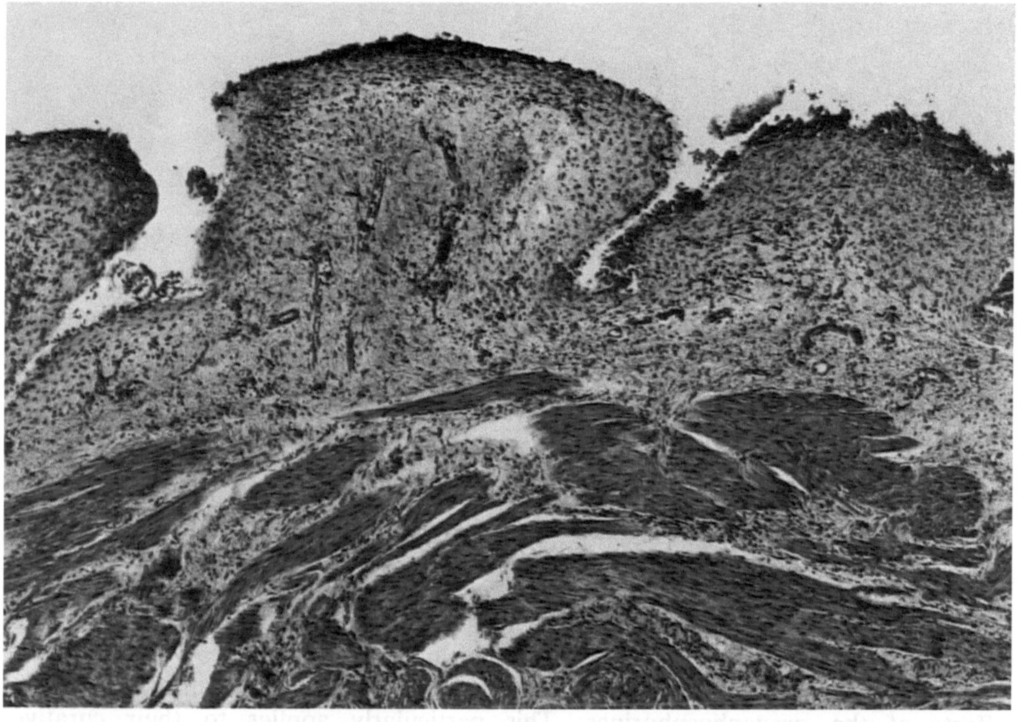

Fig. 1. Histology of the rat bladder 24 h after IV administration of 68.1 mg/kg ifosfamide. Note detachment of the urothelium, extensive edema, and necrosis in the musculature

For rapid macroscopic diagnosis, the trypan blue test has proved to be of great value. The bladders of oxazaphosphorine-treated animals show an intense blue coloration after trypan blue, whereas those of untreated animals remain unchanged. Histology fully confirms these macroscopic findings. Figure 1 shows the results of ifosfamide treatment in the rat: purulent necrotizing cystitis with submucosal edema, ulceration, and exudation of the vesical mucosa; whereas Figure 2 shows the histologic picture of a ifosfamide-mesna-treated rat whose bladder appears to be completely normal.

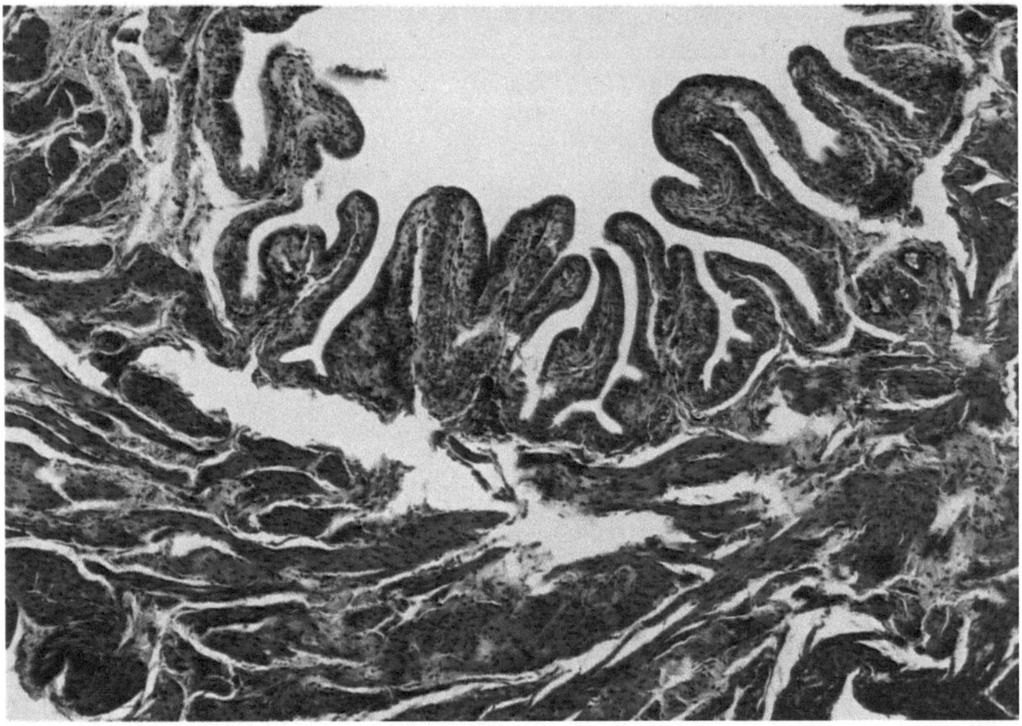

Fig. 2. Histology of the rat bladder 24 h after concurrent IV administration of 68.1 mg/kg ifosfamide and 21.5 mg/kg mesna. There was no difference compared with untreated controls

Systemic Effectiveness of Mesna

Mesna was studied in extensive pharmacologic and toxicologic assay designs, its characteristic properties and interactions being assessed in various models. From a pharmacologic viewpoint, mesna is inconspicuous and relatively nontoxic (LD_{50} in the male rat IV 2080 mg/kg). The doses needed for effective prevention of experimentally induced urotoxicity amounted to about 1% of the LD_{50}. Thus mesna has a very wide margin of safety in view of its intended clinical use.

Of particular importance is the fact that mesna does not interfere with the systemic effects of the oxazaphosphorines. This particularly applies to their curative cancerotoxic action, but also to their leukotoxic and immunosuppressive effect. Figure 3 shows the curative effect of ifosfamide on DS carcinosarcoma of the rat to persist at the same level, even on extremely high doses of mesna. These findings were confirmed in a number of different experimental tumors.

Results of Clinical Trials

In randomized studies by the Medical Unit of Cologne University Hospital and the Radiation Hospital Janker, Bonn, the pharmacologically elaborated detoxification method with mesna was compared with the standard prophylaxis during high-mas-

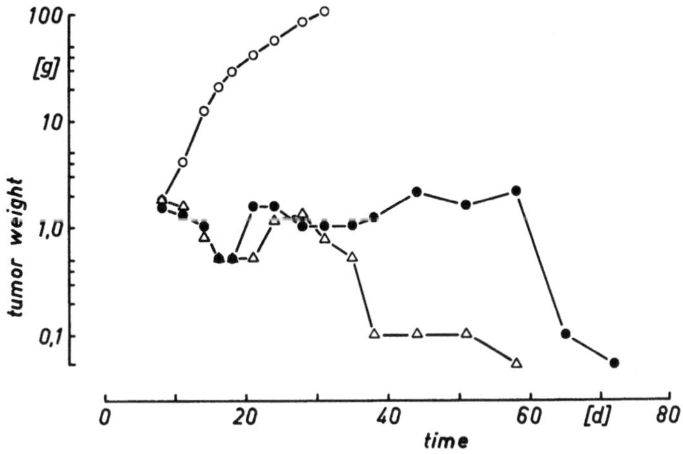

Fig. 3. Median tumor weights of solid DS carcinosarcoma of the rat; O——O untreated controls (n = 10); ●——● treatment on day 8 with a single IV dose of 215 mg/kg ifosfamide (5 of 9 cured); Δ——Δ treatment on day 8 with a single IV dose of 215 mg/kg ifosfamide and 215 mg/kg mesna (6 of 10 cured)

Table 5. RBC count in urine after massive-dose administration of ifosfamide or cyclophosphamide

Prophylactic measure	No. of patients with RBCs/µl urine		
	≤ 15	16–50	> 50
Group I (mesna)	9	2	0
Group II (standard prophylaxis)	0	1	8

sive-dose treatment with cyclophosphamide or ifosfamide (Table 5). In spite of careful administration of the standard prophylactic measures, all nine ifosfamide-treated patients showed hematuria, three even macrohematuria. In the test group which was concurrently given mesna, there was only one case of a slight rise in red cells (18/µl urine); a second patient had microhematuria at the onset of treatment, and in the other patients no red cells were detected. In two patients of the control group suffering from macrohematuria, cytostatic treatment was continued under the protection of mesna, whereby the hemorrhages were arrested within 1–2 days. In no case did mesna interfere with the therapeutic effectiveness of cytostatic treatment.

Meanwhile, extensive positive results have been obtained with mesna in cooperative studies in 242 patients from 22 hospitals. Patients with various malignant tumors were treated with high doses of cyclophosphamide, ifosfamide, and trofosfamide, sometimes in combination with other cytostatics. With adequate dosage, only three patients (1.2%) developed macrohematuria, and 12 patients (5%) microhematuria. Seven patients had macrohematuria at the onset of treatment. Under the protection of mesna, the macrohematuria receded in six cases, and remained unchanged in one case only. In these cooperative studies, the uroprotector did not exert any negative influence on the antitumor effect of the cytostatics.

After detailed studies of the elimination kinetics of the oxazaphosphorine metabolites and mesna in the urine, the IV injection of mesna at time 0 (= administration of the cytostatic), 4, and 8 h later has proved to be the best method. The mesna dose was 20% (w/w) of the respective oxazaphosphorine dose.
The clinical trials have shown that mesna is a reliably acting uroprotector which enables the safe prevention of the often therapy-limiting side effects of antitumor treatment with oxazaphosphorines. In the absence of their urotoxic side effects, these cytostatics can be given at a higher dosage so that their therapeutic benefit will be increased.

References

1 Brock N (1979) The special position of ifosfamide in the series of cytostatically active oxazaphosphorines. In: Fox BW (ed) Advances im Medical Oncology, Research and Education, vol 5, Basis for Cancer Therapy 1. Pergamon Press, Oxford New York
2 Brock N, Stekar J, Pohl J, Niemeyer U, Scheffler G (1979) Acrolein, the causative factor of urotoxic side-effects of cyclophosphamide, ifosfamide, trofosfamide and sufosfamide. Arzneim Forsch 29: 659–661
3 Brock N, Stekar J, Pohl J, Scheef W (1979) Antidot gegen urotoxische Wirkungen der Oxazaphosphorin-Derivate Cyclophosphamid, Ifosfamid und Trofosfamid. Naturwissenschaften 66: 60–61
4 Burkert H, Schnitker J, Fichtner E (1979) Verhütung der Harnwegstoxizität von Oxazaphosphorinen durch einen "Uroprotektor". Münch Med Wochenschr 121: 760–762
5 Klein HO, Christian E, Coerper C, Klein PJ, Scheef W, Brock N, (1978) Experimental and clinical investigation on the protective effect of 2-mercapto-aethan-sulfon-acid (MAS) on kidneys and urinary bladder during high-dose therapy with ifosfamide (IF) and cyclophosphamide (CPA). Medical Oncology, Abstr., 4th Annual Meeting Oncology Society, Nice, Dec 2–4, 1978
6 Scheef W, Klein HO, Brock N, Burkert H, Günther U, Hoefer-Janker H, Mitrenga D, Schnitker J, Voigtmann R (1979) Controlled clinical studies with an antidote against the urotoxicity of oxazaphosphorines: Preliminary results. Cancer Treat Rep 63: 501–505

*Cell Kinetic Factors, Single Drugs and Combination**

P. Lelieveld, J. H. Mulder, M. B. Edelstein, and L. M. van Putten

Summary

This communication focuses on the problems that exist in the application of cell kinetic information in cancer chemotherapy. From selected historical work, the following conclusions can be drawn.
1) Theoretically optimal drug sequences may fail to show the expected effect.
2) Similar drug sequences cause different effects in different tumors, even when the tumors have similar proliferation characteristics.
The unpredictability and the heterogeneity in response make the extrapolation to clinical cancer chemotherapy very difficult. Better prediction may be made from the integration of results from studies combining cell kinetic factors, cellular pharmacokinetics, and biochemistry of drug exposure.

Introduction

In the last decade, extensive studies have been performed on the relation between cell kinetics and cancer chemotherapy. From the reviews that have appeared on the more fundamental aspects of cell kinetics as related to general cytotoxicity [8, 12, 18, 23], it is evident that variations in cell kinetics can seriously influence the efficacy of cytostatic chemotherapy. In this communication we critically consider the role that cell kinetic information may have in its application in clinical chemotherapy.
In 1966, Bruce et al. [2] distinguished phase-specific and cell-cycle-specific agents. Their model studies revealed several principles that should be applied in cancer chemotherapy. We mention here that for both phase-specific and cell-cycle-specific agents, maximally tolerated doses should be given in short courses. Since the hemopoietic system often is the dose-limiting factor, a second course can be given only after full recovery of this system. Drug administration in small daily doses should be avoided. Under these circumstances, normal resting cells are drawn into the active cell cycle (recruitment), by which they become more sensitive to the next dose. These principles were supported from experimental and clinical work. DeWys et al. [3] showed that cyclophosphamide-treated hemopoietic stem cells were very sensitive to a second dose of cyclophosphamide when given before recovery of the hemopoietic system was completed. As soon as recovery was completed, however, the sensitivity was similar to that seen after the first dose. Goldie et al. [7] showed that a high dose of

* Supported by the Koningin Wilhelmina Fonds, Netherlands Organization for the Fight against Cancer, by grant number 5 PO1CA13053-05, awarded by the National Cancer Institute, DHEW, and by Premeso

methotrexate (MTX) can be given safely in the relative short period of 24 h, while much lower doses can produce severe bone marrow toxicity when given over several days. Similar phenomena were observed for other drugs.

Increasingly, drugs are used in combination since this type of treatment is often superior to single-drug treatment. Many reports have appeared on experimental models in which drug sequences and optimal time intervals have been tested. The basic cell kinetic mechanisms by which a sequence of cytotoxic agents can be optimally applied are synchronization and recruitment. A number of reviews on these two mechanisms have been published in the last few years [9, 13, 16, 22]. In addition, reviews have cautioned against the implication that all effects of modifying drug sequences in chemotherapy are due to cell kinetic mechanisms [6, 17, 24]. For these reasons, we want to summarize the data on some drug sequences in animal systems from our laboratory, and make a comparison with results obtained elsewhere in order to evaluate the extent to which cell kinetic factors may be responsible for inducing reproducible changes in chemotherapy efficacy.

Vincristine plus Cyclophosphamide

On the basis of synchronization studies by Klein et al. [11], a claim has been made that there is a cell kinetic advantage in some systems of the sequence vincristine before cyclophosphamide, but this is not always the case. An occasional failure is not unexpected; it might be explained by the fact that different tumor cell populations will be in a different cell kinetic status after an interval of 24 h. The kinetic aspect of this effect, however, is far from proven. Cyclophosphamide is effective on cells in various parts of the cycle, and recent studies [25] have indicated that an increased effectiveness in the S phase claimed for this drug [10] cannot be found in all cell lines. In addition, the data of Razek et al. [19] on the duration of increased effectiveness of cyclophosphamide after vincristine indicate that the time period of increased cell sensitivity lasts for more than a full cell cycle (from 6–18 h after vincristine injection) in AKR leukemia and for a similar period in L1210 leukemia. Such long periods of increased cell sensitivity cannot be explained by simple cell kinetic mechanisms and for this reason alternative interpretations based on a pharmacokinetic effect must also be considered. Other peculiarities of this combination are the difference in response between different L1210 lines (St. Louis, Rijswijk, Villejuif; Table 1) and the limited effect of varying drug sequences. Recently, Mulder et al. [14] investigated combination chemotherapy with vincristine and cyclophosphamide in leukemia L1210, Lewis lung carcinoma, a mouse osteosarcoma, and two experimental colon tumors. Therapeutic synergism could not be demonstrated in any of the tumor cell lines (Table 1). These results indicate that simple generalizations concerning the cell kinetic interpretation of the effect of varying drug sequences are not justified.

Methotrexate plus Cytosine Arabinoside

This is supported by the finding of similar discrepancies in other combinations such as MTX and cytosine arabinoside (ara-C) (Table 2). Theoretically, we would not expect any increase in cell killing if we combine two drugs simultaneously that are known to kill the same subpopulation. Indeed, Tattersall and Harrap showed the expected antagonism in vitro [21]. However, results from in vivo studies by Avery and Roberts

Table 1. Experimental data on the combination vincristine–cyclophosphamide in different sequences[a]

	VCR →CY	VCR + CY	CY →VCR	
Resting BM stem cells	–	–	–	St. Louis + Rijswijk [19]
Repopulating BM stem cells	–	–	–	Rijswijk
Leukemia L5222	+	NT	–	Heidelberg [26]
AKR lymphoma	+	–	–	St. Louis [19]
L1210	+	–	+	St. Louis [19]
	–	–	–	Rijswijk
	+	–	–	Villejuif [17]
Ehrlich ascites	+	–	NT	Köln [11]
Osteosarcoma C22LR	–	–	–	Rijswijk
Colon carcinoma 26	–	±	–	Rijswijk
Colon carcinoma 51	–	–	–	Rijswijk
C3H mammary tumor	–	–	–	Rijswijk
Lewis lung carcinoma	–	–	–	Rijswijk

[a] VCR, vincristine; CY, cyclophosphamide; BM, bone marrow; +, most cytotoxic sequence; –, less cytotoxic sequence or no difference; NT, not tested

Table 2. Experimental data on the combination methotrexate–cytosine arabinoside in different sequences[a]

	Ara-C →MTX	Ara-C + MTX	MTX →Ara-C	
Resting BM stem cells	–	–	–	Rijswijk
Repopulating BM stem cells	–	–	±	Rijswijk
L1210	NT	+	NT	Memphis [1]
	–	+	–	St. Louis [5]
	–	+	–	Rijswijk
AKR lymphoma	–	–	–	St. Louis [5]
L5178 in vitro	–	–	–	London [21]

[a] Ara-C, cytosine arabinoside; MTX, methotrexate; BM, bone marrow; +, most cytotoxic sequence; –, less cytotoxic sequence or no difference; NT, not tested

[1] showed the contrary. In these studies, the combination of MTX and ara-C showed maximal effectiveness if applied simultaneously. Although each of the agents alone kills almost all the cells in S phase, effectiveness increases markedly if the drugs are given simultaneously rather than sequentially. The same phenomenon was observed in St. Louis and Rijswijk for leukemia L1210, but not for AKR lymphoma and hemopoietic stem cells (Table 2).

Cytosine Arabinoside plus Daunorubicin

Studies by Edelstein et al. [4] showed that supra-additive results were obtained when daunorubicin was given after ara-C with an optimum at an interval of 16 h. The

Table 3. Experimental data on the combination cytosine arabinoside–daunorubicin in different sequences[a]

	Ara-C →Dauno	Ara-C + Dauno	Dauno →Ara-C	
Resting BM cells	–	–	–	St. Louis [4]
Repopulating BM stem cells	+	–	NT	Rijswijk
L1210	+	–	–	St. Louis [4]
	+	–	+	Rijswijk
Osteosarcoma C22LR	±	–	–	Rijswijk
C3H mammary tumor	–	–	NT	Rijswijk
Rat rhabdomyosarcoma R1	–	–	NT	Rijswijk

[a] Ara-C, cytosine arabinoside; Dauno, daunorubicin; BM, bone marrow; +, most cytotoxic sequence; –, less cytotoxic sequence or no difference; NT, not tested

explanation was simple: ara-C killed the S-phase cells and caused a block for cells entering that phase, resulting in an accumulation of cells at the G1/S border. Daunorubicin is most active on G1/S cells which, 16 h after ara-C treatment, apparently progress through the cell cycle. We could confirm these results in L1210, though the reverse sequence was also effective (Table 3). From the results presented in Table 3, we might conclude tentatively that a supra-additive effect occurs in rapidly proliferating cells and not in the slower proliferating cell types. It is also evident that the drugs should not be given simultaneously.

CCNU plus 5-Fluorouracil

Based on the concept of recruitment, Schabel [20] suggested a sequential treatment with cell-cycle-nonspecific drugs, such as CCNU, followed by a cell-cycle-specific drug. This suggestion was actually tested by Mulder et al. [15], using the combination of CCNU and 5-fluorouracil (5-FU) given either simultaneously or with a 24-h time interval. The expected most effective schedule (CCNU followed by 5-FU) appeared to be least effective on several tumor lines, but was the most toxic treatment sequence for normal resting and rapidly proliferating bone marrow stem cells. According to these observations, the reversed sequence (5-FU followed within a short time interval by CCNU) was suggested for the treatment of gastrointestinal tumors.

Discussion

These examples emphasize the caution that should be exercised in applying theoretic constructions in cell kinetics. Unless actually tested, a theoretically constructed schedule, however rational its design, cannot be trusted to make optimal use of all of the cell kinetic information presently available on the action of each of the component drugs alone; nor can a purely cell-kinetic construction predict biochemical interactions which override the cell kinetic considerations.

Two major problems in the application of cell kinetics to tumor chemotherapy are:

1) Theoretically optimal drug sequences may fail to show the predicted effect, due to the appearance of non-cell-kinetic interactions.
2) Different tumors respond differently to similar drug sequences, even when the tumors do not differ in proliferation characteristics.

The heterogeneity makes an extrapolation to the clinical situation very difficult. The major effort needed to study the validity of extrapolation of cell kinetic results to many tumor systems, as well as to many techniques, points to the desirability of collaborative studies. Results of correlated studies on different parameters in many cell lines are hard to collect in a single institute. A well-integrated collaboration may lead to much more rapid progress than can be achieved by many groups working in isolation. This does not only refer to an integration of different methods of evaluation of cell kinetic studies and different methods of evaluation of chemotherapy effectiveness; it must necessarily include integration with studies on cellular pharmacokinetics and biochemistry of drug exposure in order also to identify those interaction effects in chemotherapy sequences in which cell kinetics do not seem to play a major role.

References

1 Avery TL, Roberts D (1974) Dose-related synergism of cytosine arabinoside and methotrexate against murine leukemia L1210. Eur J Cancer 10: 425–429

2 Bruce WR, Meeker BE, Valeriote FA (1966) Comparison of the sensitivity of normal hematopoietic and transplanted lymphoma colony-forming cells to chemotherapeutic agents administered in vivo. J Natl Cancer Inst 37: 233–245

3 DeWys WD, Goldin A, Mantel N (1970) Hematopoietic recovery after large doses of cyclophosphamide: Correlation of proliferation state with sensitivity. Cancer Res 30: 1692–1697

4 Edelstein M, Vietti T, Valeriote F (1974) Schedule-dependent synergism for the combination of 1-β-D-arabinofuranosylcytosine and daunorubicin. Cancer Res 34: 293–297

5 Edelstein M, Vietti T, Valeriote F (1975) 1-β-D-Arabinofuranosylcytosine and methotrexate. Cancer Res 35: 1555–1558

6 Goldenberg GJ (1974) Drug-induced stimulation of nitrogen mustard and choline transport and other systems in L5178Y lymphoblasts in vitro. Cancer Res 34: 2511–2516

7 Goldie JH, Price LA, Harrap KR (1972) Methotrexate toxicity: Correlation with duration of administration, plasma levels, dose and excretion pattern. Eur J Cancer 8: 409–414

8 Hill BT, Baserga R (1975) The cell cycle and its significance for cancer treatment. Cancer Treat Rev 2: 159–175

9 Klein HO (1972) Synchronization of tumour cell proliferation and the timing of cytostatic drugs. Biomedicine 17: 835–838

10 Klein HO, Lennartz KJ (1974) Chemotherapy after synchronization of tumour cells. Semin Hematol 11: 203–227

11 Klein HO, Lennartz KJ, Habicht W, Eder M, Gross R (1970) Synchronisation von Ehrlich-Ascites-Tumorzellen und ihre Bedeutung bei der Anwendung eines alkylierenden Cytostaticums. Klin Wochenschr 48: 1001–1005

12 Lamerton LF (1972) Cell proliferation and the differential response of normal and malignant tissues. Br J Radiol 45: 161–170

13 Mauer AM (1973) Effects of chemotherapeutic agents on cell cycle and cellular proliferation: Basic and clinical considerations. Transplant Proc 5: 1181–1184

14 Mulder JH, Lelieveld P, Van Putten LM (1979) Lack of vincristine-cyclophosphamide potentiation in different experimental tumour lines. Eur J Cancer 15: 499–507

15 Mulder JH, Smink T, Van Putten LM (1977) Schedule dependent effectiveness of CCNU and 5-fluorouracil in experimental chemotherapy. Eur J Cancer 13: 1123–1131

16 Nicolini C (1976) The principles and methods of cell synchronization in cancer chemotherapy. BBA Rev Cancer 458: 243–283

17 Pouillart P, Hoang Thy Huong T, Brugerie E, Lheritier J (1974) Sequential administration of two oncostatic drugs: Study of modalities for pharmacodynamic potentiation. Biomedicine 21: 471–479

18 Rajewsky MF (1975) Proliferative parameters relevant to cancer therapy. In: Grundman E, Gross R (eds) The ambivalence of cytostatic therapy. Springer, Heidelberg, pp 156–171

19 Razek A, Vietti T, Valeriote F (1974) Optimum time sequence for the administration of vincristine and cyclophosphamide in vivo. Cancer Res 34: 1857–1861

20 Schabel FM Jr (1975) Synergism and antagonism among antitumor agents. In: Pharmacological basis of cancer chemotherapy. Williams and Wilkins, Baltimore, pp 595–621

21 Tattersall MHN, Harrap KR (1973) Combination chemotherapy: The antagonism of methotrexate and cytosine arabinoside. Eur J Cancer 9: 229–232

22 Tubiana M, Frindel E, Vassort F (1975) Critical survey of experimental data on in vivo synchronization by hydroxyurea. In: Grundman E, Gross R (eds) The ambivalence of cytostatic therapy. Springer, Heidelberg, pp 187–205

23 Valeriote F, Van Putten LM (1975) Proliferation-dependent cytotoxicity of anticancer agents: A review. Cancer Res 35: 2619–2630

24 Van Putten LM, Keizer HJ, Mulder JH (1976) Synchronization in tumour chemotherapy. Eur J Cancer 12: 79–85

25 Volm M, Krieg L, Mattern J, Wayss K (1977) Effect of synchronization on chemotherapy of solid transplanted tumours. Eur J Cancer 13: 1099–1108

26 Zeller WJ, Ivankovic S, Schmähl D (1975) Chemotherapy of the transplantable acute leukemia L5222 in rats. Cancer Res 35: 1168–1174

Hyperthermia and Chemotherapy: Preclinical Considerations

D. L. Kisner and B. J. Lewis

Summary

Malignant cells appear to be selectively sensitive to thermal injury. The precise mechanism of cell death after thermal exposure has not been established, but the phenomenon has been demonstrated by both in vitro and in vivo techniques. Synergy of hyperthermia and chemotherapy has been demonstrated for several agents, but in vitro results are not uniformly confirmed in vivo. In some agents (methyl-CCNU) no synergy was found in vivo. In others (adriamycin) synergy was only demonstrated at drug doses with intolerable toxicity. Studies of the effects of hyperthermia on drug pharmacokinetics are desirable for future clinical trial design.

Introduction

In recent years there has been an expanding interest in the use of localized or systemic hyperthermia as a primary cancer therapy or as an adjunct to radiotherapy or chemotherapy. The literature dealing with the subject has become voluminous, largely due to extensive preclinical and clinical studies adding hyperthermia to radiation.

Hyperthermia-drug interactions have been less extensively reported, but suggestions of synergy in animal models have been demonstrated. It is this latter body of work we intend to review here with an eye toward pharmacologic considerations. No exhaustive review of the literature is intended. Representative work will be discussed dealing with preclinical studies using hyperthermia alone, and hyperthermia with chemotherapy. Hyperthermia technology, thermal dosimetry, and clinical trials are beyond the scope of this brief review.

Hyperthermia Cytotoxicity

There have been a great many reports of a relatively selective killing of cancer cells exposed to higher than physiologic temperatures. These have been extensively reviewed elsewhere [3].

The exact mechanisms of cytotoxicity have not yet been established, though many potentially lethal lesions have been identified. An excellent treatment of this complex problem has recently been published by Strom et al. [15]. Two general categories of lesions have been identified in thermally injured cancer cells: those occurring in membrane systems and those found in the biochemistry of intracellular macromolecules.

Membrane effects include changes in permeability of cells exposed to hyperthermia [15]. Increased temperature causes a profound increase in the rate of passive diffusion of low molecular weight substances through the plasma membrane which is reversible even when cell damage is not [15]. An irreversible defect in the membrane transport of a variety other substances has been documented, including glutamate, 2-deoxyglucose, thymidine, and several ribonucleotides [14, 15]. These irreversible alterations in membrane permeability occur with a variable delay after hyperthermic exposure and may therefore be secondary to other cellular injury rather than being the primary lesions [15]. The biochemical abnormalities that occur secondary to hyperthermia are numerous and include several that may play some role in lethality.

A profound inhibition of cellular respiration (as determined by rates of oxygen consumption) has been demonstrated in a variety of malignant cell lines [3, 5, 12]. Cavaliere et al. [3] and Mondavi et al. [12] have shown that the synthesis of DNA, RNA, and protein are even more sensitive to heat exposure than is oxygen consumption in Novikoff and Morris hepatoma cell lines. In that same study a control of regenerating liver cells suffered no metabolic abnormalities under the same conditions. Irreversibility of these effects of thermal exposure has been correlated with the inability of malignant cells to subsequently replicate in vitro or to produce tumors after transplantation [5]. More detailed studies have suggested that inhibition of ribosomal RNA synthesis may be a key lesion in the thermally injured malignant cell [15], but the issue must still be considered as unsettled.

Hyperthermia – In Vitro Studies

The kinetics of malignant cell killing by thermal exposure are worthy of a few comments. Westra and Dewey [18] have demonstrated in Chinese hamster ovary (CHO) cells that cells in "S" phase or "M" phase are more susceptible to thermal injury than cells in G, or G_2. Despite this it has been demonstrated with L1210 cells in culture that exposure to 43° C for 1 h was more lethal to noncycling plateau-phase cells than to exponentially growing cells [2]. This is clearly dissimilar to the situation with most chemotherapeutic agents.

In general the survival response to thermal exposure for cells in culture is characterized by a shoulder region followed by a straight exponential portion. Figure 1 shows these data for several cell lines reported by Bhuyan et al. [2]. The existence of a shoulder in these curves may imply some ability to repair sublethal damage.

Hyperthermia – In Vivo Studies

A large number of studies using a variety of hyperthermia techniques have been performed in many animal tumor models. Only two representative examples will be discussed.

In 1963, Crile [4] reported results of local hyperthermia treatment of S180 sarcomas transplanted into the footpad of SWR mice; 7-mm tumors were routinely destroyed by immersion of the foot in a bath at 44° C, while normal tissues were not injured. Additionally he found that each increase of 1° C in the bath temperature reduced the exposure time required for tumor destruction by 50%.

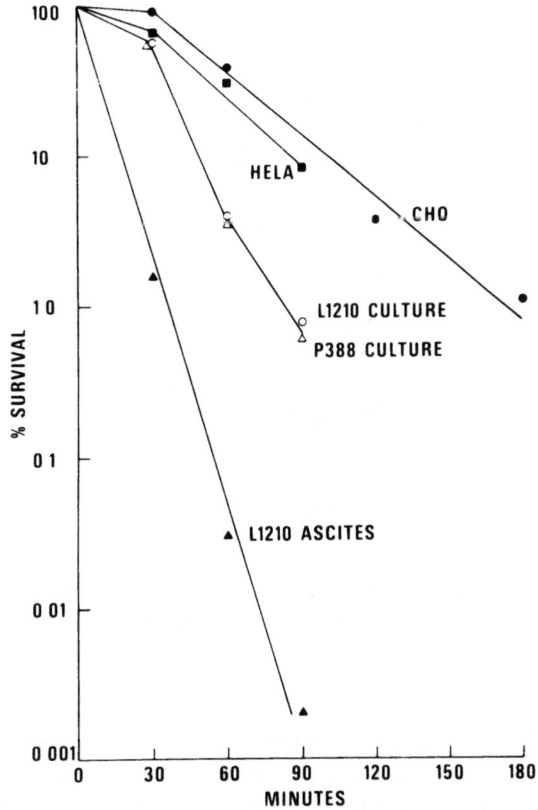

Fig. 1. Survival curves for different cell lines heated to 43° C. From BHUYAN et al. [2]

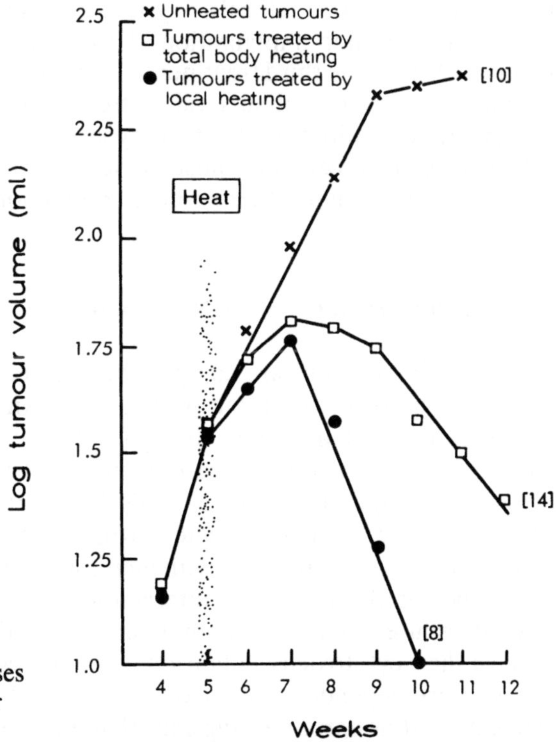

Fig. 2. Growth curve for VX2 carcinoma in rabbit following inoculation of 1 × 10^6 tumor cells into rear limb muscles, and changes in tumor volume following local and total body hyperthermia applied in fractionated doses of 1 h each on days 35, 36, and 37 after tumor implantation. From DICKSON [5]

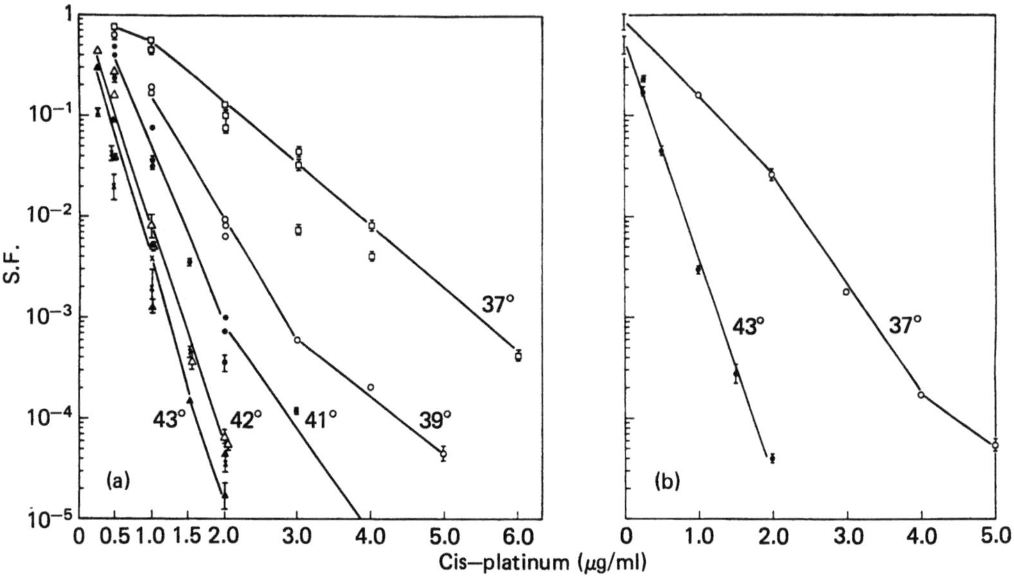

Fig. 3a, b. In vitro thermochemotherapy with cis-diamminedichloroplatinum of HA-1 Chinese hamster cells; **a** exponentially growing cells; **b** plateau-phase cells. From HAHN [6]

More recently, DICKSON [5] described treatment of a VX2 carcinoma injected into the rear limb muscles of rabbits, using local or systemic hyperthermia. Figure 2 shows results of tumor volume measurements done on treated animals and controls. Hyperthermia at 42° C (local or systemic) was applied in 1-h fractions on days 35, 36, and 37 after tumor implantation. Histologic studies revealed widespread necrosis within 24 h after the third treatment. This was followed by marked reductions in tumor volumes and prolonged survival in treated animals. These are examples of studies demonstrating antitumor effects of hyperthermia in which tumor destruction could be achieved with acceptable host toxicity. They will serve as a background for consideration of hyperthermia-drug interactions.

Thermochemotherapy – In Vitro Studies

Heat-drug interactions are complex because each class of drugs not only has its own model of cytotoxic action, but probably its own mode of interaction with heat [6]. We will attempt to characterize the type of in vitro work that has been performed. JOHNSON an PAVELAC [8] have demonstrated increased cell killing with progressive increase in temperature from 37°–43° C with thiotepa. They found this interaction to be consistent with that predicted from the kinetics of alkylation. The rate of cell inactivation was nearly linear with increasing temperature. Thiotepa is regarded as the prototype for the heat-drug interaction of the bifunctional alkylating agents [6]. The nitrosoureas and cis-diamminedichloroplatinum (DDP) have been demonstrated to have their cytotoxicity enhanced by increased temperature [6]. Figure 3 shows this temperature-dependent cytotoxicity for DDP. Note that DDP is somewhat more active against nonproliferating cells than proliferating cells. Of additional importance

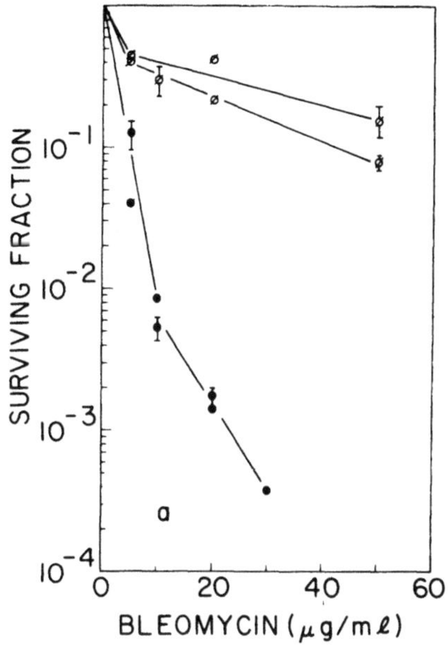

Fig. 4. Thermochemotherapy of Chinese hamster cells with bleomycin, showing threshold behavior. Exponentially growing cells. 0, 37° C; 0, 39° C; 0, 43° C. From HAHN [6]

is the progressive enhancement above 37° C with no "threshold" phenomenon. These points are true of the nitrosoureas as well [6].

Enhancement of antitumor activity of the antitumor antibiotics bleomycin, adriamycin, and actinomycin D by heating have been documented [7]. These agents show no synergism with heat between 37° C and 42° C. Above 42° C there is marked synergism, as demonstrated in Fig. 4 for bleomycin. Recently BARLOGIE et al. [1] have added mitomycin C to the list of drugs that are synergistic with heat. Significant enhancement of killing of a human LOVO colon cancer cell line occurred above 42° C, suggesting a temperature threshold for this agent as well.

Thermochemotherapy – In Vivo Studies

Thermochemotherapy studies in tumor-bearing animals are important to the design of human experiments for several reasons. The degree of enhancement of cell killing with a given drug may differ significantly between in vitro and in vivo studies. In the intact animal consideration must be given to the effects of hyperthermia or tumor and organ blood flow, as well as drug distribution, metabolism and excretion [9]. For drugs requiring activation in vivo (e.g., cyclophosphamide) the effect of temperature upon the specific organ responsible for conversion to the active compound may also be a factor in the in vivo results [6]. These factors should be considered in reviewing the in vivo studies mentioned below.

Nitrosourea

Potentiation of the antitumor effect of BCNU with localized hyperthermia in the treatment of the EMT6 and KHT mouse tumor systems have been reported by

Twentyman et al. [17] and Marmor [9]. Effects of the combined modalities were significantly greater than for either alone. Greatest potentiation occurred between 42° C and 43° C, confirming the temperature response in in vitro studies [6]. Potentiation was greatest when heat and BCNU were given simultaneously [9]. Subsequent work by Marmor and Hahn [10] utilizing local heating in the KHT tumor system have shown significant potentiation of the cytotoxicity of chlorozotocin by heat. Only minor enhancement of methyl-CCNU effect was found despite significant enhancement in the in vitro work. Strepotozotocin effects were not increased by heat.

DDP

Marmor [9] has reported enhancement of DDP cytotoxicity in the mouse KHT tumor system. Delay in doubling of mean tumor diameters was greater for the combination of heat and DDP than for either treatment alone. Unfortunately no treatment temperatures below 43° C were reported, leaving open the question of a "threshold temperature" in vivo for this agent.

Alkylators

The effect of local hyperthermia (42° C) upon the effects of mechlorethamine *N*-oxide treatment of the Yoshida sarcoma in rats has been reported by Suzuki [16]. Regressions were noted in heated tumors at a dose that did not produce regressions without heat. Local toxicity was reported to be greatest with the combined treatment.

Antitumor Antibiotics

Bleomycin has been studied together with heat in cell survival studies of the mouse EMT6 tumor [9]. Synergism was demonstrated at 42°–43° C but not at lower temperatures, which was consistent with in vitro results [7]. Tumor growth delay studies in the KHT mouse tumor system revealed potentiation of bleomycin tumor growth delay when local heating to 43° C was performed [9]. Worsened local toxicity and frequency of toxic deaths were also noted at this temperature.

Cell survival studies using in vitro cloning of cells from tumors treated in vivo have also been reported for adriamycin and heat [9]. EMT6 mouse tumors were excised 2 h after injection of adriamycin (2.5, 5.0, or 10.0 mg/kg, with and without heating to 43° C). Enhancement of adriamycin cytotoxicity was seen only at the highest dose level. Further studies using adriamycin and heat in the KHT tumor system showed no enhancement of drug effect at 2.0 or 5.0 mg/kg while doses of 10 mg/kg resulted in toxic deaths of 14 of the 25 animals [9]. The author suggests that adequate concentrations of drug may not be sustained long enough to allow heat potentiation at doses tolerated by the animal. Further animal studies using adriamycin and heat may well be warranted using a longer infusion time to maintain higher serum levels for longer periods in light of the relatively short serum half-life [11].

Hyperthermia and Drug Pharmacokinetics

The apparent disparity between the in vitro and in vivo studies with adriamycin cited above point out the need for thorough in vivo investigations with agents found in vitro to be synergistic with hyperthermia. Additionally, it suggests a need for pharmacokinetic studies to be performed in animals undergoing thermochemotherapy to assess hyperthermic effects on plasma clearance, distribution, and excretion. Relatively little has been done in this area. SHINGLETON et al. [13] demonstrated increased uptake of labeled nitrogen mustard into tumor and normal tissue under localized hyperthermic conditions in the normal dog leg and the VX2 carcinoma in rabbits. This was also accompanied by increased toxicity in the heated areas.

Pertinent to the adriamycin issue is a study reported by MIMNAUGH et al. [11] in which adriamycin serum levels and distribution were studied in normothermic and hyperthermic rabbits. Serum half-life, urinary and biliary excretion were unaffected by hyperthermia. Tissue distributions and concentrations were very similar except for larger total amounts of drug in the hearts of hyperthermic rabbits, and higher concentrations in skeletal muscle. It is unclear whether the apparently greater cardiac accumulation may have implications for clinical cardiomyopathy. Studies exposing animals to large total doses with hyperthermia would be of interest.

Conclusion

Heating malignant cells above physiologic temperature (for their host) can result in irreversible cellular damage and lethality. The precise intracellular lesions responsible for cytotoxicity have not been established, but inhibition of RNA synthesis appears to play a key role. Malignant cells are, in general, more sensitive to thermal injury than normal cells. When cells are in cycle they are more sensitive to thermal injury during mitosis and "S" phase. However, nonproliferating cells appear equally or more sensitive than exponentially proliferating cells. Thermal killing of malignant cells has been demonstrated in both in vitro and in vivo experiments.

In vitro studies combining heat and drugs have suggested synergy between heat and alkylating agents, nitrosoureas, adriamycin, bleomycin, actinomycin D, DDP, and mitomycin C. The antitumor antibiotics (adriamycin, bleomycin, actinomycin D) appear to have their cytotoxicity enhanced only at temperatures in excess of 42° C. This has been confirmed by in vivo experiments and suggests that these agents may be best tested with localized hyperthermia where these higher temperatures are better tolerated. In vivo studies have confirmed synergy of heating and alkylators, DDP, BCNU, and chlorozotocin. Methyl-CCNU and streptozotocin do not appear promising.

In general enhanced antitumor activity in vivo is accompanied by greater local or systemic toxicity.

Far too little is known about the effect of hyperthermia upon drug distribution, plasma clearance, excretion, or uptake into host and malignant tissues. Generally in the in vivo studies reviewed, the drug was given by a single route at different doses and temperatures. Further study of drug pharmacokinetics and experimentation with different schedules of administration may reveal greater synergy or reduced toxicity with hyperthermia. These studies will certainly aid in development and design of future clinical trials of thermochemotherapy.

References

1 Barlogie B, Drewinko B, Corry PM (1979) In vitro thermochemotherapy of human colon cancer (LOVO) cells with cis-dichlorodiammine platinum II (DDP) and mitomycin-C (M). Proc Am Assoc Cancer Res 20:58

2 Bhuyan BK, Day KJ, Edgerton CE, Ogunbase O (1977) Sensitivity of different cell lines and of different phases in the cell cycle to hyperthermia. Cancer Res 37:3780–3784

3 Cavaliere R, Ciocatto CC, Giovanella BC, Heidelberger C, Johnson RO, Margottini M, Mondovi B, Moricca G, Rossi-Fanelli A (1967) Selective heat sensitivity of cancer cells. Cancer 20:1351

4 Crile G (1963) The effects of heat and radiation on cancers implanted on the feet of mice. Cancer Res 23:372–380

5 Dickson JA (1977) The effects of hyperthermia in animal tumor systems. Recent Results Cancer Res 59:43–111

6 Hahn GM (1979) Potential for therapy of drugs and hyperthermia. Cancer Res 39:2264–2268

7 Hahn GM, Braun J, Har-Kedar I (1975) Thermochemotherapy: Synergism between hyperthermia (42–43° C) and adriamycin (or bleomycin) in mammal cell inactivation. Proc Natl Acad Sci USA 72:937–940

8 Johnson HA, Pavelac M (1973) Thermal enhancement of thiotepa cytotoxicity. J Natl Cancer Inst 50:903–908

9 Marmor J (1979) Interactions of hyperthermia and chemotherapy in animals. Cancer Res 39:2269–2276

10 Marmor JB, Hahn GM (1979) Effect of four nitrosoureas with local hyperthermia on primary tumor and metastases. Proc Am Assoc Cancer Res 20:67

11 Mimnaugh EG, Waring RW, Sikic BI, Magin RL, Drew R, Litterst CL, Gram TE, Guarino AM (1978) Effect of whole-body hyperthermia on the disposition and metabolism of adriamycin in rabbits. Cancer Res 38:1420–1425

12 Mondavi B, Strom R, Rotilio G, Finazzi-Agro S, Cavaliere R, Rossi-Fanelli A (1969) The biochemical mechanism of selective heat sensitivity of cancer cells. I. Studies on cellular respiration. Eur J Cancer 5:129

13 Shingleton WW, Bryan F, O'Quinn W, Krueger LC (1962) Selective heating and cooling of tissue in cancer chemotherapy. Ann Surg 156:408–416

14 Strom R, Caiafa P, Mondavi B, Rossi-Fanelli A (1970) Temperature dependency of transcellular migration of glutamate in normal and neoplastic cells. In: Keynes RD, Loewenstein WR, Pethica BA (eds) Permeability and function of biological membranes. North-Holland, Amsterdam, p 333

15 Strom R, Crifo C, Rossi-Fanelli A, Mondavi B (1977) Biochemical aspects of heat sensitivity of tumour cells. Recent Results Cancer Res 59:7–35

16 Suzuki K (1967) Application of heat to cancer chemotherapy. Nagoya J Med Sci 30:1–21

17 Twentyman PR, Morgan JE, Donaldson J (1978) Enhancement by hyperthermia of the effect of BCNU against the EMT6 mouse tumor. Cancer Treat Rep 62:439–443

18 Westra A, Dewey WC (1971) Variation in sensitivity to heat shock during the cell cycle of Chinese hamster cells in vitro. Int J Radiat Biol 19:467–477

The Disposition of Intraperitoneal Bleomycin, Melphalan, and Vinblastine in Cancer Patients

D. S. Alberts, H.-S. G. Chen, S. Y. Chang, and Y. M. Peng

Summary

We have studied the disposition of bleomycin, melphalan, or vinblastine after intraperitoneal (IP) instillation in 14 cancer patients. Although IP bleomycin had a somewhat longer terminal-phase plasma half-life than after intravenous (IV) administration (5.5 vs 4.0 h, respectively), its systemic absorption averaged only 44%–52% of the administered dose. IP melphalan's mean terminal-phase half-life of 1.3 h was similar to that seen after IV drug administration. Melphalan's systemic absorption from the IP space averaged only 39% of the administered dose. In contrast, vinblastine plasma levels remained elevated for longer than 24 h after IP instillation. Its use was associated with life-threatening adynamic ileus in two patients. Bleomycin's and melphalan's reduced systemic availability after IP dosing suggests that their dose could be increased safely by a factor of two over their standard IV doses.

Introduction

Intraperitoneal (IP) anticancer drug administration may be the most effective way to treat advanced ovarian cancer. This malignancy is usually confined to the IP space [15]. By administering drugs IP, it may be possible to increase the concentration of the drug at the tumor site while decreasing systemic availability and, thus, normal tissue toxicity [7].

Recently, bleomycin [3], methotrexate [10], 5-fluorouracil [14], and adriamycin [12] have all been studied pharmacokinetically after IP dosing. Investigators at the National Cancer Institute, Bethesda, Maryland, have used a peritoneal dialysis technique to maintain a constant concentration of an anticancer drug in the IP space of ovarian cancer patients [7, 10, 12, 14]. In contrast, we have chosen to administer the anticancer drug of interest as a single bolus IP injection [3]. This report presents a preliminary description of the systemic disposition of bleomycin, melphalan, and vinblastine after IP dosing in our patients.

Materials and Methods

Patients. After intraperitoneal (IP) administration, bleomycin disposition was studied in nine cancer patients, melphalan was studied in three, and vinblastine in two. Patient characteristics are summarized in Table 1. All patients had advanced cancer at the time

Table 1. Characteristics of patients receiving intracavitary anticancer drugs

Patient	Tumor type	Sex	Age (years)	BSA (M^2)	Creatinine clearance (ml/min)	Drug	Drug dose (mg/m^2)[a]
EL	Ovary	F	63	1.63	56.0[b]	Bleomycin	61.3
JP	Endometrial	F	64	1.60	107.6	Bleomycin	60.0
PE	Hepatoma	M	50	2.00	0.7	Bleomycin	15.0
AS	Hepatoma	M	79	1.60	23.4	Bleomycin	60.0
MC	Ovary	F	55	2.00	53.0	Bleomycin	60.0
EP	Ovary	F	50	1.75	74.0[b]	Bleomycin	60.0
VP	Ovary	F	77	1.67	34.4[b]	Bleomycin	60.5
DO	Ovary	F	29	1.80	128.4[b]	Bleomycin	59.0
TW	Ovary	F	73	1.50	50.0	Bleomycin	53.0
EP_2	Ovary	F	50	2.00	74.0[b]	Mephalan	35.0
LZ	Ovary	F	55	1.63	132.8[b]	Mephalan	36.8
VL	Ovary	F	72	1.71	88.1[b]	Mephalan	35.1
VO	Ovary	F	22	1.38	85.8[b]	Vinblastine	7.0
EH	Ovary	F	61	1.45	113.8[b]	Vinblastine	7.0

[a] For bleomycin, mg = units
[b] Creatinine clearance estimated from serum creatinine, lean body weight, and age. From Mawer et al.

of study. The serum creatinine was normal in 13 of 14 patients. Patient PE (Table 1) had a serum creatinine of 2.9 mg/100 ml. None of the patients received other anticancer drugs within 3 weeks of these pharmacokinetic studies. An attempt was made to stop all routine-type drugs at least 3 days prior to the anticancer drug disposition studies.

Treatment. All patients given IP bleomycin received approximately 60 U/m^2, except one (PE, Table 1) who received only 15 U/m^2. Bleomycin in doses of 30–110 U was diluted in 100 ml normal saline and injected in bolus form into the peritoneal cavity after near maximal evacuation of the effusion fluid (i.e., approximately 1 l residual ascites). All patients given melphalan received 1 mg/kg body weight in 100 ml normal saline as a single bolus IP injection. Again, the drug was injected into a residual of approximately 1 l of actites fluid following paracentesis. Finally, vinblastine was injected as a 7 mg/m^2 dose in 100 ml saline into the IP space of two ovarian cancer patients.

Biological Fluid Sampling. Blood samples (6–10 ml) were obtained from a heparin lock and collected in tubes containing 100 IU heparin. Samples were taken just before the start of therapy and in most cases at 5, 15, 30, 45, and 60 min and at 2, 3, 4, 6, 8, 12, and 24 h after drug administration. Fractional urine collections were taken for the first 8 h after drug injection and then at known intervals throughout the 24 h, and stored in sterile containers at −20° C. Blood samples were kept on ice until centrifugation at 4° C and then frozen at −20° C. Repeated 10-ml samples of ascites fluid were obtained at varying intervals up to 24 h after IP drug administration in two patients (VP and VL, Table 1). The samples were centrifuged to remove cellular components and frozen at −20° C.

Assay Procedure. The bleomycin concentrations in plasma and urine were determined by means of the antiserum and radioimmunoassay techniques developed by BROUGHTON and STRONG [4]. Melphalan was measured in plasma and urine samples by using a high-pressure liquid chromatographic assay developed by CHANG et al. [5]. Vinblastine was assayed in plasma only by using a radioimmunoassay developed by Dr. M. A. ROOT of the Eli Lilly Co., Indianapolis, Indiana.

Data Analysis. Bleomycin, melphalan, and vinblastine plasma concentration versus time data obtained from each patient were fitted by computer to a multiexponential equation according to a nonlinear regression program NONLIN [9]. Preliminary parameter estimates were obtained by means of a computer method [13]. Calculations of plasma terminal-phase half-lives and areas under the plasma concentration versus time curves (CXT) after IP drug administration have been described in detail in a previous publication [3].

Results

Bleomycin Plasma and Urine Disposition. In Tables 2 and 3 are the mean pharmacokinetic parameters of IP and intravenous (IV) bleomycin, respectively, in groups of nine patients. For six patients with adequate renal function (i.e., creatinine clearance ≥ 50 ml/min), bleomycin's mean terminal-phase plasma half-life (± SD) after IP instillation of 5.5 ± 2.6 h was significantly longer the that previously reported [2] IV plasma half-life of 4.0 ± 0.6 h ($P < 0.01$). In these patients, bleomycin urinary excretion during the first 24 h was significantly lower following IP than following IV administration (23.5 ± 9.5% vs 44.8 ± 12.6%, respectively) ($P < 0.005$). The mean plasma CXT of 135 ± 87 mU · min/ml (normalized for a $t^{\beta}_{1/2}$ = 4.0 h and dose = 15 U/m^2) for the IP patients was significantly lower ($P < 0.001$) than that for the IV patients (i.e., 307 ± 60 mU · min/ml).
In one (EP, Table 2) of nine patients receiving IP bleomycin, the malignant effusion disappeared for more than 30 days. There was no obvious relationship between clinical response and length of bleomycin plasma half-life or size of plasma CXT. Aside from fevers of up to 39° C in six of the nine patients receiving IP bleomycin, there were no other serious clinical toxicities. These short-lived fevers were easily controlled with antihistamines and, if necessary, oral steroids.

Melphalan Plasma and Urine Disposition. In Tables 2 and 3 are the mean pharmacokinetic parameters of IP and IV [1] melphalan in groups of three and nine patients, respectively. Representative IP melphalan plasma disappearance curves in two patients are shown in Fig. 1. Peak melphalan plasma concentrations after 1 mg/kg in three patients varied between 0.34 and 0.71 µg/ml. The mean terminal-phase plasma half-life for the patients treated with IP and IV drug were similar (i.e., 1.3 and 1.4 h, respectively). The normalized plasma CXT (59 ± 36 µg · min/ml) and 24-h urinary excretion (5.1 ± 7.9%) resulting from IP melphalan instillation (Table 2) were significantly lower ($P < 0.05$) than those seen after IV dosing (Table 3). Two (EP_2 and LZ, Table 1) of three patients treated with IP melphalan responded with disappearance of malignant ascites for 4 and 6+ months, respectively. In one patient (VL, Table 1), it was too early to evaluate the result. Two (EP_2 and VL, Table 1) had moderately severe nausea and vomiting on the day of treatment. Bone marrow toxicity

Table 2. Mean pharmacokinetic parameters of bleomycin, melphalan, and vinblastine after intraperitoneal administration

Drug	$t_{1/2}^{\beta}$ (h)	CXT[a] (μG · min/ml)	Normalized CXT[b]	24-h Urinary excretion (% dose)	Response to therapy (%)[c]
Bleomycin	5.5 ± 2.6	904 ± 767	135 ± 87	23.5 ± 9.5[d]	11
Mephalan	1.3 ± 0.7	77 ± 27	59 ± 36	5.1 ± 7.9	67
Vinblastine	–	21[e]	–	–	0

[a] CTX concentration · time product of anticancer drugs in plasma. For bleomycin, CTX was measured in mU · min/ml

[b] CTX normalized in bleomycin patients for a $t_{1/2}^{\beta}$ = 4.0 h and bleomycin dose = 15 U/m²; normalized in melphalan patients for a $t_{1/2}^{\beta}$ = 1.4 h and melphalan dose = 0.6 mg/kg

[c] Response: disappearance of malignant effusion for > 30 days

[d] Mean urinary excretion data for only six of nine bleomycin-treated patients

[e] CXT for vinblastine calculated on basis of mean bolus IV plasma $t_{1/2}^{\beta}$ of 17.1 h [8, 11]

Table 3. Mean pharmacokinetic parameters of bleomycin and melphalan after bolus intravenous administration

Drug	$t_{1/2}^{\beta}$ (h)	Ctx[a] (μG · min/ml)	24-h Urinary excretion (% dose)
Bleomycin[b]	4.0 ± 0.6	307 ± 60	44.8 ± 12.6
Melphalan[c]	1.4 ± 0.8	151 ± 67	13.0 ± 5.4

[a] Bleomycin CXT was measured in mU · min/ml and was normalized for a $t_{1/2}^{\beta}$ = 4.0 h and bleomycin dose = 15 U/m²

[b] Data taken from ALBERTS et al. [2]

[c] Data taken from ALBERTS et al. [1]

was mild (nadir WBC > 3000/mm³ and platelets > 125,000/mm³) in all three patients.

Vinblastine Plasma Disappearance. As seen in Fig. 2, after the IP instillation of vinblastine, 7 mg/m², in patient EH peak plasma concentrations of 7–9 ng/ml were achieved within 30 min. These concentrations remained stable for up to 24 h when the last plasma samples were obtained. Although a plasma half-life could not be calculated, using a $t_{1/2}^{\beta}$ = 17.1 h, derived from IV data [8, 11], a plasma CXT for the IP drug was determined to be 21 μg · min/ml.

IP vinblastine was extremely toxic in both patients. Both developed severe adynamic ileus within 24 h of drug administration. Patient VO (Table 1) required exploratory laparotomy to relieve bowel obstruction related to ileus. Patient EH also experienced prolonged, although reversible, ileus and later died of progressive disease without response.

Systemic Availability of Intraperitoneal (IP) Bleomycin and Melphalan. In Table 4 are the ratios of IP to IV plasma terminal-phase half-life, CXT, and urinary excretion for

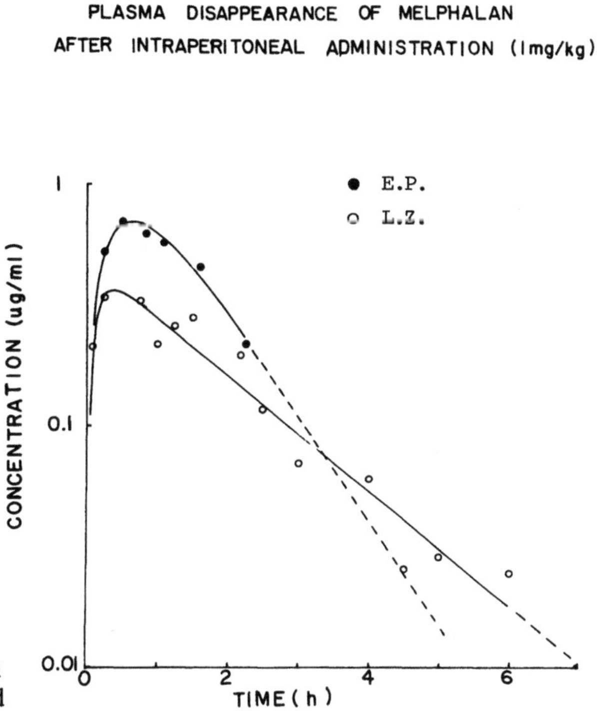

Fig. 1. Representative plasma disappearance curves in two patients (EP and LZ) who received IP melphalan as a single bolus injection into approximately 1 l of ascites fluid

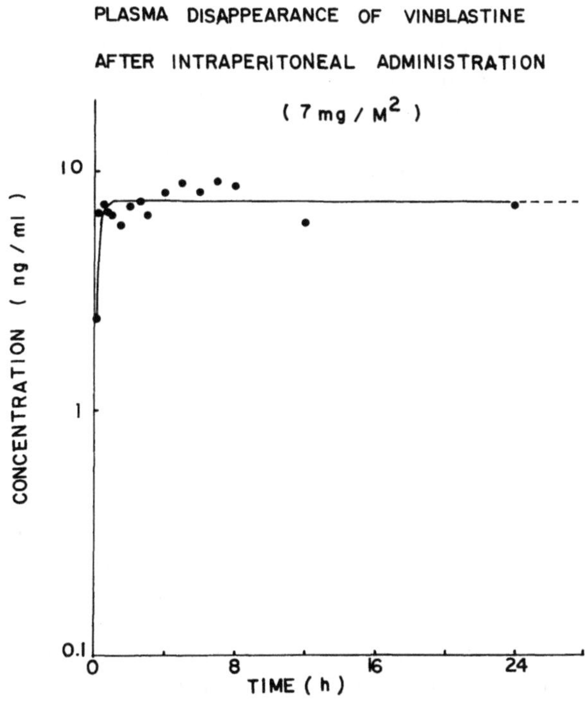

Fig. 2. Plasma disappearance curve in one patient (EH, Table 1) who received vinblastine as a single bolus IP dose

Table 4. Systemic availability of bleomycin and melphalan after intraperitoneal administration

Drug	Intraperitoneal–intravenous ratio		
	$t^{\beta}_{1/2}$	CXT[a]	Urinary excretion
Bleomycin	1.36	0.44	0.52
Melphalan	0.92	0.39	0.39

[a] CXT data for bleomycin normalized for a $t^{\beta}_{1/2} = 4.0$ h and dose = 15 U/m^2 and for a $t^{\beta}_{1/2} = 1.4$ h and dose = 0.6 mg/kg

bleomycin and melphalan. On the basis of these data, bleomycin appears to have a 44%–52% systemic availability and melphalan a 39% availability after IP administration.

Discussion

We have shown that both bleomycin and melphalan have limited systemic availability following IP bolus instillation. Absorption into the systemic circulation averaged 44%–52% for bleomycin and 39% for melphalan (Table 4). In ovarian cancer patients, the disease is usually limited to the IP space [15]. Thus, IP bleomycin and melphalan administration result in high concentrations of these drugs at the tumor site and decreased concentrations systemically at their targets of normal tissue toxicity.

Since total bleomycin dosage is limited by an increasing incidence of life-threatening pulmonary toxicity at approximately 500 U [6], the IP administration route may be the most advantageous for ovarian cancer patients. The same argument can be advanced for the IP use of melphalan in this patient population. It may be possible to double the standard, monthly dose of melphalan (i.e., 1 mg/kg) to 2 mg/kg if it is used IP. The resulting melphalan-induced bone marrow toxicity should approximate that associated with a 1-mg/kg IV dose, but the antitumor activity of the IP bolus may be increased.

Although vinblastine was only used IP in two patients, it was associated with life-threatening ileus in both. The greatly prolonged vinblastine plasma levels seen in one of these patients (EH, Table 2) may help to explain this excessive toxicity. As a result of this severe, but reversible, bowel disorder, we have terminated IP vinblastine trials.

The peritoneal dialysis technique for anticancer drug administration in ovarian cancer patients has many merits [7, 10, 12, 14]. It allows maximal exposure of IP tumor to high drug concentrations under tightly controlled conditions. However, it requires a highly trained medical staff, which currently is available only in a few institutions. The standard, IP bolus administration technique for anticancer drug treatment of ovarian cancer currently has more general applicability and can be highly effective. In the last analysis, clinical trials will establish which IP technique is of greatest utility.

Acknowledgments. We thank Dr. M. A. Root of the Eli Lilly Co., Indianapolis, Indiana for performing the vinblastine assays in plasma and Drs. Sydney E. Salmon,

Thomas E. Moon, and Joseph F. Gross for their scientific advice, and Thomas Evans, Nancy Mason, Kathy Griffith, Patricia Dombrowski, and Aurelia Chester for their technical assistance. This research was supported by grants CA-17094 and T32-GM007533 from the National Institutes of Health, U.S. Public Health Service, Department of Health, Education, and Welfare, and donations by Burroughs-Wellcome Co., Research Triangle Park, N.C., and The Phi Beta Sci National Sorority, Lima, Ohio.

References

1 Alberts DS (1979) Pharmakinetics of melphalan in man: intravenous administration. Clin Pharmacol Therap 26: 73–80

2 Alberts DS, (1978) Bleomycin pharmacokinetics in man. I. Intravenous administration. Cancer Chemother Pharmacol 1: 177–181

3 Alberts DS, Chen H-SG, Mayersohn M, Perrior D, Moon TE, Gross JF (1979) Bleomycin pharmacokinetics in man. II. Intracavitary administration. Cancer Chemother Pharmacol 2: 127–132

4 Broughton A, Strong JE (1976) Radioimmunoassay of bleomycin. Cancer Res 36: 1418–1421

5 Chang SY, Alberts DS, Melnick LR, Walson PD, Salmon SE (1978) High-pressure liquid chromatographic analysis of melphalan in plasma. J Pharm Sci 67: 679–681

6 Comis RL (1978) Bleomycin pulmonary toxicity. In: Carter SK, Crooke ST, Umezawa H (eds) Bleomycin: Current status and new developments. Academic Press, New York, pp 279–291

7 Dedrick RL, Myers CS, Bungay PM, DeVita VT Jr (1978) Pharmacokinetic rationale for peritoneal drug administration in the treatment of ovarian cancer. Cancer Treat Rep 62: 1–11

8 Lu K, Yep HY, Watts S, Loo TL (1979) Comparative clinical pharmacology of vinblastine (VBL) in patients with advanced breast cancer: Single versus continuous infusion. Proc Am Assoc Cancer Res and Am Soc Clin Oncol 20: C-333

9 Metzler CM (1969) NONLIN: A computer program for parameter estimation in nonlinear situations. Upjohn Co., Kalamazoo, Michigan (Technical Rep 7292/69/7292/005)

10 Myers C, Jones R, Londer H, Hubbard S, Brennan M, Balow J, Dedrick R, Ozols R, DeVita V (1978) Pharmacology of high-dose methotrexate (MTX) administered via peritoneal dialysis. Proc Am Assoc Cancer Res and Am Soc Clin Oncol 19: C-333

11 Owellen RJ, Hartke CA, Hains FO (1977) Pharmacokinetics and metabolism in vinblastine in humans. Cancer Res 37: 2597–2602

12 Ozols R, Grotzinger K, Myers C, Yong RC (1979) Ovarian cancer (OC): Intraperitoneal (I.P.) therapy with adriamycin (ADR). Proc Am Assoc Cancer Res and Am Soc Clin Oncol 20: 978

13 Sedman AJ, Wagner JG (1976) CSTRIP: A Fortran IV computer program for obtaining initial polyexponential parameter estimates. J Pharm Sci 65: 1006–1010

14 Speyer JL, Collins JM, Dedrick RL, Brennan H, Londer H, DeVita VT, Jr, Myers CE (1979) Phase I and pharmacological studies of intraperitoneal (I.P.) 5-fluorouracil (5.Fu). Proc Am Assoc Cancer Res and Am Soc Clin Oncol 19: C-333

15 Tobias JS, Griffiths CF (1976) Management of ovarian carcinoma. Current concepts and future prospects. Part 1. N Engl J Med 294: 818–822

Clinical Correlations of Drug Sensitivity in the Human Tumor Stem Cell Assay

S. E. Salmon, D. S. Alberts, B. G. M. Durie, F. L. Meyskens, S. E. Jones, B. Soehnlen, H.-S. G. Chen, and T. Moon

Summary

We have applied an in vitro soft-agar tumor-colony assay (which is now applicable to a variety of human cancers) to measurement of in vitro sensitivity to drugs and prediction of clinical response to cancer chemotherapy. The assay predicts drug resistance with 96% accuracy and sensitivity (in heavily pretreated patients) with 62% accuracy. On a pharmacokinetic basis the zone in vitro sensitivity for any given drug was only 5%–10% of the clinical concentration-time product (Cxt) achievable. This suggests that intratumoral drug concentrations in vivo may be lower than those in the plasma, and/or that > 2 log kills of tumor stem cells (not measurable in the assay) are required for clinical response. Serial in vitro studies showed that acquisition of drug resistance is a common clinical phenomenon which can be directly detected and quantitated in vitro.

Introduction

Of the various cells comprising a malignant tumor, the key replicative units appear to be the small fraction of clonogenic tumor cells or tumor stem cells [10, 14]. Studies of transplantable murine tumors had shown that the chemosensitivity of tumor stem cells was predictive of the in vivo therapeutic response to specific anticancer drugs [1, 9], again suggesting that these cells were highly relevant to the neoplastic process. Tumor stem cells appear to be central to the metastatic process, as they retain the capability to form secondary colonies at distant sites in the body (assuming that they can gain access to the circulation and find "fertile soil" for colonization [12]). The colony-forming capability of human tumor stem cells has recently been exploited through the development of simple in vitro colony assays in soft agar or other semisolid media. Our group at the University of Arizona Cancer Center initiated studies of human myeloma stem cells in 1975. The program was based on development by Hamburger and Salmon [4, 5] of a simple two-layer agar colony assay. Subsequently, our program was broadened considerably and enlarged in scale as the assay proved suitable to fresh biopsies of a variety of solid tumors as well as myelomas and lymphomas [3–7]. Ovarian carcinoma [6] and melanoma [8] are two solid tumors which have been particularly easy to study with this system, as tissue for biopsy is often readily available, and excellent in vitro tumor-colony growth is obtained frequently. Table 1 summarizes the range of tumors which we have successfully cultured with this assay. Von Hoff et al. at the National Cancer Institute recently reported independent validation of this assay system [15].

Table 1. Human tumor types successfully cultured directly from biopsies with the bioassay for tumor stem cells (of Hamburger and Salmon)[a]

Carcinomas	Sarcomas and other neoplasms
(Adeno, squamous and undifferentiated variants for carcinomas of various sites)	Chronic lymphocytic leukemia
	Diffuse lymphomas
Adrenal	Ewing's tumor
Bladder	Fibrosarcoma
Breast	Hodgkin's disease
Colon	Liposarcoma
Kidney	Macroglobulinemia
Lung	Melanoma (melanotic and amelanotic)
Ovary	Multiple myeloma
Pancreas	Nephroblastoma (Wilms' tumor)
Prostate	Neuroblastoma
Thyroid	Nodular lymphomas
Upper airways (head and neck)	Rhabdomyosarcoma
Uterus (corpus and cervix)	
Unknown primary (squamous)	

[a] Summary as of May, 1979; more than 500 biopsy samples tested, including primary tumors and metastases

In June 1978, we published our first report on the use of the human tumor assay system for measurement of drug sensitivity in 18 patients with myeloma or ovarian cancer [13]. That report provided preliminary evidence that the assay system might prove useful for prediction of clinical response as well as playing a role in new drug development. The purpose of this report is to update our experience to May 1979. Thus, it includes the 32 clinical correlations reported previously [13].

Materials and Methods

Detailed descriptions of the methods of cell culture and measurement of drug sensitivity have been reported previously [3, 4, 6, 13]. In brief, a single cell suspension is prepared from the tumor biopsy using mechanical dissociation techniques. Aliquots of cells are exposed for 1 h at 37° C to at least three concentrations of each of a series of 6–10 anticancer drugs. Drugs are studied in vitro only at low concentrations generally ranging up to 1.0 μg/ml, with emphasis on concentration-time exposures (Cxt) which are in a range which would be pharmacologically achievable in vivo. Subsequently, the cells are washed twice by centrifugation, and suspended at a concentration of 500,000 cells/ml in an enriched tissue culture medium containing 0.3% molten agar; 1 ml of this mixture is plated in each 35-ml plastic Petri dish on top of a 0.5% agar feeder layer containing various nutrients and growth stimulants. All drug assay points are plated in triplicate and incubated at 37° C in a humidified CO_2 incubator for 2–3 weeks and evaluated serially by inverted phase microscopy and counted when a sufficient number of colonies (consisting of > 30 cells) have developed to permit measurement of a 1–2 log reduction in survival of colony-forming units. A sensitivity index is computed from the area under survival-concentration curves using a linear scale out to an upper limit which is defined by clinically achievable dosage exposures. For any given drug, patients are ranked with respect to the in vitro sensitivity index (area under the curve) and the initial spread of clinical responses used to create a training set to determine boundaries between sensitivity and resistance. Proof of the neoplastic nature of the colonies is routinely obtained using a newly developed dried-slide technique [11] which provides exellent morphology for pathology review.

While such drug sensitivity assays have been carried out on more than 200 biopsy samples, the current report relates only to studies in 66 patients who (a) had sensitivity to multiple agents measured in vitro and (b) had retrospective or prospective data available for independent clinical evaluation of therapeutic response in vivo. Drugs studies in vitro included melphalan, doxorubicin, BCNU, methotrexate, vinblastine, cisplatinum, bleomycin, fluorouracil, actinomycin, dacarbazine, and m-AMSA. Clinical trials generally included either single-agent chemotherapy or simple two-drug combinations. Prospective selection of specific agents for clinical trial on the basis of marked in vitro sensitivity proved feasible in ten instances. Aside from these instances, prospective trials were initiated independently of the in vitro assay results. Standard criteria of response were employed as reported previously [13].

Results and Discussion

A total of 148 clinical correlations of in vitro and in vivo sensitivity or resistance could be made in the 66 patients reported. Many of these patients could be analyzed for one retrospective correlation and one or more prospective correlations in relation to clinical trials carried out subsequent to the in vitro assay. Each correlation was based on single clinical trial (generally 6 weeks in duration) with a single agent or simple drug combination. The overall results of these studies are summarized in Table 2. The predominant tumor categories included were myeloma, ovarian carcinoma, and melanoma, with the miscellaneous category consisting of patients with diffuse histiocytic lymphoma, oat cell carcinoma of the lung, or hypernephroma.

Despite the fact that many of these patients had been heavily pretreated, a total of 42 correlations could be made when the in vitro assay showed sensitivity. In 26 (62%) of these instances, the patient also showed a clinical response to treatment. Drugs uncommonly used for certain tumors were sometimes identified and proved effective. Examples include cis-platinum or actinomycin for melanoma, and bleomycin or vinblastine for ovarian cancer. All responses were at least partial responses except for two of the four melanoma patients who had mixed responses (one to BCNU-dacarbazine, and the second to m-AMSA). This suggests that more clonal heterogeneity of metastases might be present in melanoma, and necessitate multiple biopsies for assay when feasible. Patients who achieved clinical responses with the agents to which they showed sensitivity in vitro uniformly manifested exquisite in vitro sensitivity. Thus, the Cxt required in vitro to fall in the sensitive zone on the sensitivity index rankings was only 5%–10% of the pharmacologically achievable Cxt or peak concentration achievable in vivo.

We would propose that two separate explanations may be related to this requirement for exquisite in vitro sensitivity. Firstly, the intratumoral drug concentrations achieved in vivo may be far lower than those measurable in the plasma. Secondly, while the in vitro assay has a sensitivity limit of 1–2 logs in vitro (based on assay design), clinical response may require a 3 or more log reduction in survival of tumor stem cells, and hence require a Cxt of the drug in vivo which is ten times that which can be measured in

Table 2. Update of correlations of in vitro and in vivo sensitivity to anticancer drugs (May 1979)

Tumor type	No. of points	No. of clinical trials for correlations	Tumor sensitive both in vitro and in vivo	Tumor sensitive in vitro and resistant in vivo	Tumor resistant in vitro and sensitive in vivo	Tumor resistant both in vitro and in vivo
Ovarian	25	72	9	7	1	55
Myeloma	20	48	12	6	1	29
Melanoma	18	24	4[a]	3	2	15
Misc.[b]	3	4	1	0	0	3
Total	66	148	26 (62% true positive)	16	4	102 (96% true negative)

[a] Mixed responses
[b] The miscellaneous category includes one patient each with oat cell carcinoma (sensitive in vitro and in vivo) and one each with hypernephroma and lymphoma both of whom were resistant. With the Fisher exact test [2] the association of in vitro and in vivo results was highly significant ($P < 0.000001$)

vitro with this assay. Both explanations may well apply in many instance. A total of 106 correlations were obtained where in vitro resistance was observed. In 96% of the correlations where in vitro resistance was manifest, the patients also failed to respond to this treatment in vivo. Thus, this assay has extraordinary power to predict which drugs will only cause toxicity, and to indicate that they can be deleted from clinical trial. Patients who failed to respond to agents in vivo sometimes had in vitro survival-concentration curves showing resistance to levels of drug which exceeded the clinically achievable Cxt by a factor of 10 or more with no evidence of drug-induced lethality over the entire dose range tested. More frequently, however, the in vitro response was one suggesting an admixture of sensitive and resistant tumor stem cells within the biopsy sample. Such in vitro survival curves showed an initial steep slope with lethality to 40%–60% of the tumor colony-forming units at low doses of the drug, but with a plateau of resistant cells whose survival was not decreased even at drug doses above the normal range (10–100 μg/ml). Such curves were observed even with cycle-nonspecific drugs such as melphalan, doxorubicin, and cis-platinum. Our overall experience with prediction of sensitivity or resistance with the assay is extremely good. Using the Fisher exact test [2] the probability that the correlations shown in Table 1 could be due to chance alone is less than one in one million ($P < 0.000001$). Serial studies of in vitro drug sensitivity proved feasible in seven patients who recieved treatment with the drug tested between the two serial assays. These results are summarized in Table 3. Twelve individual comparisons could be made. In six instances the in vitro sensitivity index (expressed as area under the curve) did not change between assays. Two of these were patients who were sensitive and responded to treatment, relapsed of treatment and could be subsequently reinduced into remission again (e.g., myeloma with melphalan). Four patients who were initially resistant in vitro remained so when retested in vitro after failing to respond to the same agent in vivo.

Table 3. Serial in vitro sensitivity studies in seven patients

Sensitivity index[a]	No. of instances	Circumstance
No change	6	2 s→s (sensitive on both tests) 4 r→r (resistant on both tests)
Increase	6	3 s→r (conversion from sensitive to resistant) 3 r→R (increasing resistance)
Decrease	0	

[a] Area under the in vitro survival concentration curve

In six instances, the sensitivity index (area under the curve) increased by at least 50%. In three of these, the patients converted from sensitive to resistant in vitro after having had an initial response followed by a relapse on treatment as well. Three patients who failed to respond to treatment also had an increased area under the curve as well indicating increasing drug resistance of the tumor stem cells. In no instance did a patient show evidence of increasing in vitro sensitivity (decreased sensitivity index) on serial testing. Based on this relatively small experience to date with serial testing, the general pattern appears to be one of progressive acquisition of increasing drug resistance to single agents with which the patients were treated. Thus, the acquisition of drug resistance is a common phenomenon which can be directly detected and quantitated in vitro.

While the focus of this report has been on clinical drug testing and prediction of response, it is clear to us from our various studies that the in vitro assay may have many other uses. Not only should such a system be useful for a variety of investigations of cancer biology [e.g., 12]. It also could greatly simplify preclinical screening of cytotoxic, hormonal, and immunotherapeutic agents as well as for studying potential new and innovative treatment modalities. We are currently working on automated technique for tumor-colony counting which should greatly facilitate such applications of the assay system.

Acknowledgments. The authors wish to acknowledge the scientific input of ANNE HAMBURGER, Ph.D., RONALD BUICK, Ph.D., GENE GERNER, Ph.D., JEFF TRENT, Ph.D., and STEPHEN E. JONES, M.D. in these culture studies; the laboratory skills of Ms. LAURIE YOUNG and Ms. YVETTE FRUTIGER; the computer systems efforts of Ms. DALE CURTIS; and the helpful patient referrals from a large number of Arizona physicians. This research was supported in part by grants CA 17094, CA 21839, and CA 23074 from the U.S. Public Health Service, Bethesda, Maryland.

References

1 Bruce WR, Meeker BE, Valeriote FA (1966) Comparison of the sensitivity of normal hematopoietic and transplanted lymphoma colony-forming cells to chemotherapeutic agents administered in vivo. J Natl Cancer Inst 37: 233–245
2 Fisher RA (1960) The design of experiments, 7th edn. Hafner, New York
3 Hamburger AW, Kim MB, Salmon SE (1979) The nature of cells generating human myeloma colonies in vitro. J Cell Physiol 98: 371–376

4 Hamburger A, Salmon SE (1977) Primary bioassay of human myeloma stem cells. J Clin Invest 60: 846–854
5 Hamburger AW, Salmon SE (1977) Primary bioassay of human tumor stem cells. Science 197: 461–463
6 Hamburger AW, Salmon SE, Kim MB, Trent SM, Soehnlen BJ, Alberts DS, Schmidt HJ (1978) Direct cloning of human ovarian carcinoma cells in agar. Cancer Res 38: 3438–3443
7 Jones SE, Hamburger AW, Kim MB, Salmon SE (1979) Development of a bioassay for putative human lymphoma stem cells. Blood 53: 294–303
8 Meyskens FL, Salmon SE (1979) Inhibition of human melanoma colony formation by retinoids. Cancer Res 40: 4055–4057
9 Ogawa M, Bergsagel DE, McCulloch EA (1973) Chemotherapy of mouse myeloma: Quantitative cell culture predictive of response in vivo. Blood 41: 7–15
10 Park CH, Bergsagel DE, McCulloch EA (1971) Mouse myeloma tumor stem cells: A primary cell culture assay. J Natl Cancer Inst 46: 411–422
11 Salmon SE (1980) Morphologic studies of tumor colonies. In: Salmon SE (ed) Cloning of human tumor stem cells. Alan Liss, New York
12 Salmon SE, Hamburger AW (1978) Immunoproliferation and cancer: A common macrophage-derived promoter substance. Lancet 1: 1289–1290
13 Salmon SE, Hamburger AW, Soehnlen BJ, Durie BGM, Alberts DS, Moon TC (1978) Quantitation of differential sensitivities of human tumor stem cells to anticancer drugs. N Engl J Med 298: 1321–1327
14 Steel CG (1973) Cytokinetics of neoplasia. In: Holland JF, Frei E III (eds) Cancer medicine. Lea and Febiger, Philadelphia
15 Von Hoff DD, Johnson GE (1979) Secretion of tumor markers in the human tumor stem cell system. Proc Am Assoc Cancer Res 20: (abstr 206)

Comments on the Carcinogenic, Mutagenic, and Teratogenic Properties of Anticancer Drugs

F. M. Muggia and J. Ziegler

Summary

Relevance of the carcinogenic effects of anticancer agents has arisen in the context of three circumstances: (a) when patients who have a favorable outlook *without* treatment receive chemotherapy, (b) when several alternate therapies with varying carcinogenic potential are available, and (c) when considering the introduction of a new drug into clinical investigation and/or clinical practice. Teratogenic effects require special attention when dealing with women in their reproductive years. Techniques to evaluate the mutagenic effects have opened up new areas of research and will be increasingly applied to the study of anticancer drugs.

Introduction

Since anticancer agents most often exert their cytotoxic action by interaction with macromolecules transmitting genetic information, it is not surprising that many of them are mutagenic and carcinogenic. The teratogenic properties of these drugs may be related to their effects on proliferating and differentiating tissues, such as those in the developing embryo. Indirect mutagenic effects on germ cells may also result in teratogenesis. Because of their somewhat specialized interest, teratogenic effects will not be discussed further.

Concern about the mutagenic and carcinogenic effects of established anticancer drugs after successful cancer treatment arises in three possible contexts: (a) when chemotherapy is applied to individuals with expected long-term survival, (b) when the choice of several effective therapies exists, and (c) when considering the introduction of a new agent. Following description of the experience with carcinogenic and mutagenic properties of current anticancer drugs, each one of these situations will be reviewed separately.

Experience with Current Anticancer Drugs

Studies of lymphocyte mutants lacking hypoxanthine-guanine phosphoribosyl transferase (as determined by their resistance to 6-thioguanine) indicate the selective emergence of cell populations following prolonged exposure to chemotherapy [11]. The biologic significance of such mutants is currently speculative. Nevertheless, the identification of genetic abnormalities among normal cell populations exposed to chemotherapeutic agents constitutes an important area of future study. For example, males with Hodgkin's disease have shown a high incidence of aspermia and sterility following MOPP chemotherapy [12], but women have conceived normally following similar therapy. Evaluation of offspring of individuals who have been cured of childhood cancer and the long-term follow-up of these patients are other important areas for study [7].

There has been increasing awareness of the carcinogenic potential of current anticancer therapy. Such concern once again has arisen primarily from studies of surviving patients with Hodgkin's disease [3, 4]. The risk of developing acute leukemia increases progressively with time after chemotherapy, and is particularly high after combined chemo- and radiotherapy. The chemotherapeutic agents implicated have been nitrogen mustard and procarbazine in the MOPP combination. Alkylating agents such as L-phenylalanine mustard (L-PAM), chlorambucil, and cyclophosphamide have also been implicated in the development of acute leukemia following treatment of multiple myeloma [10]. These and thiotepa have also contributed to the risk of acute leukemia following successful chemotherapy of advanced ovarian cancer, which also often occurred in association with prior irradiation [9]. Treosulfan, hydroxybusulfan, and other drugs related to busulfan have also been implicated in the leukemia associated with this disease. A common finding in the development of leukemia has been the occurrence of prolonged bone marrow suppression. Short-term administration of alkylating agents, such as the NSABP studies with thiotepa in breast cancer adjuvant, have not yielded definite evidence of leukemogenesis [6].

The type of agents used is undoubtedly important. Alkylating agents and procarbazine are leukemogenic to other mammals [2]. Methylnitrosourea and chlorethylnitrosoureas are also highly carcinogenic to animals [1], but information from clinical studies in the USSR and USA, respectively, with regard to leukemogenesis have not been forthcoming. Other antineoplastic agents such as streptozotocin (related to methylnitrosourea) and adriamycin also show considerable carcinogenicity in animal systems, but such effects in man are not yet supported by clinical data. A number of case reports exist linking busulfan to the development of epithelial malignancies. The association of cytologic dysplasia with busulfan has also been prominent. The development of secondary neoplasms from prolonged administration of azathioprine and steroids, with or without alkylating agents, has also been noted in renal transplant recipients and other patients receiving drug regimens as immunosuppressives. These neoplasms have been predominantly epithelial and lymphoreticular in origin, particularly malignant lymphoma and Kaposi sarcoma [13].

On the other hand, carcinogenesis has not been associated with antimetabolites such as 5-fluorouracil and methotrexate, although thorough and systematic clinical studies have not been performed. The Environmental Epidemiology Branch of the NCI is now carrying out prospective surveillance of various clinical trials with regard to long-term complications (Table 1). Of interest is an analysis by the National Wilms Tumor Study Group indicating a lower incidence of second tumors in patients receiving both actinomycin D and radiation, than in those receiving radiation alone [5]. In addition, in some conditions, such as stage I lung cancer, a higher incidence of second primary malignancies has been reported in those patients not receiving adjuvant therapy than in those receiving cyclophosphamide.

Table 1. Studies of secondary malignancy risks by the environmental epidemiology branch (NCI)

Type of cancer (group)	Therapy	Trial years	Type of study (no. of patients)
Cervix (International Cervical Cancer Study)	Radium vs X-ray vs X-ray + radium vs surgery	1960–1969	Retrospective (4,200, 2,400, 20,700, 2,700)
Ovarian stages IA or IB (GOG-1)	Melphalan vs survery vs radiation	1971–present	Retrospective, prospective (96, 52, 44)
Ovarian (Princess Margaret)	Chlorambucil + RT vs RT	1971–1974	Retrospective (71, 120)
Breast			
(NSABP-5)	Melphalan vs placebo	1972–present	Prospective (179, 169)
(NSABP-7)	Melphalan vs melphalan + 5-Fu	1975–present	Prospective (306, 299)
(NSABP-4)	Radical mastectomy vs total vs total + radiation	1971–present	Prospective (355, 344, 282)
Colorectal (VASAG)	Thiotepa vs control 5-FUDR vs control	1957–1961 1962–1964	Retrospective (470, 530) Retrospective (276, 300)
Colon (GITSG 6,175)	5-FU + MeCCNU + MER; MER alone; surgery alone	1975–present	Prospective (> 600)
Colon (ECOG 2,276)	5-FU + MeCCNU vs 5-FU	1976–present	Prospective (> 600)
Rectum (GITSG 7,175)	RT + 5-FU + MeCCNU; 5-FU + MeCCNU alone; surgery alone	1975–present	Prospective (> 600)
Rectum (ECOG 4,276)	Same as above except for surgery alone	1976–present	Prospective (> 450)
Ewing's sarcoma (NCI)	5,000 rad + chemotherapy	1964–1979	Retrospective (135)
Non-Hodgkin's lymphoma (NCI)	Chemotherapy	1950–1979	Retrospective (600)

Future Considerations

Circumstances Associated with Long-Term Survival

The importance of carcinogenicity of anticancer drugs emerges primarily in those circumstances where therapy is applied to patients with potentially long-term survival. In general, however, other side effects of treatment pose an even greater threat to these patients. For example, adjuvant therapy in osteogenic sarcoma may be given to 25% of patients who would presumably be cured by surgical resection alone. Patients with stages I and II breast cancer normally may expect 65% and 25% 10-year survival, respectively. The carcinogenic risk of adjuvant chemotherapy must be balanced against the potential benefit in those patients who will relapse.

Similar considerations arise when very effective chemotherapy is introduced in patients whose disease stage is already associated with reasonable survival. Illustrative in this regard are the early stages of Hodgkin's disease and testicular carcinoma. In these and other circumstances, careful clinical studies should balance the relative effectiveness and risk of such initial treatment strategy as opposed to effective "salvage" therapy [8].

The threat of exposing cured cancer patients to the carcinogenic insult of chemotherapy may be overstated. Risks such as immunosuppression and specific organ toxicity as well as recurrence of the disease itself probably pose a greater threat than induction of a second cancer in most instances. Witness, for example, the results from lung and colon cancer or melanoma adjuvant studies of the last two decades. Nevertheless, caution is required when designing therapies for these and the above circumstances. Also, the more effective the adjuvant therapy, the less would be the concern for these secondary effects, except when such therapy is just as effective when given as "salvage" in the event of relapse.

Carcinogenicity as Determinant in Treatment Selection

Efficacy is the major consideration in selection of therapy. However, as our knowledge of carcinogenic risks increases, it will be possible to select therapies under specific circumstances which reduce these risks. In fact, combination regimens for Hodgkin's disease are being examined critically in light of the enhanced risk of leukemia. The individual components of the MOPP combination are undergoing scrutiny in determining their contribution to this enhanced risk. Requiring confirmation and longer follow-up is the report of a reduced risk for combined radiation and ABVD [15]. By the same token, trials using nitrosoureas in this disease must be followed carefully.

A major concern in the selection of appropriate agents and regimens associated with lower carcinogenic risks arises with the adjuvant treatment of breast cancer. Combinations of antimetabolites have been given to stage I patients in order to avoid carcinogenic drugs; the clinical value of such adjuvant therapy remains unproven. There has been concern in current programs containing alkylating agents and adriamycin administered to patients with stage I breast cancer, because of the relatively good outlook for these patients. Proponents of such therapy, however, justify it by pointing to the relatively high relapse rate in untreated patients, the poor results of salvage therapy upon recurrence, and the lessened risk of carcinogenesis since chemotherapy duration may be appropriately shortened in this favorable group. The current generation of adjuvant trials in stage II breast cancer are only now reaching the fifth year median duration of follow-up, and it is too early even to estimate the carcinogenic potential of such regimens. Nevertheless, current concepts favor the shortest possible intensive course of adjuvant therapy consistent with maximal efficacy. Low-dose attenuated chemotherapy is theoretically unsound, since it exposes the patient to carcinogenic risks without the likelihood of effective tumoricidal treatment.

Carcinogenicity as a Factor in Drug Development

Since many effective anticancer drugs are carcinogenic, such a feature must be regarded as undesirable in the selection of new drugs. Moreover, carcinogenicity and mutagenicity are an expected consequence of the interaction of many of these compounds with DNA and other cellular macromolecules. The relationship between carcinogenicity and antitumor effects is the subject of investigations within the Division of Cancer Treatment [1, 2].

The development of simplified tests for mutagenicity (Ames test) has added a new dimension in the evaluation of all chemicals introduced for human use. Remarkable differences may be seen in mutagenic potential within the same class of agents. For example, studies indicate that the newly introduced anthracycline antibiotic aclacinomycin A is markedly less mutagenic than adriamycin in these systems [14]. The relevance of these findings to the clinical application of these analogues cannot be presently ascertained, nor can mutagenicity be predictive of carcinogenicity in man.

Only rarely has the threat of carcinogenicity curtailed development of an anticancer agent. The antibiotic sterigmatocystin was shown to induce liver neoplasms in drug concentrations that were within the range of its antitumor effects (R. H. Adamson, unpublished work). This potent organ-specific phenomenon plus its relatively narrow spectrum of effectiveness in experimental systems led to discontinuation of its development toward the clinic.

Conclusion

Carcinogenic and mutagenic effects of anticancer drugs are the subject of increasing practical concern as the outlook of patients receiving such drugs improves. Although these effects are not the primary consideration in therapeutic trials, efforts to document possible risks are important and in specific circumstances may lead to modifications in trial design or to the pursuit of other therapeutic alternatives. For instance, in the treatment of Hodgkin's disease, the enhanced risk of combined radiation and chemotherapy regimens must be considered in relation to the lesser efficacy of single modalities. The success of "salvage" therapy renders less efficacious but "safer" primary treatments just as optimal. Breast cancer represents a different circumstance. The rationale for adjuvant therapy is well founded, but various treatment alternatives differ considerably in their carcinogenic potential. The main objective remains superior efficacy, but as more data on carcinogenic risks accumulate, adjuvant regimens may be altered. Still another example is osteosarcoma, where the relative efficacy of adjuvant chemotherapy is in doubt; up to 40% of patients may require no therapy other than surgery, and chemotherapy in advanced stages has been only modestly effective [8]. This dilemma can only be resolved through careful monitoring of such studies and related clinical experience.

Finally, it is also important to begin investigating the *active* prevention of second cancers, through administration of compounds capable of interrupting the progression from a carcinogenic insult to overt neoplasia. In this regard, clinical trials are beginning with 13-cisretinoic acid or related compounds for populations at high risk of developing malignancies. Such a concept must also be extended in the future to those patients receiving treatment with anticancer drugs.

References

1 Adamson RH, Krolikowski FJ, Correa P, Sieber SM, Dalgard DW (1977) Carcinogenicity of 1-methyl-1-nitrosourea in nonhuman primates. J Natl Cancer Inst 59: 415–419

2 Adamson RH, Sieber SM (1977) Carcinogenic potential of cancer chemotherapy agents in man. Cancer Bull 29: 179–183

3 Arsenau JC, Canellos GP, Johnson R, DeVita VT Jr (1977) Risks of new cancers in patients with Hodgkin's disease. Cancer 40: 1912–1916

4 Coleman NC, Williams CJ, Flint A, Glatstein EJ, Rosenberg SA, Kaplan HS (1977) Hematologic neoplasia in patients treated for Hodgkin's disease. N Engl J Med 297: 1249–1257

5 D'Angio GJ, Meadows AT, Miké V, Harris C, Evans A, Jaffe N, Newton W, Schweisguth O, Sutow W, Morris-Jones P (1976) Decreased risk of radiation-associated second malignant neoplasms in actinomycin-D-treated patients. Cancer 37: 1177–1185

6 Greene MH, Boice JD, Keehn RJ, Higgins GA, Fraumeni JF (1979) Late effects of low dose adjuvant chemotherapy in colorectal cancer. Proc Am Assoc Cancer Res and Am Soc Clin Oncol 20: 413

7 Li FP (1977) Second malignant tumors after cancer in childhood. Cancer 40: 1899–1902

8 Muggia F, Catane R, Lee YJ, Rozencweig M (1979) Factors responsible for therapeutic success in osteosarcoma: A critical analysis of adjuvant trial results. In: Salmon S, Jones SE (eds) Adjuvant therapy in man. Elsevier/North-Holland, Amsterdam, pp 383–390

9 Reimer RR, Hoover R, Fraumeni JF Jr, Young RC (1977) Acute leukemia after alkylating-agent therapy of ovarian cancer. N Engl J Med 297: 177–181

10 Rosner F (1976) Acute leukemia as a delayed consequence of cancer chemotherapy. Cancer 37: 1033–1036

11 Scott D, Bridges BA, Sobels FH (1977) Progress in genetic toxicology. Elsevier/North-Holland, Amsterdam

12 Sherins RJ, DeVita VT Jr (1973) Effect of drug treatment for lymphoma on male reproductive capacity. Ann Intern Med 79: 216–220

13 Stribling J, Weitzner S, Smith GV (1978) Kaposi's sarcoma in renal allograft recipient. Cancer 47: 442–446

14 Sugimura T, Matsushima T, Sawamura M, Seino Y, Yahagi T, Nagao M (1978) Predication of risk of a second tumor and use of the mutation test for monitoring improvement of drugs. In: Carter SK, Goldin A, Kuretani K, Mathé G, Sakurai Y, Tsukagoshi S, Umezawa H (eds) Advances in cancer chemotherapy

15 Valagussa P, Kenda R, Fossati Bellani F, Franchi F, Banfi A, Rilke F, Bonadonna G (1979) Incidence of second malignancies in Hodgkin's disease (HD) after various forms of treatment. Proc Am Assoc Cancer Res and Am Soc Clin Oncol 20: 360

Long-Term Sequelae of Cancer Chemotherapy

J. Ziegler and F. M. Muggia

Summary

Long-term sequelae of therapy of neoplastic disease have become an important topic, since many patients exposed to anticancer drugs will have prolonged survival. The advances which have been made in the treatment of pediatric malignancies, in fact, give particular relevance to a study of these complications. Moreover, clues as to the mechanism of action and molecular pharmacology of these agents may emerge from such studies. Herein we review both the *specific organ dysfunction* and the *generalized effects* which may become apparent as late consequences of chemotherapy.

Introduction

Successful therapy has resulted in an increasing number of cures among cancer victims. The cure rate is particularly notable among patients under age 35, where considerable strides have been made in lowering the death rate. These advances have been achieved mainly through the introduction of chemotherapy and its integration with surgery, radiation, or both local modalities. As a consequence, we have become increasingly concerned with long-term complications of therapy. Identification of specific toxicities may provide an indication of occasionally subtle drug effects which would otherwise go unrecognized. This review describes long-term complications of anticancer drugs which have become apparent in the last few years, and which have been revealed by surveillance of cancer patients who are long survivors after treatment with chemotherapy.

Sequelae from Specific Organ Dysfunction

Cardiac Toxicity. Both daunorubicin and adriamycin induce dose-dependent cardiotoxicity manifested by congestive heart failure and cardiomyopathy. Such a complication occurs variably after interruption of therapy and is somewhat unpredictable [12]. Efforts have been ongoing in defining susceptibility factors and in monitoring toxicity. Furthermore, the development of analogues lacking cardiac toxicity, as well as protective measures which may avert cardiac damage, has been investigated recently [1]. In addition, study of this phenomenon promises to shed some light on the mechanism of cytotoxicity of these drugs. Research on anthracycline toxicity is particularly important because of the widespread therapeutic role these drugs have acquired.

Liver Toxicity. Methotrexate has been known to induce cirrhosis, and this prompted its withdrawal from use in patients with psoriasis. Long-term administration was believed to predispose to these hepatic lesions [5]. 6-Mercaptopurine and related antimetabolites have also been associated with liver dysfunction and, more recently, are incriminated in veno-occlusive disease leading to a Budd-Chiari-type syndrome. It is very difficult to separate drug-induced liver dysfunction in patients with leukemia from complications which arise from the disease itself, from associated infections, or from administration of blood products or other measures of support which frequently accompany the treatment of leukemia [6].

Renal Toxicity. Renal damage caused by drugs may lead to cumulative long-term renal dysfunction. Both streptozotocin and cisplatin may be associated with chronic renal disease, following acute damage. In fact, a recent Southwest Oncology Group study indicates progressive renal function impairment after repeated courses of 75 mg/m^2 of cisplatin every 3 weeks given to 76 patients with genitourinary or gynecologic tumors [8]. In 11 patients, the mean creatinine clearance was 123 ml/min prior to the first course and 60 ml/min prior to the sixth course ($P = 0.01$).

A recent report indicates that chloroethyl nitrosoureas may lead to silent, but progressive, manifestations of renal failure. These have been known to occur upon repeated administration of relatively high doses of at least two nitrosoureas [3, 11]. This observation raises concern regarding the use of these drugs for adjuvant chemotherapy. An extensive case review is ongoing to establish the relative risk for patients so treated.

Central Nervous System (CNS) Toxicity. CNS toxicity of chemotherapy is reported with increasing frequency. A syndrome of dementia, blindness, and progressive invalidism ascribed to progressive multifocal leukoencephalopathy occurs as a result of methotrexate treatment. The interaction of radiation and chemotherapy as commonly employed in the prophylaxis of meningeal leukemia greatly increases the frequency of this manifestation [4]. The clinician must be alert to other possible deleterious drug-radiation interactions resulting in CNS disease.

More subtle manifestations of CNS disease have been uncovered through serial computerized tomography examination and tests of intellectual functions [7]. Prospective studies directed toward the recognition of long-term sequelae are an important area of clinical research.

Another form of CNS toxicity is chronic peripheral neuropathy, which occurs after prolonged vincristine administration. Although usually reversible, some manifestations may persist for years. Such patients also have increased susceptibility to the development of neuropathy following administration of other drugs [13].

Gonadal Toxicity. Germ cells in the mature male have been susceptible to damage from a number of cytotoxic agents. Oligospermia and testicular biopsies documenting tubular atrophy with absent to near-absent spermatogenesis have been observed frequently after administration of alkylating agents. Endocrine abnormalities include elevations of follicle-stimulating hormone (FSH) with normal testosterone levels. In adolescents receiving MOPP, however, possible damage to Leydig cell function resulting in gynecomastia and elevated luteinizing hormone (LH) levels has been described [10]. Women frequently manifest amenorrhea and elevations of FSH under similar therapies. However, resumption of menses and successful pregnancies after prolonged cytotoxic therapy have been reported. The entire field of reproductive malfunction in patients receiving chemotherapy requires more thorough and systematic prospective study.

Miscellaneous Organ Toxicities. Bladder fibrosis and severe dysfunction may result from prolonged administration of cyclophosphamide, particularly in children [2]. On occasion, "recall' cystitis may occur on exposure to other drugs. Bladder cancer has also been reported to arise from these irreversibly damaged bladders [15]. Dysfunction of endocrine organs, special senses, gastrointestinal tracts, and lungs has not been considered among late sequelae in the absence of preceding acute manifestations. Pulmonary toxicity is usually preceded by acute manifestations, but may appear as a late consequence of treatment with certain drugs [14]. Enhanced bone resorption occurs with glucocorticoids, but the contribution of other drugs has not been adequately studied.

Generalized Effects

Impairment of Growth and Development. Definite evidence of growth changes attributed to chemotherapy has not been reported. A recent report, however, indicates a decrease in lung volume, and narrowed thoracic diameter was present in children treated with cyclophosphamide [14]. Hormonal replacement therapy is, of course, necessary to maintain normal sexual development if damage to the gonads has been produced, as reported in adolescent males [9].

Impairment of Hemopoiesis and Immunity. The bone marrow is a major site of acute drug toxicity from chemotherapeutic agents. Prolonged dysfunction may result which can be related to the type of drug used, the intensity of treatment, the previous integrity of the target organ, and the efficiency of repair mechanisms. Such dysfunction has been linked to the predisposition toward subsequent acute leukemia.
Another prominent consequence of cytotoxic drugs is prolonged lymphocytopenia and impairment of immune function. Predisposition to a variety of infections, particularly of viral and fungal etiology, results from chronic immune deficiency in such patients. Additional detailed studies on this subject are needed.

Teratogenesis. Although teratogenic effects have been amply demonstrated in pregnant animals, data in human studies are scanty. Series describing the outcome of pregnancy in women given aminopterin, 6-mercaptopurine, azathioprine, and alkylating agents have been reported. Fortunately, malformations have rarely been reported. Consequences of germ cell damage in men and women have not been documented.

Second Cancers. This area has received the most attention. The preceding paper has focused on this aspect of drug treatment.

Generalized Disability and Emotional Impairment. It is beyond the scope of this review to discuss long-term emotional effects of cancer and its treatment. The mental health of long-term survivors, however is as important as their physical well being. In addition, recognition must be given to the discrimination in employment, insurance, and other loss of opportunities that may result from an otherwise successful battle against cancer.

Conclusions

Prolonged survival after administration of chemotherapy has become more than an occasional phenomenon. Attention to long-term sequelae is increasing. Prospective studies evaluating complications at regular intervals after treatment are singularly important in this regard. Physicians in the practice of oncology must seriously consider this aspect as they administer cytotoxic agents to patients exclusive of study situations. It is time that we carefully assess long-term sequelae with all of our clinical trials where treatment is given for curative intent.

References

1 Doroshow JH, Locker GY, Myers CE (1979) Experimental animal models of adriamycin cardiotoxicity. Cancer Treat Rep 63: 855–860

2 Hansen HH, Muggia FM, Saini N (1971) Cyclophosphamide and the urinary bladder. N Engl J Med 284: 1043–1044

3 Harmon WE, Cohen HJ, Schneeberger EE, Grupe WE (1979) Chronic renal failure in children treated with methyl CCNU. N Engl J Med 300: 1200–1203

4 Muggia FM, Cortes-Funes H, Wasserman TH (1978) Radiotherapy and chemotherapy in combined clinical trials: Problems and promise. Int J Radiat Oncol Biol Phys 4: 161–171

5 Muller SA, Farrow GM, Martalock DL (1971) Cirrhosis caused by methotrexate in the treatment of psoriasis. Arch Dermatol 100: 523–530

6 Penta JS, Von Hoff DD, Muggia FM (1977) Hepatotoxicity of combination chemotherapy for acute myelocytic leukemia. Ann Intern Med 87: 247–248

7 Peylan-Ramu N, Poplack DG, Pizzo PA, Adornato BT, DiChiro G (1978) Abnormal CT scans of the brain in asymptomatic children with acute lymphocytic leukemia after prophylactic treatment of the central nervous system with radiation and intrathecal chemotherapy. N Engl J Med 298: 815–818

8 Rossof AH, Talley RW, Stephens R, Thigpen T, Samson MK, Groppe C Jr, Eyre HJ, Fisher R (to be published) Phase II evaluation of cis-diamminedichloroplatinum (II) in advanced malignancies of the genitourinary and gynecologic organs. Cancer Treat Rep 63: 1557–1563

9 Schein PS, Winokur SH (1975) Immunosuppressive and cytotoxic chemotherapy. Long-term complications. Ann Intern Med 82: 84–95

10 Sherins RJ, Olweny CLM, Ziegler JL (1978) Gynecomastia and gonadal dysfunction in boys treated with chemotherapy. N Engl J Med 299: 12–16

11 Silver HKB, Morton DL (1979) CCNU nephrotoxicity following sustained remission in oat cell carcinoma. Cancer Treat Rep 63: 226–227

12 Von Hoff DD, Layard M, Rozencweig M, Muggia M (1977) Time relationship between last dose of daunomycin and congestive heart failure. Cancer Treat Rep 61: 1411–1413

13 Weiss HD, Walker MD, Wiernik PH (1974) Neurotoxicity of commonly used antineoplastic agents. N Engl J Med 291: 75–81 (part 1), 127–133 (part 2)

14 Weiss RB, Muggia FM (1980) Cytotoxic drug-induced pulmonary disease: Update 68: 259–266

15 Worth PHL (1971) Cyclophosphamide and the bladder. Br Med J 3: 182

Recent Results in Cancer Research

Sponsored by the Swiss League against Cancer. Editor in Chief: P. Rentchnick, Genève

For information about Vols. 1–9, please contact your bookseller of Springer-Verlag

10 Nelson, R. S.: Radioactive Phosphorus in the Diagnosis of Gastrointestinal Cancer.
11 Freeman, R. G. and J. M. Knox: Treatment of Skin Cancer.
12 Lynch, H. T.: Hereditary Factors in Carcinoma.
13 Tumours in Children, 2nd Edition. Edited by H. B. Marsden and J. K. Steward.
14 Odartchenko, N.: Production Cellulaire Erythropoïétique.
15 Sokoloff, B.: Carcinoid and Serotonin.
16 Jacobs, M. L.: Malignant Lymphomas and Their Management.
17 Normal and Malignant Cell Growth. Edited by R. J. M. Fry, M. L. Griem, and W. H. Kirsten (Symposium).
18 Anglesio, E.: The Treatment of Hodgkin's Disease.
19 Bannasch, P.: The Cytoplasm of Hepatocytes during Carcinogenesis. Electron- and Lightmicroscopical Investigations of the Nitrosomorpholineintoxicated Rat Liver.
20 Rubidomycin. A new Agent against Cancer. Edited by J. Bernard, R. Paul, M. Boiron, C. Jacquillat, and R. Maral.
21 Scientific Basis of Cancer Chemotherapy. Edited by G. Mathé (Symposium).
22 Koldovský, P.: Tumor Specific Transplantation Antigen.
23 Fuchs, W. A., J. W. Davidson, and H. W. Fischer: Lymphography in Cancer. With contributions by G. Jantet and H. Rösler.
24 Hayward, J.: Hormones und Human Breast Cancer. An Account of 15 Years Study.
25 Roy-Burman, P.: Analogues of Nucleic Acid Components. Mechanisms of Action.
26 Tumors of the Liver. Edited by G. T. Pack and A. H. Islami.
27 Szymendera, J.: Bone Mineral Metabolism in Cancer.
28 Meek, E. S.: Antitumour and Antiviral Substances of Natural Origin.
29 Aseptic Environments and Cancer Treatment. Edited by G. Mathé (Symposium).
30 Advances in the Treatment of Acute (Blastic) Leukemias. Edited by G. Mathé (Symposium).
31 Denoix, P.: Treatment of Malignant Breast Tumors. Indications and Results.
32 Nelson, R. S.: Endoscopy in Gastric Cancer.
33 Experimental and Clinical Effects of L-Asparaginase. Edited by E. Grundmann and H. F. Oettgen (Symposium).
34 Chemistry and Biological Actions of 4-Nitroquinolin 1-Oxide. Edited by H. Endo, T. Ono, and T. Sugimura.
35 Penn, I.: Malignant Tumors in Organ Transplant Recipients.
36 Current Concepts in the Management of Lymphoma and Leukemia. Edited by J. E. Ultmann, M. L. Griem, W. H. Kirsten, and R. W. Wissler (Symposium).
37 Chiappa, S., R. Musumeci, and C. Uslenghi: Endolymphatic Radiotherapy in Malignant Lymphomas. With contributions by G. Bonadonna, B. Damascelli, G. Fava, F. Pizzetti, U. Veronesi.
38 Koller, P. C.: The Role of Chromosomes in Cancer Biology.
39 Current Problems in the Epidemiology of Cancer and Lymphomas. Edited by E. Grundmann and H. Tulinius (Symposium).
40 Langley, F. A. and A. C. Crompton: Epithelial Abnormalities of the Cervix Uteri.
41 Tumours in a Tropical Country. A Survey of Uganda (1964–1968). Edited by A. C. Templeton.
42 Breast Cancer: A Challenging Problem. Edited by M. L. Griem, E. V. Jensen, J. E. Ultmann, and R. W. Wissler (Symposium).
43 Nomenclature, Methodology and Results of Clinical Trials in Acute Leukemias. Edited by G. Mathé, P. Pouillart, L. Schwarzenberg (Symposium).
44 Special Topics in Carcinogenesis. Edited by E. Grundmann (Symposium).
45 Koldovský, P.: Carcinoembryonic Antigens.
46 Diagnosis and Therapy of Malignant Lymphoma. Edited by K. Musshoff (Symposium).
47 Investigation and Stimulation of Immunity in Cancer Patients. Edited by G. Mathé and R. Weiner (Symposium).
48 Platinum Coordination Complexes in Cancer Chemotherapy. Edited by T. A. Connors and J. J. Roberts (Symposium).
49 Complications of Cancer Chemotherapy. Edited by G. Mathé and R. K. Oldham (Symposium).
50 Cancer Registry, Edited by E. Grundmann and E. Pedersen (Symposium).
51 Gliomas. Current Concepts in Biology, Diagnosis and Therapy. Edited by J. Hekmatpanah (Symposium).

52 The Ambivalence of Cytostatic Therapy. Edited by E. GRUNDMANN and R. GROSS (Symposium).

53 A. CLARYSSE, Y. KENIS, and G. MATHÉ: Cancer Chemotherapy.

54 Malignant Bone Tumors. Edited by E. GRUNDMANN.

55 MATHÉ, G.: Cancer Active Immunotherapy, Immunoprophylaxis, and Immunorestoration.

56 Lymphocytes, Macrophages, and Cancer. Edited by G. MATHÉ, I. FLORENTIN, and M.-C. SIMMLER (Symposium).

57 Breast Cancer: A Multidisciplinary Approach. Edited by G. ST. ARNEAULT, P. BAND, and L. ISRAËL (Symposium).

58 B. S. SCHOENBERG: Multiple Primary Malignant Neoplasms.

59 Selective Heat Sensitivity of Cancer Cells. Edited by A. ROSSI-FANELLI, R. CAVALIERE, B. MONDOVI, and G. MORICCA.

60 Tumors of the Male Genital System. Edited by E. GRUNDMANN and W. VAHLENSIECK (Symposium).

61 D. METCALF: Hemopoietic Colonies.

62 Tactics and Strategy in Cancer Treatment. Edited by G. MATHÉ (Symposium).

63 Antitumor Antibiotics. Edited by S. K. CARTER, H. UMEZAWA, J. DOUROS, and Y. SAKURAI (Symposium).

64 Lymphoid Neoplasias I: Classification, Categorization, Natural History.

65 Lymphoid Neoplasias II: Clinical and Therapeutic Aspects. Lymphoid Neoplasias I & II. Proceedings of the 1977 CNRS-EORTC International Colloquium. Editors: G. MATHÉ, M. SELIGMANN, M. TUBIANA. Devided into two volumes.

66 Carcinogenic Hormones. Edited by C. H. LINGEMAN.

67/68 Adjuvant Therapies and Markers of Post-Surgical Minimal Residual Disease I & II. Proceedings of the 1978 Annual Plenary Meeting of the EORTC. Editors: G. BONADONNA, G. MATHÉ, S. E. SALMON. Divided into two volumes.

67 Markers and General Problems of Cancer Adjuvant Therapies.

68 Adjuvant Therapies of the Various Primary Tumors.

69 Strategies in Clinical Hematology. Edited by R. GROSS and K.-P. HELLRIEGEL.

70 New Anticancer Drugs. Edited by S. K. CARTER

71 Endocrine Treatment of Breast Cancer. Edited by B. HENNINGSEN, F. LINDER, C. STREICHELE.

72 CAWLEY, J. C., BURNS, G. F., HAYHOE, F. G. J.: Hairy-Cell Leukaemia.

73 Thyroid Cancer. Edited by W. DUNCAN.

74 Cancer Chemo- and Immunopharmacology. 1. Chemopharmacology. Edited by G. MATHÉ and F. M. MUGGIA.

75 Cancer Chemo- and Immunopharmacology. 2. Immunopharmacology, Relations and General Problems. Edited by G. MATHÉ and F. M. MUGGIA.

MIX
Papier aus verantwortungsvollen Quellen
Paper from responsible sources
FSC® C105338

If you have any concerns about our products,
you can contact us on
ProductSafety@springernature.com

In case Publisher is established outside the EU,
the EU authorized representative is:
Springer Nature Customer Service Center GmbH
Europaplatz 3, 69115 Heidelberg, Germany

Printed by Libri Plureos GmbH
in Hamburg, Germany